THE ADRENERGIC RECEPTORS

THE RECEPTORS

KIM A. NEVE, SERIES EDITOR

The Adrenergic Receptors

In the 21st Century

Edited by

Dianne M. Perez

Department of Molecular Cardiology
The Lerner Research Institute,
The Cleveland Clinic Foundation, Cleveland, OH

HUMANA PRESS ✳ TOTOWA, NEW JERSEY

Cover design by Patricia F. Cleary

Cover illustration: Fluorescent ligand (QAPB, also known as BODIPY FL-prazosin, 30 n*M*) binding to α_1-adrenoceptors in isolated smooth muscle cells. The data is displayed as an isosurface model in which the cell membrane is rendered with a transparent "blue" surface. Intracellular fluorescent regions, indicating ligand-receptor binding, are colored orange and green in the two cells. Bright "clusters" of fluorescence are shown as red in both cells. Alternative views and explanations of the data are given in Chapter 6 by McGrath and Daly.

This publication is printed on acid-free paper. ⊚

ANSI Z39.48-1984 (American National Standards Institute) Permanence of Paper for Printed Library Materials

Library of Congress Cataloging-in-Publication Data

The adrenergic receptors : in the 21st century / edited by Dianne M. Perez.
    p. cm. -- (The receptors)
 Includes bibliographical references and index.
 ISBN 1-58829-423-4 (alk. paper)
 1. Adrenaline--Receptors. 2. Pharmacogenetics. I. Perez, Dianne M. II.Series.
 QP364.7.A375 2005
 612.4'5--dc22
                                    2005008529

Preface

Our understanding of adrenergic function has advanced considerably in the 15 years since three adrenergic receptor books were published in *The Receptors* series. In the late 1980s, many of the adrenergic subtypes had not yet been cloned. Most of the studies during that time focused on traditional pharmacological approaches in selected tissues and cell lines. We learned about structure–function relationships through the manipulation of the drug, not the receptor. We understood that there were multiple subtypes within each class of adrenergic receptors, but the functions of the subtypes were unclear because they seemed to control the same signal transduction and biological processes. Molecular cloning of the receptors led to the realization that there were many different subtypes, some not previously described by the tissue pharmacology. With the genes of these receptors in hand, the field has now advanced with more precise experiments and questions, but it has still suffered from the lack of highly selective ligands and antibodies. Foreseeing that these limitations would not be overcome any time in the near future, scientists in the adrenergic receptor field—using modern genetic approaches—started to redirect their work to answer questions about structure and function and the possible physiological and patho-physiological pathways that would be regulated by adrenergic receptors. *The Adrenergic Receptors: In the 21st Century* focuses on these modern approaches and was written by the scientists who developed them to elucidate adrenergic receptor function.

Dianne M. Perez

Contents

Contributors

LIZA BARKI-HARRINGTON • *Division of Cardiology, Duke University Medical Center, Durham, NC*

DAVID B. BYLUND • *Department of Pharmacology, University of Nebraska Medical Center, University of Nebraska, Omaha, NE*

CRAIG J. DALY • *Autonomic Physiology Unit, Institute of Biomedical and Life Sciences, Division of Neuroscience and Biomedical Systems, University of Glasgow, Glasgow, Scotland, UK*

ANDREA D. ECKHART • *Center for Translational Medicine, Thomas Jefferson University, Philadelphia, PA*

ANGELA M. FINCH • *Molecular Cardiology Program, Victor Chang Cardiac Research Institute, Darlinghurst, New South Wales, Australia*

MARY LOLIS GARCÍA-CAZARIN • *Department of Molecular and Biomedical Pharmacology, The University of Kentucky College of Medicine, Lexington, KY*

ROBERT M. GRAHAM • *Molecular Cardiology Program, Victor Chang Cardiac Research Institute, Darlinghurst, New South Wales, Australia*

PAUL A. INSEL • *Department of Pharmacology and Medicine, University of California San Diego, San Diego, CA*

BRIAN KOBILKA • *Department of Molecular and Cellular Physiology, Stanford Medical Center, Stanford University, Palo Alto, CA*

WALTER J. KOCH • *Center for Translational Medicine, Thomas Jefferson University, Philadelphia, PA*

STEPHEN B. LIGGETT • *Cardiopulmonary Research Center, University of Cincinnati College of Medicine, Cincinnati, OH*

LEE E. LIMBIRD • *Department of Pharmacology, Vanderbilt University Medical Center, Vanderbilt University, Nashville, TN*

JOHN C. MCGRATH • *Autonomic Physiology Unit, Institute of Biomedical and Life Sciences, Division of Neuroscience and Biomedical Systems, University of Glasgow, Glasgow, Scotland, UK*

MARTIN C. MICHEL • *Department of Pharmacology, University of Amsterdam, Amsterdam, The Netherlands*

KENNETH P. MINNEMAN • *Department of Pharmacology, Emory University, Atlanta, GA*

DIANNE M. PEREZ • *Department of Molecular Cardiology, The Lerner Research Institute, The Cleveland Clinic Foundation, Cleveland, OH*

CINZIA PERRINO • *Division of Cardiology, Duke University Medical Center, Durham, NC*

MICHAEL T. PIASCIK • *Department of Molecular and Biomedical Pharmacology, The University of Kentucky College of Medicine, Lexington, KY*

STEVEN R. POST • *The Department of Molecular and Biomedical Pharmacology, The University of Kentucky College of Medicine, Lexington, KY*

HOWARD A. ROCKMAN • *Division of Cardiology, Duke University Medical Center, Durham, NC*

BOYD RORABAUGH • *Department of Pharmacology, College of Pharmacy, Ohio Northern University, Ada, OH*

VALERIE SARRAMEGNA • *Molecular Cardiology Program, Victor Chang Cardiac Research Institute, Darlinghurst, New South Wales, Australia*

PAUL C. SIMPSON • *Cardiology Division, San Francisco VA Medical Center, and the CVRI and Department of Medicine, University of California, San Francisco, CA*

CHRISTOPHER M. TAN • *Department of Pharmacology, Merck Research Laboratories, Merck Frosst Centre for Therapeutic Research, Kirkland, Quebec, Canada*

YANG XIANG • *Department of Molecular and Cellular Physiology, Stanford Medical Center, Stanford University, Palo Alto, CA*

JUNE YUN • *The Department of Physiology and Pharmacology, Northeastern Ohio Universities College of Medicine, Rootstown, OH*

Color Plates

Color Plates follow p. 148.

Color Plate 1. Confocal imaging of human aortic smooth muscle cells transfected with an adenovirus (*Fig. 1, Chapter 4; see* full caption and discussion on pp. 117–118).

Color Plate 2. Classical AR signaling (*Fig. 1, Chapter 11; see* full caption and discussion on p. 294).

Color Plate 3. Major mechanisms involved in β-AR desensitization and internalization (*Fig. 2, Chapter 11; see* full caption on p. 296 and discussion on p. 295).

Color Plate 4. Histopathological characteristics of left ventricular specimens taken from mice overexpressing the human β_1-AR (*Fig. 5, Chapter 11; see* full caption on p. 307 and discussion on pp. 306–308).

Color Plate 5. Phylogenetics of β_2-AR haplotypes (*Fig. 2, Chapter 13; see* full caption on p. 342 and discussion on pp. 340–341).

Part I

Historical Perspectives

1

Adrenergic Receptors

Historical Perspectives From the 20th Century

David B. Bylund

Summary

During the 20th century, extraordinary progress was made in our understanding of adrenergic receptors. This progress was the result of the hard work and insightful thinking of a remarkable cadre of investigators throughout the world. A summary of some of the more important developments is presented two ways: as a summary listing by decade and as four major, overlapping eras—biochemical, physiological, pharmacological, and molecular.

Key Words: α_1-Adrenergic receptor; α_2-adrenergic receptor; β-adrenergic receptor; classification; function; history; molecular cloning; pharmacology; radioligand binding; structure.

1. Introduction

Adrenergic receptors mediate the central and peripheral actions of the neurohormones norepinephrine and epinephrine. Both of these catecholamine messengers play important roles in the regulation of diverse physiological systems; thus, adrenergic receptors are widely distributed throughout the body. Stimulation of adrenergic receptors by catecholamines released from the sympathetic branch of the autonomic nervous system results in a variety of effects, such as increased heart rate, regulation of vascular tone, and bronchodilation. In the central nervous system, adrenergic receptors are involved in many functions, including memory, learning, alertness, and the response to stress.

During the 20th century, extraordinary progress was made in our understanding of receptors in general and of adrenergic receptors in particular. The century

From: *The Receptors: The Adrenergic Receptors: In the 21st Century*
Edited by: D. Perez © Humana Press Inc., Totowa, NJ

dawned with the crystallization of the receptor concept and closed with the crystallization and determination of the three-dimensional structure of rhodopsin. At the start of the century, epinephrine and norepinephrine had not yet been isolated; by its end, knockout mice were available for all nine adrenergic receptor subtypes, and clinically relevant polymorphisms were being elucidated. This progress was the result of the hard work and insightful thinking of a remarkable cadre of investigators throughout the world. A few of these are mentioned in this chapter, although most (unfortunately) remain unnamed.

A summary listing by decade of some of the more important developments in our understanding of adrenergic receptors is given in Table 1. The accomplishments are indeed impressive. I have chosen to divide the century into four major, overlapping epochs or eras, each named to represent the dominant focus of a given time period. The century started with the biochemical era, which lasted until the mid-1960s and resulted in the isolation of many small compounds, such as norepinephrine, epinephrine, and the second messenger cyclic adenosine 5′-monophosphate (AMP). This was followed by what I term the physiological era, from about 1960 to the early 1980s; it was characterized by elegant use of isolated tissue preparations to elucidate the general characteristics of adrenergic receptors. The pharmacological era, lasting from the mid-1970s to the early 1990s, included not only the use the physiological techniques of the previous era, but also, perhaps more important, radioligand-binding techniques to classify, localize, and characterize the types and subtypes of adrenergic receptors based on their interactions with a rich variety of agonists and antagonists. The molecular era, which is just now ending, started in the mid-1980s and has seen the characterization of receptors by the molecular biological techniques of cloning, site-directed mutagenesis, and genetic engineering.

2. The Biochemical Era (1901–1960)

"Tentatively the first kind of receptor has been called the alpha adrenotropic receptor and the second kind the beta receptor." (Ahlquist, 1948)

John Jacob Abel, a newly appointed professor of pharmacology at Johns Hopkins in Baltimore, Maryland, started work on the isolation of epinephrine about 1896 and by 1901 had a relatively pure preparation. He is generally credited with isolating the first hormone *(1)*. Starting in the 1920s, Cannon attempted to identify the chemical transmitter of the sympathetic nervous system (which he called sympathin) and mistakenly concluded in 1933 that there were two sympathins, sympathin E (excitatory) and sympathin I (inhibitory) *(2)*. This was partly because he was using a natural preparation, adrenaline, which at that time was a variable mixture of epinephrine and norepinephrine. It was not until the late 1940s that von Euler finally established that norepinephrine was the predominant postganglionic neurotransmitter of the sympathetic nervous system *(3)*.

Table 1
Progress in Understanding Adrenergic Receptors
by Decade of the 20th Century

1901–1910	• Langley proposes that cells have "receptive substances" • Dale refers to "receptive mechanism for adrenalin" • Abel isolates epinephrine from the adrenal medulla, the first hormone to be isolated
1911–1920	
1921–1930	
1931–1940	
1941–1950	• von Euler demonstrates that norepinephrine is the sympathetic neurotransmitter • Ahlquist defines α– and β-types of adrenergic receptors
1951–1960	• Sutherland discovers cyclic AMP, leading to the second messenger concept
1961–1970	• Sir James Black develops propranolol, the first clinically useful β-antagonist • Lands defines β_1- and β_2-subtypes
1971–1980	• Langer defines α_1 as postsynaptic and α_2 as presynaptic • Pettinger defines α_1- and α_2-receptors functionally • Snyder and Lefkowitz develop radioligand binding assays for most adrenergic receptors • Lefkowitz develops the ternary complex model for G protein-coupled receptors
1981–1990	• Khorana clones bacteriorhodopsin, the first of the seven transmembrane receptors • Nathans and Hogness clone rhodopsin, the first of the G protein-coupled receptors • Arch defines the β_3-receptor using pharmacological criteria • Bylund defines α_1, α_2, and β as the three types of adrenergic receptors • Dixon, Strader, and Lefkowitz clone the β_2-adrenergic receptor • Creese proposes α_{1A}- and α_{1B}-subtypes based on radioligand binding • Bylund defines α_{2A}-, α_{2B}-, and α_{2C}-subtypes using pharmacological criteria • Lefkowitz clones β_1-, α_{2A}-, α_{2B}-, α_{2A}-, α_{1A}-, and α_{1B}-receptors • Strosberg clones the β_3-receptor
1991–2000	• Strader's laboratory and other laboratories use site-directed mutagenesis to define ligand-binding site and signaling mechanisms • Graham and Perez clone α_{1D} • Transgenic mice developed by several laboratories • Lefkowitz works out desensitization mechanism involving β-adrenergic receptor kinase and β-arrestin • Lowell generates β_3-knockout mice • Kobilka generates β_1-, β_2-, α_{2A}-, α_{2B}-, and α_{2C}-knockout mice • Cotecchia generates α_{1B}-knockout mice • Liggett describes clinically relevant polymorphisms in α_2- and β-receptors • Crystal structure of rhodopsin, a G protein-coupled receptor, determined

This listing represents some of the more important developments (in my opinion) in the understanding of adrenergic receptors. For purposes of clarity, no attempt was made to be comprehensive in the citing of laboratories. It is understood that many additional laboratories were instrumental in the remarkable progress that was made during the 20th century.

Although the concept of receptors as physical entities that receive and transduce information from hormones, neurotransmitters, and drugs to the cell is axiomatic at present, it was not always so. Our current receptor concept had its beginnings in the work of Langley, who was investigating the action of curare on skeletal muscle *(4)*. Dale was probably the first to make significant use of the receptor concept in connection with the sympathetic nervous system. In his classical article on the sympatholytic action of the ergot alkaloids, he recognized that what he called the "sympathetic myoneural junction" to denote "the structure which can be excited either by adrenaline or by impulses" could also be called "the receptive mechanism for adrenaline." He used this mechanism to explain the fact that the ergot alkaloids prevented only the motor (excitatory) actions of epinephrine and had no effect on the inhibitory actions of epinephrine *(5)*.

Throughout most of the 20th century, adrenergic receptors were considered to be "those hypothetical structures or systems located in, on or near the muscle or gland cell effected by epinephrine" *(6)*. In 1964, de Jongh wrote, "To most modern pharmacologists the receptors is like a beautiful but remote lady. He has written her many a letter and quite often she has answered those letters. From these answers the pharmacologist has built himself an image of this fair lady. He cannot, however, truly claim ever to have seen her, although one day he may do so" *(7)*. Remarkably, this view that receptors were more of a concept than a reality held until well into the 1980s. "Until receptor structure can be defined by physicochemical methods, it might be wise to remember that receptors are fictions of the human brain, based on observations of biological effects, elicited by various substances!" *(8)*.

In the 1950s, Sutherland was studying the effect of epinephrine on glycogen phosphorylase activity in dog liver slices. He found that if he incubated a particulate fraction from liver homogenate with epinephrine, a heat-stable factor was produced that could activate phosphorylase when added back to the supernatant fraction. He further showed that this heat-stable factor was an adenine ribonucleotide *(9)*, which was subsequently identified as cyclic AMP. These studies led to the concept of the hormone (epinephrine) as the first messenger and cyclic AMP as the second messenger. "The first messenger in this concept is the hormone or neurohormone, which is released by stimuli which may be varied and complex ... this first messenger travels to effector cells and causes the release therein of a second messenger. The only second messenger identified to date is cyclic 3'5'-AMP, but possibly other second messengers exist, even for the same hormones that stimulate adenyl cyclase" *(10)*.

Although I have called this time period the biochemical era, one of the most important developments of the era was the truly seminal studies of Ahlquist using isolated tissues. He introduced the concept of α- and β-adrenergic receptors in 1948 as a result of studying the effects of catecholamines on a variety of physiological responses *(6)*. These included contraction and relaxation of the uterus, dilation of the pupil, and stimulation of myocardial contraction. He demonstrated that norepinephrine, epinephrine, isoproterenol, methylnorepinephrine, and methylepinephrine could cause either contraction or relaxation of smooth muscle, depending on the dose and the site of action. For instance, Ahlquist reported that isoproterenol and norepinephrine caused smooth muscle relaxation and contraction, respectively, whereas epinephrine could cause both contraction and relaxation of smooth muscle.

Based on these observations, Ahlquist proposed that the effects of the amines were mediated by two distinct receptors, designated α- and β-adrenergic receptors. The β-receptors were defined by the catecholamine potency series isoproterenol > epinephrine > norepinephrine, whereas α-receptors were defined by the series epinephrine = norepinephrine > isoproterenol. The critical concept here was that receptor subtypes are defined by their pharmacological characteristic, which is the rank order of agonist (and later antagonist) potencies. Until this time, the attempts at receptor classification were based on functional criteria such as contraction vs relaxation. The proposal of receptor subtypes was in stark contrast to the earlier proposal of sympathin E and sympathin I as distinct transmitter substances. Ahlquist's studies laid the foundation for both of the next two eras, the physiological and pharmacological eras.

3. The Physiological Era (1961–1984)

"What we are allowed to see of a molecule's properties is totally dependent on the techniques of bioassay we use." (Sir James W. Black, Nobel Lecture, 1988)

Ahlquist's classification of adrenergic receptors into two kinds or types stimulated Black to develop substances with selective β-receptor blocking properties in a systematic way. Using the isoproterenol molecule as a starting point, Black and coworkers succeeded in developing the first clinically useful β-receptor antagonist propranolol in 1964 *(11)*. In addition to the classical Langendorff preparation, the isolated spontaneously beating guinea pig heart, they developed a new in vitro assay based on guinea pig cardiac papillary muscle as a way of measuring the contractile effects of isoproterenol independent of changes in heart rate. They were astonished to find that, in this preparation, dichloroisoproterenol acted as a pure antagonist, whereas in the Langendorff preparation, it was a full agonist. This was a remarkable early demonstration that the efficacy of partial agonists can vary dramatically with the assay system.

The paradigm used by Ahlquist for classifying receptors based on their pharmacological characteristics (i.e., rank order of potency of agonists) was further developed by Lands and colleagues with the subdivision of the β-adrenergic receptors into β_1- and β_2-subtypes *(12)*. The β_1-adrenergic receptor, the dominant receptor in heart and adipose tissue, was equally sensitive to epinephrine and norepinephrine, whereas the β_2-adrenergic receptor, responsible for relaxation of vascular, uterine, and airway smooth muscle, was less sensitive to norepinephrine compared to epinephrine. At the same time, Furchgott also proposed the presence of various types of β-adrenergic receptors *(13)*. These studies determined the dissociation constant for an α- (phentolamine) and β- (pronethalol) adrenergic receptor blocker in several isolated tissues. "The results will, I believe, … show that there may be various types of beta receptors within the general class of such receptors."

In the mid-1950s, Brown and Gillespie measured the levels of sympathin (norepinephrine) in the venous blood from the cat spleen following nerve stimulation. In the presence of α-adrenergic antagonists (dibenamine or dibenzyline), the amount of sympathin released was greatly increased *(14)*. This study was misinterpreted at that time as showing that the adrenergic receptor served as an important site in the loss of norepinephrine. In the early 1970s, based on studies in several laboratories utilizing tritiated norepinephrine, both Langer and Starke and coworkers correctly concluded that these drugs increased the output of norepinephrine elicited by nerve stimulation *(15,16)*. Starke then quickly showed that phenylephrine caused a dose-dependent inhibition of norepinephrine release from the isolated rabbit heart, leading to the conclusion of presynaptic regulation of norepinephrine release mediated by α-adrenergic receptors *(17)*. A few months later, Langer formalized the concept *(18)*: "These presynaptic receptors would regulate the transmitter released by nerve stimulation. A negative feedback inhibition can be envisaged in which noradrenaline released by nerve stimulation would itself inhibit further release once a threshold concentration of the transmitter is achieved in the neighborhood of the nerve ending. Block of these receptors would lead to an increase in release of the transmitter by nerve stimulation."

This work in turn led to a proposal for the subclassification of the α-adrenergic receptors based on their anatomical location *(19)*. "These results are compatible with the view that the pre- and the post-synaptic α receptors are not identical. Perhaps the postsynaptic α receptor that mediates the response of the effector organ should be referred to as α-1, while the presynaptic α receptor that regulates transmitter release should be called α-2." It was, however, quickly realized that not all α-receptors with α_2 pharmacological characteristics were presynaptic. Thus, a functional classification of α-adrenergic receptors was proposed with the excitatory receptors as α_1 and the inhibitory receptors as α_2 *(20)*. It was noted, however, that there was a different agonist potency order for the two subtypes. Although the functional aspect of their proposal turned out not to be generally applicable, the pharmacological definition based on the rank order of potency of agonists has prevailed.

It also became apparent that not all of the β-adrenergic receptor-mediated responses could be classified as either β_1 or β_2, suggesting the existence of at least one additional β subtype, generally referred to as the "atypical" β-adrenergic receptor. Arch and colleagues *(21)* in the early 1980s developed a series of β-adrenergic receptor agonists that selectively stimulated lipolysis in brown adipocytes, thus showing that the "β adrenergic receptors in rat brown adipocytes are of neither the β-1 nor β-2 subtype."

4. The Pharmacological Era (1976–1993)

"The absence of an α_{1C}-adrenoceptor, as with the absence of the 5-HT$_{1C}$ receptor, may serve as a reminder that the classification of receptors is a nasty business." (D. E. Clarke, 1994)

A major new technique of the pharmacological era was the radioligand-binding technique for characterization of receptors. In the early 1970s, based on success with labeling the nicotinic cholinergic receptor from the electric organs of the fish *Electrophorus (22)* and *Torpedo (23)*, which have an extraordinarily high receptor density, Goldstein et al. *(24)* attempted to label the opioid receptor in mouse brain. He was, however, able to demonstrate only 2% specific binding, as it turned out, because of the low specific activity of the radioligand. Soon thereafter, using tritiated and iodinated radioligands of higher specific activity, Snyder, Lefkowitz, and others demonstrated stereoselective labeling of many neurotransmitter receptors, including the β-adrenergic receptor in the turkey erythrocyte *(25)* and in rat and monkey brain *(26,27)* and α-adrenergic receptors in rat brain *(28)* and uterus *(29)*.

The radioligand-binding technique became a relatively simple and powerful tool for studying adrenergic and other G protein-coupled receptors, particularly when vacuum filtration was used to separate bound from free. It was used to determine the affinity of numerous drugs for these receptors and to characterize regulatory changes in receptor number and in subcellular localization. As a result, this assay was widely used by investigators in a variety of ways, including drug screening by pharmaceutical companies. Although the typical assay used membrane preparations from tissues and cell lines, the basic technique was also used to label and thus study receptors in intact cells, solubilized receptors, receptors in tissue slices (by receptor autoradiography), or receptors in intact animals.

One of the most important uses of the radioligand-binding technique was in the area of receptor classification and the identification of new subtypes. The quantitative analysis of both β_1- and β_2-adrenergic receptors in single tissues in the late 1970s nicely confirmed the β_1/β_2 classification scheme *(30)*. Similarly, radioligand-binding studies confirmed the pharmacological definition of α_1- and α_2-adrenergic receptors (for review, *see* ref. *31*). In the mid-1980s, Morrow and Creese *(32)* suggested the existence of α_{1A} and α_{1B} subtypes based on their differential affinities for adrenergic agents such as WB4101 and phentolamine in radioligand-binding assays. This suggestion was confirmed by additional

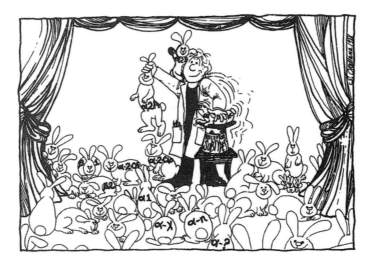

Fig. 1. A cartoon from 1988 indicating the frustration some investigators felt at the seemingly endless proliferation of adrenergic receptor subtypes. (From ref. *40*; © 1988, with permission from Elsevier.)

radioligand-binding studies showing that the two subtypes had differential sensitivities to the site-directed alkylating agent chloroethylclonidine *(33)*.

The evidence for α_2-receptor subtypes came from binding studies in various tissues and cell lines *(34)*. The α_{2A} and α_{2B} subtypes were initially defined based on their differential affinities for adrenergic agents such as prazosin and oxymetazoline *(35)*, and their existence was confirmed by functional studies *(36)*. The third subtype, α_{2C}, was identified originally in an opossum kidney cell line using radioligand-binding studies *(37)*. A fourth pharmacological subtype, the α_{2D}, was identified in the rat and cow *(38,39)*. Subsequently, it was shown that this pharmacological subtype was a species orthologue of the human α_{2A} subtype, and thus it is not considered a separate genetic subtype.

During the second half of the 1980s, when new receptor subtypes were proposed regularly, there was considerable opposition to this seemingly endless proliferation of subtypes. One reviewer chided the author on this point in the review of one of his papers in 1987: "Shall we expect proposals for further equally trivial revisions each time a new ligand is found with very high selectivity between receptors for which all previously known ligands had only modest selectivity?" Perhaps the mood at this time is accurately reflected in the cartoon (Fig. 1) from my 1988 review of α-adrenergic receptor classification *(40)*. In this cartoon, it should be noted that the investigator is trying to push the "subtypes" back into the hat, or at least prevent them from popping out, rather than happily pulling them out.

The mechanism of action of adrenergic receptors includes the activation of guanine nucleotide regulatory binding proteins (G proteins), and thus members of this receptor superfamily are also known as G protein-coupled receptors. Building on work of Rodbell on the effect of guanine nucleotides on the glucagon receptor *(41)*, the Lefkowitz and Gilman labs found that guanine nucleotides affected the binding of agonists but not antagonists to the β-adrenergic receptor *(42,43)*. Extensive radioligand-binding studies led to the ternary complex model for adrenergic receptors *(44)*, which was extended to other G protein-coupled receptors. "This model provides a general scheme for the activation by agonists of adenylate cyclase-coupled receptor systems and also of other systems where the effector might be different."

Although adrenergic receptors were originally divided into two major types, α and β, Bylund suggested in the mid-1980s that the classification scheme should be revised to accommodate three major types: α_1, α_2, and β *(40)*. Each of these three receptor types was further divided into two or three subtypes: α_{1A}, α_{1B}; α_{2A}, α_{2B}, α_{2C}; β_1, β_2. The justification for this new classification scheme was based on three independent lines of evidence *(40)*. The first was that the pharmacological differences among the main receptor types (α_1, α_2, and β) were much greater than among the subtypes (β_1 vs β_2; α_{1A} vs α_{1B}; etc.). Second, each of the three types coupled to their effectors through a different family of G proteins: α_1 through G_q to stimulate phosphatidylinositol hydrolysis; α_2 through G_i to inhibit adenylate cyclase; and β through G_s to stimulate adenylate cyclase. Finally, the data from the molecular cloning of some of the adrenergic receptor subtypes that were just beginning to emerge clearly indicated that, at the molecular level, the α_2-receptors were no more similar to the α_1 receptors than they were to the β-receptors. This classification scheme is now generally accepted.

5. The Molecular Era (1987–2002)

"Studies of transfected receptors tell us what can happen, not what does happen." (Lee Limbird, 1990s)

The application of the techniques of molecular biology starting in the mid-1980s provided for rapid advances in our understanding of adrenergic receptors. The cloning of the various subtypes confirmed and extended the classification schemes worked out by pharmacological techniques, and site-directed mutagenesis greatly enhanced our insights into the molecular mechanisms of receptor action. Importantly, the β_2-adrenergic receptor quickly became the prototypic G protein-coupled receptor.

Bacteriorhodopsin was cloned in 1981 *(45)* and was found to contain seven putative transmembrane (TM) regions composed of hydrophobic amino acids, thus making it the first known seven TM protein *(46)*; however, it is a light-driven proton pump, not a G protein-coupled receptor. The opsin apoprotein of bovine rhodopsin was subsequently cloned and also found to have seven putative membrane-spanning regions *(47)*. In 1986, Dixon, Strader, Lefkowitz, and colleagues cloned the β_2-adrenergic receptor using olignucleotide probes based on the sequence of a CNBr peptide obtained from the β_2-receptor purified to homogeneity from hamster lung *(48)*. They noted that its predicted amino acid sequence had significant homology with bovine rhodopsin and suggested that, like the rhodopsins, the β_2-adrenergic receptor possessed multiple membrane-spanning regions, later shown to be seven. It is now recognized that adrenergic receptors are seven TM receptors, which consist of a single polypeptide chain with seven hydrophobic regions that are thought to form α-helical structures and span or transverse the membrane.

Lefkowitz and colleagues quickly realized the potential existence of a large family of these seven TM receptors and started cloning other receptors by homology screening. Using the human β_2-adrenergic receptor as a probe, they isolated a genomic clone called G-21, the first of the "orphan" receptors *(49)*, which was subsequently shown to be the 5-HT$_{1A}$ receptor *(50)*. This clone in turn was used as a probe to clone the human β_1-adrenergic receptor *(51)*. The β_3-receptor, which had been pharmacologically defined in 1984 *(21)*, was cloned in 1989 by Strosberg's lab *(52)*. A β_4-receptor has also been postulated and was even "canonized" by the Adrenergic Receptor Subcommittee of the IUPHAR Committee on Receptor Nomenclature and Drug Classification in 1998 *(53)*. It has not been cloned, however, and thus definitive evidence of its existence is lacking. The putative β_4-receptor is now thought to be a "state" of the β_1-adrenergic receptor *(54)*.

The α_{2A}-receptor from the human platelet was cloned in 1987 by Lefkowitz's group based on the same strategy they used for the β_2-adrenergic receptor *(55)*. The gene was found to be located on chromosome 10, and thus it was subsequently called α_2-C10. A Southern blot of human genomic deoxyribonucleic acid (DNA) blotted with a probe from this receptor indicated the existence of genes homologous to α_{2A} receptor on chromosomes 2 and 4 and suggested that these might represent other pharmacologically defined α_2-receptor subtypes.

A second subtype was cloned two years later from a human kidney complementary DNA (cDNA) library using the gene for the human α_{2A}-adrenergic receptor as a probe *(56)*. The gene for this subtype was shown to be located on human chromosome 4 and thus became known as α_2-C4; it was initially identified as the α_{2B}-pharmacological subtype, although this was later shown to be in error.

A third α_2-subtype was cloned first from a rat kidney cDNA library screened with an oligonucleotide complementary to a highly conserved region found in all biogenic amine receptors that had been described up to that time *(57)*. It was called the α_2-RNG (for rat nonglycosylated) and was correctly identified as the

α_{2B}-subtype. A short time later, the human α_{2B} was cloned from a human genomic spleen library using the human 5-HT$_{1A}$ receptor gene (G-21) as a probe *(58)* and was subsequently shown to be located on chromosome 2, and hence termed α_2-C2. The confusion that existed regarding the relationship of the three cloned subtypes with the three pharmacologically defined subtypes was put to rest with a collaboration between the Bylund and Lefkowitz labs in which the binding characteristics of the three cloned receptors expressed in COS cells were compared in the same assays with the pharmacologically defined native receptors, which confirmed that C10 was α_{2A}, C2 was α_{2B}, and C4 was α_{2C} *(59)*.

In 1988, just a year after the first α_2-receptor was cloned and two years after the first β-receptor, the α_{1B}-receptor was cloned by the same strategy of isolating a peptide from the purified receptor (from hamster DDT cells) and screening a hamster genomic library with the corresponding oligonucleotides *(60)*. A couple of years later, a second α_1-receptor was cloned by first screening a human genomic library with a probe from the hamster α_{1B}-receptor. Using a probe isolated from that screening, a bovine brain cDNA library was screened, and a full length clone was obtained *(61)*. Although it was noted that this clone had some pharmacological characteristics similar to the α_{1A}-receptor, the authors felt it was a novel subtype and subsequently identified it as the α_{1c}-subtype.[1] A year later, they isolated a third subtype from a rat cerebral cortex cDNA library, which they mistakenly identified as the α_{1a}-subtype *(62)*. That same year, Perez and Graham cloned a receptor from the rat and correctly identified it as an α_{1D}-subtype (although it was essentially identical to the α_{1a}-subtype cloned by Lomasney et al.) because it had pharmacological characteristics different from both the α_{1A}- and α_{1B}-subtypes *(63)*.

Of the nine adrenergic receptor subtypes, the α_{1D} is the only one to be identified by cloning before characterization pharmacologically. Subsequently, it was shown that the so-called α_{1c}-receptor was actually the pharmacological α_{1A} *(64,65)*, and this was formalized by the IUPHAR Adrenergic Receptor Subcommittee *(66)*. The current classification scheme includes the α_{1A}, α_{1B}, and α_{1D}, but there is no α_{1C}. A fourth pharmacological subtype, the α_{1L}, has been identified in vascular tissues from several species *(67)* but may represent a conformational state of the α_{1A}-receptor *(68)*.

A second technique of molecular biology that proved enormously useful in understanding adrenergic receptor mechanisms was site-directed mutagenesis,

---

[1] The convention established by IUPHAR was that lowercase letters were used to denote subtypes identified by cloning (if the pharmacological subtype was not obvious), whereas uppercase letter were used to denote the pharmacologically defined subtypes. Once there was general acceptance of the correspondence between the two, the use of the lowercase letters was discontinued.

which allows for the alteration or deletion of specific amino acids in a receptor (*see* Chapter 2). The first application of this technique, which was then used by many workers to define ligand-binding site and signaling mechanism, was by the Strader lab in 1987 *(69)*. Based on a series of deletion mutants of the hamster β_2-adrenergic receptor that showed that most of the hydrophilic residues are not directly involved in ligand binding, they concluded that the binding site must involve residues within the hydrophobic TM domain. They then went on to show the importance of Asp 113 in TM III in agonist binding to the receptor *(70)* and of the serine residues 204 and 207 in TM V in the activation of the β_2 receptor *(71)*.

The third extremely useful technique of molecular biology was the use of transgenic animals, particularly gene targeting to disrupt the expression of a specific receptor to generate so-called knockout mice (*see* Chapters 8–11). Interestingly, the first adrenergic receptor to be knocked out was the β_3-receptor in 1995 by Lowell's lab *(72)*. These mice had only modestly increased lipid stores but lacked the physiological responses to administered β_3-agonists observed in wild-type mice. The next year, Kobilka's lab generated mice lacking the β_1-adrenergic receptor *(73)*. In addition to developmental defects, these mice lacked both chronotropic and inotropic responses to administered β-agonists. The β_2-knockout mice, generated several years later by Kobilka, showed that this subtype primarily influences the smooth muscle relaxant properties of several tissues *(74)*. Simple breeding experiments have allowed for the generation of the three combinations of double β-receptor knockouts, as well as the triple knockout *(75)* (*see* Chapter 10).

Mice lacking the α_{1B}-adrenergic receptor were generated by the Cotecchia lab in 1997 *(76)*. Whereas basal blood pressure was not altered in these animals, the hypertensive response to α_1-agonists was significantly blunted. Subsequently, the α_{1A}- *(77)* and α_{1D}-knockouts *(78)* were generated. All three α_1-subtypes play important roles in the cardiovascular system, and the α_{1B} may be particularly important in the central nervous system (reviewed in ref. *79*) (*see* Chapter 8).

In 1996, the Limbird lab genetically modified the α_{2A}-receptor by the hit-and-run technique, which essentially is site-specific mutagenesis in vivo *(80)* (*see* Chapter 9). Mice homozygous for the D79N substitution lack the profound hypotension normally induced by α_2-agonists. Concurrently, the Kobilka lab produced α_{2B}- and α_{2C}-knockouts *(81)* and then a few years later the α_{2A}-knockout *(82)*. These studies indicated that primarily the α_{2A}-subtype mediates most of the classical α_2-adrenergic functions, such as hypotension, sedation, analgesia, and hypothermia. The α_{2B}-subtype is the principal mediator of the hypertensive response to α_2-agonists, whereas the α_{2C}-subtype appears to be involved in many central nervous system functions (reviewed in ref. *83*).

The fourth molecular technique of note to be applied to the adrenergic receptors was the determination of receptor polymorphisms in human populations. Polymorphisms are frequently occurring genetic variants (by contrast with rarer occurring mutations). A working hypothesis was developed suggesting that polymorphisms in neurotransmitter receptors might underlie individual variability in both propensity for disease and therapeutic response. In 1993, the Liggett lab showed that the β_2-adrenergic receptor is highly polymorphic and evaluated the extent to which these polymorphisms contributed to the development of asthma *(84)*. Subsequently, their lab and many others studied the association of adrenergic receptor polymorphisms with various disorders, and the molecular mechanisms involved have been partially elucidated *(85)* (*see* Chapter 13).

At least three other notable advances occurred during the last decade of the 20th century. One was the determination of the ground-state structure of rhodopsin at 2.8-Å resolution by X-ray crystallography *(86)*. This milestone has significantly advanced our understanding of the structure and activation of the adrenergic receptors as well as other members of the seven TM receptor superfamily. The second was the delineation of the molecular mechanisms of adrenergic receptor desensitization by the Lefkowitz lab *(87)* and many others. Desensitization results from the actions of the G protein-coupled receptor kinases and the arrestins, as well as protein kinases A and C, can lead to the activation of additional signaling pathways via a growing list of "scaffolded" complexes *(88)* (*see* Chapter 3). The third notable advance was the understanding of the concepts of inverse agonists and constitutive activity as they apply to G protein-coupled receptors (*see* Chapter 2). This was made possible by overexpressing receptors both in vitro and in vivo and by the generation of constitutively active receptor mutants. Both of these techniques allowed for the inhibition by inverse agonists of basal activity, that is, activity that occurs without added agonist *(89)*.

6. Conclusions

> *"Discovery consists in seeing what everyone else has seen and thinking what nobody else has thought." (Albert Szent-Gyorgyi, 1962)*

What lessons can be learned from reviewing the history of adrenergic receptors during the 20th century? Perhaps first and foremost is that the major advances have often been technique driven. As newly developed techniques, or existing techniques utilized in new ways, were thoughtfully and carefully applied to the study of adrenergic receptors, important new insights began to emerge. Second, progress came as insights made in other systems, such as the visual system, were appropriately applied to the adrenergic receptors. Finally, these advances were possible only by building on the foundation of innumerable carefully performed studies by equally innumerable dedicated workers using established techniques.

If indeed the molecular era is drawing to a close, what is the appropriate label for the emerging era? Several possibilities come to mind, including the cross-talk era, the genomic era, or the proteomic era. Only time will tell. My hope is that perhaps the emerging era will come to be known as the integrative/systems era as we take what we are learning about these magnificent receptors and more fully integrate that knowledge into better understanding of how they function in the whole animal in relation to other neurohormonal systems as components of various physiological systems. This in turn, we all expect, will lead to better therapeutics as we more rationally use existing drugs for selected populations and develop new drugs with greater selectivity, efficacy, and fewer side effects.

References

1. Davenport HW. Epinephrin(e). Physiologist 1982;25:76–82.
2. Cannon WB, Rosenbueth A. Studies on the conditions of activity in endocrine organs: 24. Sympathin E and sympathin I. Am J Physiol 1933;104:557–574.
3. von Euler US. The nature of adrenergic nerve mediators. Pharmacol Rev 1951;3: 247–277.
4. Langley JN. On the reaction of cells and of nerve-endings to certain poisons, chiefly as regards the reaction of striated muscle to nicotine and to curari. J Physiol (Lond) 1905;33:374–413.
5. Dale HH. On some physiological actions of ergot. J Physiol (Lond) 1906;34: 163–206.
6. Ahlquist RP. A study of adrenotropic receptors. Am J Physiol 1948;153:586–600.
7. de Jongh DK. Some introductory remarks on the conception of receptors. In: Ariens EJ, editor. Molecular Pharmacology. New York: Academic Press, 1964: xiii–xvi.
8. Kobinger W. Rudolf Buchheim lecture. Drugs as tools in research on adrenoceptors. Naunyn Schmiedebergs Arch Pharmacol 1986;332:113–123.
9. Sutherland EW, Rall TW. Fractionation and characterization of a cyclic adenine ribonucleotide formed by tissue particles. J Biol Chem 1958;232:1077–1091.
10. Sutherland EW, Robison GA. The role of cyclic-3',5'-AMP in responses to catecholamines and other hormones. Pharmacol Rev 1966;18:145–161.
11. Black JW, Crowther AF, Shanks RG, Smith LH, Dornhorst AC. A new adrenergic β-receptor antagonist. Lancet 1964;283:1080–1081.
12. Lands AM, Arnold A, McAuliff JP, Luduena FP, Brown TG. Differentiation of receptor systems activated by sympathomimetic amines. Nature 1967;214:597–598.
13. Furchgott RF. The pharmacological differentiation of adrenergic receptors. Ann N Y Acad Sci 1967;139:553–570.
14. Brown GL, Gillespie JE. The output of sympathetic transmitter from the spleen of the cat. J Physiol 1957;138:81–102.
15. Langer SZ. The metabolism of [^{3}H]noradrenaline released by electrical stimulation from the isolated nictitating membrane of the cat and from the vas deferens of the rat. J Physiol 1970;208:515–546.
16. Starke K, Montel H, Schumann HJ. Influence of cocaine and phenoxybenzamine on noradrenaline uptake and release. Naunyn Schmiedebergs Arch Pharmakol 1971;270:210–214.
17. Starke K. Influence of α-receptor stimulants on noradrenaline release. Naturwissenschaften 1971;58:420.

18. Enero MA, Langer SZ, Rothlin RP, Stefano FJ. Role of the α-adrenoceptor in regulating noradrenaline overflow by nerve stimulation. Br J Pharmacol 1972;44: 672–688.
19. Langer SZ. Presynaptic regulation of catecholamine release. Biochem Pharmacol 1974;23:1793–1800.
20. Berthelsen S, Pettinger WA. A functional basis for classification of α-adrenergic receptors. Life Sci 1977;21:595–606.
21. Arch JRS, Ainsworth MA, Cawthorne MA, et al. Atypical β-adrenoceptors on brown adipocytes as a target for anti-obesity drugs. Nature 1984;309:163–165.
22. De Robertis E. Molecular biology of synaptic receptors. Science 1971;171:963–971.
23. Miledi R, Molinoff P, Potter LT. Isolation of the cholinergic receptor protein of *Torpedo* electric tissue. Nature 1971;229:554–557.
24. Goldstein A, Lowney LI, Pal BK. Stereospecific and nonspecific interactions of the morphine congener levorphanol in subcellular fractions of mouse brain. Proc Natl Acad Sci USA 1971;68:1742–1747.
25. Aurbach GD, Fedak SA, Woodard CJ, Palmer JS, Hauser D, Troxler F. β-adrenergic receptor: stereospecific interaction of iodinated β-blocking agent with high affinity site. Science 1974;186:1223–1224.
26. Alexander RW, Davis JN, Lefkowitz RJ. Direct identification and characterisation of β-adrenergic receptors in rat brain. Nature 1975;258:437–440.
27. Bylund DB, Snyder SH. β-Adrenergic receptor binding in membrane preparations from mammalian brain. Mol Pharmacol 1976;12:568–580.
28. Greenberg DA, U'Prichard DC, Snyder SH. α-Noradrenergic receptor binding in mammalian brain: differential labeling of agonist and antagonist states. Life Sci 1976;19:69–76.
29. Williams LT, Lefkowitz RJ. α-Adrenergic receptor identification by [^{3}H]dihydroergocryptine binding. Science 1976;192:791–793.
30. Minneman KP, Hegstrand LR, Molinoff PB. Simultaneous determination of β_1 and β_2 adrenergic receptors in tissues containing both receptor subtypes. Mol Pharmacol 1979;16:34–46.
31. Bylund DB, U'Prichard DC. Characterization of α_1- and α_2-adrenergic receptors. Int Rev Neurobiol 1983;24:343–431.
32. Morrow AL, Creese I. Characterization of α_1 adrenergic receptor subtypes in rat brain: A reevaluation of [^{3}H]WB4101 and [^{3}H]prazosin binding. Mol Pharmacol 1986;29:321–330.
33. Minneman KP, Han C, Abel PW. Comparison of α_1-adrenergic receptor subtypes distinguished by chloroethylclonidine and WB4101. Mol Pharmacol 1988; 33:509–514.
34. Bylund DB. Heterogeneity of α_2-adrenergic receptors. Pharmacol Biochem Behav 1985;22:835–843.
35. Bylund DB, Ray-Prenger C, Murphy TJ. α_{2A} and α_{2B} adrenergic receptor subtypes: antagonist binding in tissues and cell lines containing only one subtype. J Pharmacol Exp Ther 1988;245:600–607.
36. Bylund DB, Ray-Prenger C. α_{2A} and α_{2B} adrenergic receptor subtypes: attenuation of cyclic AMP production in cell lines containing only one receptor subtype. J Pharmacol Exp Ther 1989;251:640–644.

37. Murphy TJ, Bylund DB. Characterization of α_2 adrenergic receptors in the OK cell, an opossum kidney cell line. J Pharmacol Exp Ther 1988;244:571–578.
38. Michel AD, Loury DN, Whiting RL. Differences between α_2 adrenoceptor in rat submaxillary gland and the α_{2A} and α_{2B} adrenoceptor subtypes. Br J Pharmacol 1989;98:890–897.
39. Simonneaux V, Ebadi M, Bylund DB. Identification and characterization of α_{2D}-adrenergic receptors in bovine pineal gland. Mol Pharmacol 1991;40:235–241.
40. Bylund DB. Subtypes of α_2-adrenoceptors: Pharmacological and molecular biological evidence converge. Trends Pharmacol Sci 1988;9:356–361.
41. Rodbell M, Krans HM, Pohl SL, Birnbaumer L. The glucagon-sensitive adenyl cyclase system in plasma membranes of rat liver. IV. Effects of guanylnucleotides on binding of ^{125}I-glucagon. J Biol Chem 1971;246:1872–1876.
42. Lefkowitz RJ, Mullikin D, Caron MG. Regulation of β-adrenergic receptors by guanyl-5'-yl imidodiphosphate and other purine nucleotides. J Biol Chem 1976; 251:4686–4692.
43. Maguire ME, Van Arsdale PM, Gilman AG. An agonist-specific effect of guanine nucleotides on binding to the β-adrenergic receptor. Mol Pharmacol 1976; 12:335–339.
44. De Lean A, Stadel JM, Lefkowitz RJ. A ternary complex model explains the agonist-specific binding properties of the adenylate cyclase-coupled β-adrenergic receptor. J Biol Chem 1980;255:7108–7117.
45. Dunn R, McCoy J, Simsek M, et al. The bacteriorhodopsin gene. Proc Natl Acad Sci USA 1981;78:6744–6748.
46. Engelman DM, Goldman A, Steitz TA. The identification of helical segments in the polypeptide chain of bacteriorhodopsin. Meth Enzym 1982;88:81–88.
47. Nathans J, Hogness DS. Isolation, sequence analysis, and intron-exon arrangement of the gene encoding bovine rhodopsin. Cell 1983;34:807–814.
48. Dixon RAF, Kobilka BK, Strader DJ, et al. Cloning of the gene and cDNA for mammalian β-adrenergic receptor and homology with rhodopsin. Nature 1986; 321:75–79.
49. Kobilka BK, Frielle T, Collins S, et al. An intronless gene encodes a potential member of a family of receptors coupled to guanine nucleotide regulatory protein. Nature 1987;329:75–79.
50. Fargin A, Raymond SR, Lohse MJ, Kobilka BK, Caron MG, Lefkowitz RJ. The genomic clone G-21 which resembles α β-adrenergic receptor sequence encodes the 5-HT$_{1A}$ receptor. Nature 1988;335:358–360.
51. Frielle T, Collins S, Daniel KW, Caron MG, Lefkowitz RJ, Kobilka BK. Cloning of the cDNA for the human β_1-adrenergic receptor. Proc Natl Acad Sci USA 1987; 84:7920–7924.
52. Emorine LJ, Marullo S, Briend-Sutren MM, et al. Molecular characterization of the human β_3-adrenergic receptor. Science 1989;245:1118–1121.
53. Bylund DB, Bond RA, Clarke DE, et al. Adrenoceptors. In: Vanhoutte PM, et al., editors. The IUPHAR Compendium of Receptor Characterization and Classification. London: IUPHAR Media, 1998:58–74.
54. Granneman JG. The putative β_4 adrenergic receptor is a novel state of the β_1 adrenergic receptor. Am J Physiol Endocrinol Metab 2001;280:E199–E202.

55. Kobilka BK, Matsui H, Kobilka TS, et al. Cloning, sequencing, and expression of the gene encoding for the human platelet α_2-adrenergic receptor subtype. Science 1987;238:650–656.

56. Regan JW, Kobilka TS, Yang-Feng TL, Caron MG, Lefkowitz RJ, Kobilka BK. Cloning and expression of a human kidney cDNA for an α_2-adrenergic receptor subtype. Proc Natl Acad Sci USA 1988;85:6301–6305.

57. Zeng D, Harrison JK, D'Angelo DD, et al. Molecular characterization of a rat α_{2B}-adrenergic receptor. Proc Natl Acad Sci USA 1990;87:3102–3106.

58. Weinshank RL, Zgombick JM, Macchi M, et al. Cloning, expression, and pharmacological characterization of a human α_{2B}-adrenergic receptor. Mol Pharmacol 1990;35:681–688.

59. Bylund DB, Blaxall HS, Iversen LJ, Caron MG, Lefkowitz RJ, Lomasney JW. Pharmacological characteristics of α_2-adrenergic receptors: comparison of pharmacologically defined subtypes with subtypes identified by molecular cloning. Mol Pharmacol 1992;42:1–5.

60. Cotecchia S, Schwinn DA, Randall RR, Lefkowitz RJ, Caron MG, Kobilka BK. Molecular cloning and expression of the cDNA for the hamster α_1-adrenergic receptor. Proc Natl Acad Sci USA 1988;85:7159–7163.

61. Schwinn DA, Lomasney JW, Lorenz W, et al. Molecular cloning and expression of the cDNA for a novel α_1 adrenergic receptor subtype. J Biol Chem 1990;265: 8183–8189.

62. Lomasney J, Cotecchia S, Lorenz W, et al. Molecular cloning and expression of the cDNA for the α_{1A}-adrenergic receptor: the gene for which is located on human chromosome 5. J Biol Chem 1991;266:6365–6369.

63. Perez DM, Piascik MT, Graham RM. Solution-phase library screening for the identification of rare clones: isolation of an α_{1D} adrenergic receptor cDNA. Mol Pharmacol 1991;40:876–883.

64. Ford APDW, Williams TJ, Blue DR, Clarke DE. α_1-Adrenoceptor classification: sharpening Occam's razor. Trends Pharmacol Sci 1994;15:167–170.

65. Perez DM, Piascik MT, Malik N, Gaivin R, Graham RM. Cloning, expression, and tissue distribution of the rat homolog of the bovine α_{1C}-adrenergic receptor provide evidence for its classification as the α_{1A} subtype. Mol Pharmacol 1994;46: 823–831.

66. Hieble JP, Bylund DB, Clarke DE, et al. International Union of Pharmacology. 10. Recommendation for nomenclature of α_1-adrenoceptors: consensus update. Pharmacol Rev 1995;47:267–270.

67. Muramatsu I, Murata S, Isaka M, et al. α_1 Adrenoceptor subtypes and two receptor systems in vascular tissues. Life Sci 1998;62:1461–1465.

68. Daniels DV, Gever JR, Jasper JR, et al. Human cloned α_{1A}-adrenoceptor isoforms display α_{1L}-adrenoceptor pharmacology in functional studies. Eur J Pharmacol 1999;370:337–343.

69. Dixon RA, Sigal IS, Rands E, et al. Ligand binding to the β-adrenergic receptor involves its rhodopsin-like core. Nature 1987;326:73–77.

70. Strader CD, Sigal IS, Candelore MR, Rands E, Hill WS, Dixon RA. Conserved aspartic acid residues 79 and 113 of the β-adrenergic receptor have different roles in receptor function. J Biol Chem 1988;263:10,267–10,271.

71. Strader CD, Candelore MR, Hill WS, Sigal IS, Dixon RA. Identification of two serine residues involved in agonist activation of the β-adrenergic receptor. J Biol Chem 1989;264:13,572–13,578.

72. Susulic VS, Frederich RC, Lawitts J, et al. Targeted disruption of the β₃ adrenergic receptor gene. J Biol Chem 1995;270:29,483–29,492.

73. Rohrer DK, Desai KH, Jasper JR, et al. Targeted disruption of the mouse β₁-adrenergic receptor gene: Developmental and cardiovascular effects. Proc Natl Acad Sci U S A 1996;93:7375–7380.

74. Chruscinski AJ, Rohrer DK, Schauble E, Desai KH, Bernstein D, Kobilka BK. Targeted disruption of the β₂ adrenergic receptor gene. J Biol Chem 1999;274: 16,694–16,700.

75. Bachman ES, Dhillon H, Zhang CY, et al. β-AR Signaling required for diet-induced thermogenesis and obesity resistance. Science 2002;297:843–845.

76. Cavalli A, Lattion AL, Hummler E, et al. Decreased blood pressure response in mice deficient of the α₁ᵦ adrenergic receptor. Proc Natl Acad Sci USA 1997;94: 11,589–11,594.

77. Rokosh DG, Simpson PC. Knockout of the α₁ₐ/c-adrenergic receptor subtype: The α₁ₐ/c is expressed in resistance arteries and is required to maintain arterial blood pressure. Proc Natl Acad Sci USA 2002;99:9474–9479.

78. Tanoue A, Nasa Y, Koshimizu T, et al. The α₁ᴅ-adrenergic receptor directly regulates arterial blood pressure via vasoconstriction. J Clin Invest 2002;109: 765–775.

79. Tanoue A, Koshimizu T, Shibata K, Nasa Y, Takeo S, Tsujimoto G. Insights into α₁ adrenoceptor function in health and disease from transgenic animal studies. Trends Endocrinol Metab 2003;14:107–113.

80. Macmillan LB, Hein L, Smith MS, Piascik MT, Limbird LE. Central hypotensive effects of the α₂ₐ-adrenergic receptor subtype. Science 1996;273:801–803.

81. Link RE, Desai K, Hein L, et al. Cardiovascular regulation in mice lacking α₂-adrenergic receptor subtypes b and c. Science 1996;273:803–805.

82. Altman JD, Trendelenburg AU, Macmillan L, et al. Abnormal regulation of the sympathetic nervous system in α₂ₐ-adrenergic receptor knockout mice. Mol Pharmacol 1999;56:154–161.

83. Kable JW, Murrin LC, Bylund DB. in vivo gene modification elucidates sub-type-specific functions of α₂-adrenergic receptors. J Pharmacol Exp Ther 2000; 293:1–7.

84. Reihsaus E, Innis M, MacIntyre N, Liggett SB. Mutations in the gene encoding for the β₂ adrenergic receptor in normal and asthmatic subjects. Am J Respir Cell Mol Biol 1993;8:334–339.

85. Small KM, McGraw DW, Liggett SB. Pharmacology and physiology of human adrenergic receptor polymorphisms. Annu Rev Pharmacol Toxicol 2003;43: 381–411.

86. Palczewski K, Kumasaka T, Hori T, et al. Crystal structure of rhodopsin: a G protein-coupled receptor. Science 2000;289:739–745.

87. Kohout TA, Lefkowitz RJ. Regulation of G protein-coupled receptor kinases and arrestins during receptor desensitization. Mol Pharmacol 2003;63:9–18.

88. Ahn S, Nelson CD, Garrison TR, Miller WE, Lefkowitz RJ. Desensitization, internalization, and signaling functions of β-arrestins demonstrated by RNA interference. Proc Natl Acad Sci U S A 2003;100:1740–1744.

89. Bond RA, Leff P, Johnson TD, et al. Physiological effects of inverse agonists in transgenic mice with myocardial overexpression of the β$_2$-adrenoceptor. Nature 1995;374:272–276.

Part II
Structure–Function

2

Ligand Binding, Activation, and Agonist Trafficking

Angela M. Finch, Valerie Sarramegna, and Robert M. Graham

Summary

Adrenergic receptors are critical mediators of sympathetic nervous system-regulated physiological responses. Activated by the neurotransmitter and neurohormone, norepinephrine and epinephrine, released from sympathetic nerve endings and the adrenal medulla, respectively, they play a central role in this evolutionarily ancient defense system that regulates many physiological functions, including those involved in circulatory, metabolic, respiratory, and central nervous system homeostasis. In addition, alterations in the regulation and molecular structure of adrenergic receptors have been implicated in a variety of diseases, and drugs targeting these receptors are important and widely used therapeutics. The molecular cloning of the first adrenergic receptor in 1986 revealed structural homology with the functionally related rhodopsin visual transduction system—a finding that led to the realization that these receptors formed a new superfamily of proteins, now known as G protein-coupled receptors. Since that time, a plethora of structure–function studies have provided major insights into the molecular determinants of adrenergic receptor ligand-binding, activation, and signaling, many of which are relevant not only to the adrenergic receptor family but also, more generally, to the broader superfamily of G protein-coupled receptors. These advances in our understanding of adrenergic receptor activation, regulation, and functioning are reviewed in this chapter.

Key Words: Activation; adrenergic receptor; agonist trafficking; ligand binding; mechanism; mutagenesis; structure–function.

From: *The Receptors: The Adrenergic Receptors: In the 21st Century*
Edited by: D. Perez © Humana Press Inc., Totowa, NJ

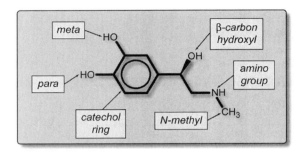

Fig. 1. Chemical structure of (–)-epinephrine. Individual moieties, including the *meta-* and *para*-hydroxyls, catechol ring, protonated amine, alcoholic chiral β-carbon hydroxyl, and *N*-methyl group are indicated.

1. Adrenergic Receptor Ligand-Binding Sites

1.1. Binding Contacts of the Endogenous Ligands

In the early 1930s, Easson and Stedman proposed that receptor binding of a compound possessing a chiral center involved interactions between three contact points on the receptor and three moieties of the ligand *(1)*. On the basis of experimental data on the activity of the enantiomers of epinephrine, they proposed that epinephrine's triad consisted of the basic group (the amide), the aromatic ring with its hydroxyl groups, and the alcoholic chiral, β-carbon hydroxyl group *(1)* (Fig. 1). The importance of these three chemical groups and their interaction with the adrenergic receptors (ARs) has been borne out by numerous mutagenesis and biochemical studies along with modeling studies performed since the first of the ARs, the mammalian β_2- and turkey β-AR, were cloned in 1986 *(2,3)*.

However, as discussed in more detail later in this section, distinct interactions were also defined for both the aromatic ring and its hydroxyls, giving a total of at least four critical receptor/ligand moiety contacts. These studies also defined the binding site for endogenous agonists to be contained within a pocket formed by the clustering of the seven putative transmembrane (TM) helical bundles of the receptor and to be located approx 11 Å below the extracellular surface *(4)*. The key interactions (Table 1) are (1) an ionic interaction between the amino group of the catechol with the carboxylate side chain of D3.32[1] of helix 3, (2) hydrogen bonding between the catechol *meta-* and *para*-hydroxyl groups and serine residues in helix 5, (3) an aromatic–aromatic interaction between the phenyl ring of agonists and aromatic residues in helix 6, and (4) hydrogen bonding between the chiral benzylic β-hydroxyl of agonists and a residue in helix 6, which accounts for the stereoselectivity of adrenergic ligands (Fig. 2).

---

[1] *See* the Appendix on page 65 for residue numbering.

Table 1
Binding Contacts of Adrenergic Receptors With Endogenous Ligands [a,b]

Receptor	Amine	*para-*Hydroxyl	*meta-*Hydroxyl	Catechol Ring	β-Carbon Hydroxyl	*N*-methyl
			Moieties of Endogenous Catecholamine Ligands			
α_{1A}	D3.32	S5.46	S5.42	F4.62, F5.41		
α_{1B}	D3.32	S5.42	S5.42	F6.51		
α_{2A}	D3.32	S5.46	—	F6.52, Y6.55	*D3.32,* S2.61, S7.46	*F7.38, F7.39*
β_2	D3.32	S5.46	S5.42, S5.43	F6.51, F6.52	N6.55, *D3.32,* T4.56	

[a] Interaction demonstrated experimentally.

[b] Residues in italics are those that have been proposed to interact based only on molecular modeling studies.

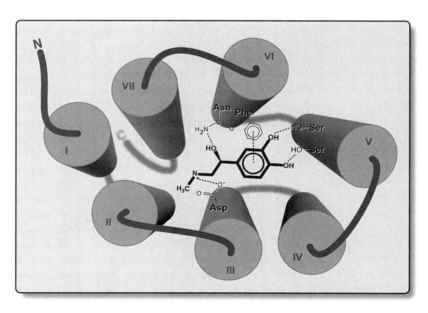

Fig. 2. Major interactions between (−)-epinephrine and its β-adrenergic receptor binding site: (a) ionic interaction between the amino group of epinephrine and the carboxylate side chain of an aspartic acid (Asp) in helix III; (b) hydrogen bonding between the catechol *meta-* and *para-*hydroxyl groups and serine (Ser) residues in helix V; (c) an aromatic–aromatic interaction between the phenyl ring of agonists and an aromatic residue (Phe) in helix VI, and (d) hydrogen bonding interaction between the chiral benzylic β-hydroxyl of epinephrine and a residue (Asn) in helix VI, which accounts for the stereoselectivity of adrenergic ligands. Transmembrane helices are indicated by Roman numerals.

Studies of the structure–activity relationship of adrenergic ligands have established the essential nature of the amine moiety for interaction with ARs *(5)*. It was proposed that a counterion within the receptor was the site of interaction with this moiety. In attempts to identify the residue that provides this counterion, aspartyl and glutamyl residues conserved across all of the receptors that bind cationic amine ligands were identified, including the highly conserved D2.50. However, it was only the loss of D3.32 that dramatically affected the binding of ligands to the β_2-AR *(6)*. D3.32 is conserved across all receptors that bind amine ligands. D3.32N or D3.32G[2] mutants of the β_2-AR had agonist binding below detectable levels; however, agonists were still fully efficacious at these mutated receptors despite their greatly decreased potency (as evidenced by an increase in the half maximal response (EC_{50}) by 300- to 40,000-fold) *(7)*. Mutation of D3.32 to Leu in the β_3-AR also resulted in loss of ligand binding *(8)*. When D3.32 was mutated to Ser, the receptor could not be activated by amine-containing ligands. However, compounds in which the amine was replaced by a moiety that can serve as a hydrogen bond acceptor, such as a catechol ester or a ketone, which do not activate the wild-type receptor, activated the D3.32S mutant receptor *(9)*. This finding demonstrated that an interaction between D3.32 and the agonist is required for both optimal binding and receptor activation, but that the nature of this interaction is not critical because it can be either ionic or hydrogen bonding. Subsequently, the salt bridge between the protonated amine of the ligand and the carboxylate side chain of D3.32 was shown to be essential for the binding of the endogenous catechols in all the AR subtypes *(6,7,9–11)*. Of all the interactions involving the receptor and its endogenous ligands, this interaction has been demonstrated as the most important energetically *(9)*.

Seryl residues in TM segment 5 (TM V) are the interaction sites for the hydroxyl groups of the catecholamines, although the exact hydrogen-bonding interactions formed between the agonist hydroxyls and the various TM V seryl residues differ among the various AR subtypes. The α_{1A}-AR has only two TM V serines (S5.42, S5.46), and both of these form hydrogen bonds with the catechol hydroxyls of endogenous ligands. The contribution of these serines to ligand binding is equal, and each is able to compensate for the loss of the other because mutation of either to alanine does not affect the affinity of epinephrine; however, mutation of both leads to a marked loss of epinephrine affinity *(12)*. S5.42 has been shown to bind the *meta*-hydroxyl of the ligand; the *para*-hydroxyl bonds with S5.46 *(13)*. Although the α_{1B}-AR has three serines available to interact with the hydroxyl moieties of the catechol ring of the endogenous ligands, only S5.42 has been demonstrated to be involved in ligand binding; in

---

[2] The nomenclature indicates that the aspartate has been mutated to asparagine or glycine, respectively.

this instance, it forms hydrogen bonds with both the *meta-* and *para*-hydroxyls *(10)*. The α_{2A}-AR also only utilizes one of the TM V serines (S5.46) to bind the endogenous ligands. Mutation of S5.46 of α_{2A}-AR suggests a possible role for this serine in hydrogen bond interactions with the *para*-hydroxyl group of the catechol ring *(14,15)*. Mutation of S5.42 of α_{2A}-AR suggested that this residue does not directly participate in receptor–agonist interactions, in contrast with the corresponding serine residue in the α_{1A}- and β_2-ARs, which has been postulated to interact with the *meta*-hydroxyl group of catecholamines *(15)*. The interaction of the β_2-AR with the *meta*-hydroxyl of a catecholamine agonist has been postulated to occur via a bifurcated hydrogen bond between the hydroxyl and both S5.42 and S5.43 *(16)*. As in all the other ARs (with the exception of α_{1B}), the *para*-hydroxyl of the endogenous ligands binds to S5.46 of the β_2-AR *(17)*. Binding of catechol agonists with the serines of TM V has also been proposed to play an important role in the orientation of the ligand within the binding pocket *(11,12,16)*. Based on the differences in the serines used to interact with the *meta-* and *para*-hydroxyls of the ligand, it has been predicted that the catechol ring lies parallel to the extracellular surface of the α-ARs; it is rotated 120° from this planar orientation in the β-ARs *(12,16)*.

The third proposed component of the interaction between the endogenous ligands and the ARs is the interaction of the catechol ring with aromatic residues of the receptor. Pharmacophore mapping indicates that the catechol ring is essential for ligand binding *(18)*. Phenylalanines in helices 4, 5, and 6 have been postulated to interact with the catechol ring. In the case of the α_{1A}-AR, F4.62 and F5.41 have been shown to be involved in independent aromatic interactions with the catechol ring of endogenous ligands *(19)*. Molecular modeling studies of the α_{1B}-AR, in which ligand has been docked, indicated that the F6.51 side chain is well positioned to interact with the catechol ring *(20)*. There is experimental evidence that the side chain of F6.51 is both solvent accessible and directed into the agonist-binding pocket *(21)*. Direct evidence for the involvement of F6.51 in an aromatic–aromatic interaction with catechol agonists comes from detailed mutagenesis studies coupled with binding and activation studies using a variety of agonists *(21)*. These studies provided compelling evidence that not only is the interaction between F6.51, but not F6.52, and the phenyl ring critical for ligand binding and for positioning the ligand in the correct orientation, but also that F5.61 is a critical switch involved in receptor activation *(20)*. In the α_{2A}-AR, it has been proposed that the phenyl group of the ligand interacts with Y6.55 and F6.52 in a π–π stacking interaction *(11)*. Both F6.51 and F6.52 have been proposed to stabilize the catechol ring of the β_2-AR, along with Y7.53 *(21,22)*, in contrast to the α_{1B}-AR, in which only F6.51 interacts with the aromatic ring *(20)*.

ARs show marked stereoselectivity for the (–)-enantiomers of epinephrine and norepinephrine, in terms of both binding affinity and agonist potency *(23,24)*.

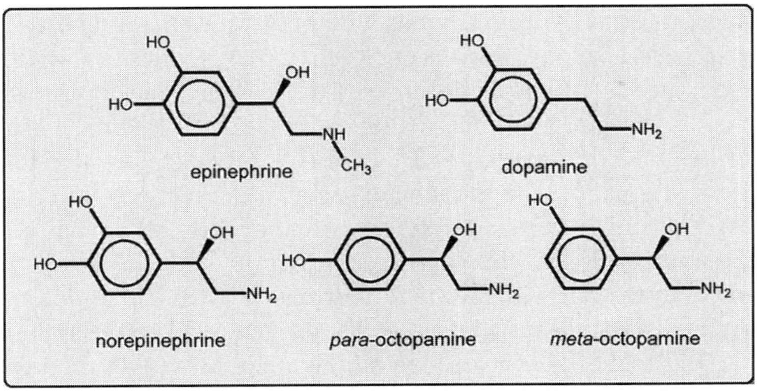

Fig. 3. Chemical structure of endogenous catecholamines.

This stereoselectivity is the underlying basis for the Easson and Stedman hypothesis *(1)*. Nevertheless, the receptor contact responsible for this stereoselectivity has not been clearly identified. Early molecular modeling of the β_2-AR proposed S4.57 as the site of interaction between the chiral β-hydroxyl and the receptor *(25,26)*. Mutation of T4.56, the residue directly N-terminal to S4.57, to an isoleucine provided supporting evidence for the involvement of S4.57 in binding the chiral β-hydroxyl *(27)*. This mutant displayed an approximately fourfold reduction in the affinity of epinephrine and norepinephrine for the receptor but had no effect on the affinity of dopamine (which lacks the chiral hydroxyl) (Fig. 3) *(27)*. The authors suggested that this effect is not caused by a loss of a direct interaction between T4.56, but instead that the mutation results in a conformational change that prevents the interaction of the β-hydroxyl with S4.57. In this study, direct evidence for the involvement of S4.57 could not be obtained because its mutation to an alanine resulted in a receptor that failed to be expressed in the plasma membrane, possibly because of global misfolding *(17)*. However, in another study expression of the S4.57 mutant was obtained, and this mutant retained stereoselectivity isoproterenol (Fig. 4) binding *(24)*, hence, eliminating S4.57 as the binding partner for the chiral β-hydroxyl.

Molecular modeling, using membStruk (a computational method to predict atomic level tertiary structure using only primary sequence) and a *de novo* model, has predicted that, in the (−)-enantiomer, the β-hydroxyl interacts with N6.55 *(28,29)*, a prediction that was not confirmed with a homology model based on the crystal structure of rhodopsin *(29)*. Mutation of N6.55 to a leucine resulted in a receptor with a sixfold decrease in its stereoselectivity of the receptor of (−)-isoproterenol vs (+)-isoproterenol *(24)*. However, this loss of binding stereoselectivity was confined to agonists, with the N6.55L mutant showing no change in its stereospecific recognition of neutral antagonists or partial agonists *(24)*. The role of N6.55 has also been examined in the β_3-AR. Mutation of N6.55 to

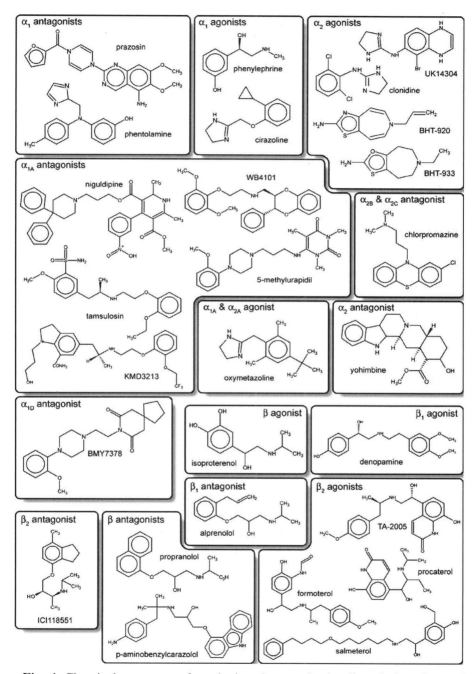

Fig. 4. Chemical structures of synthetic subtype-selective ligands for adrenergic receptors.

alanine did not alter the stereoselectivity of the binding of partial agonists but did result in these compounds displaying reduced efficacy while not altering the efficacy of the full agonists, norepinephrine and isoproterenol *(8)*.

Another molecular model of the β_2-AR also predicts an interaction not only between N6.55 and the β-hydroxyl, but also between the β-hydroxyl and D3.32 *(28)*. This last interaction has also been suggested in a model of norepinephrine binding to the α_{2A}-AR *(30)*, which proposed that a bidendate hydrogen bond is formed between oxygen atoms of the D3.32 side chain and both the β-hydroxyl and amide groups of the ligand. However, direct evaluation of D3.32 in stereoselectivity of ligand binding has been hindered by the poor expression of an alanine substitution mutant *(31,32)*.

Two seryl residues, S2.61 and S7.46, have also been suggested to play a role in stereoselective ligand recognition by the α_{2A}-AR because their mutation to alanine resulted in marked reduction in (–)-norepinephrine affinity, with little change in affinity for the (+)-enantiomer or for dopamine *(23)*. However, involvement of S2.61 was not supported by the modeling data of Nyronen et al. *(11)*. In the study of Hieble et al. *(23)*, evidence was obtained to indicate that S4.57, T6.54, Y6.55, and T6.56 are not involved in determining stereoselectivity of agonist binding.

Interactions between ARs and their ligand moieties, distinct from those proposed by Easson and Stedman, have been suggested. For example, molecular modeling of the interaction of the α_{2A}-AR with epinephrine has indicated that its *N*-methyl group may bond with F7.38 and F7.39 *(11)*. However, experimental support for this interaction from mutagenesis studies is lacking.

1.2. Structural Basis of Subtype Selectivity and Antagonist Binding

The ARs, particularly those of a particular type (e.g., α_1, α_2, β) share a high degree of amino acid homology, especially within the TM forming the ligand-binding pocket (68–77% identity for α_1-, 79–82% for α_2-, and 63–73% for β-ARs). Nevertheless, although all amide-containing ligands bind to D3.32 and many also bind to the serines of TM V, ligand-binding residues unique to each receptor have been identified (Fig. 5) that confer subtype selectivity. In some instances, it has been possible to identify residues responsible for subtype selectivity (Fig.5); in other cases, the lack of ligands that are sufficiently selective for particular subtypes has limited such analyses.

In a detailed study of the residues responsible for subtype selectivity, Hwa et al. *(33)* demonstrated that just 2 of the approx 172 residues forming the TM segments of the α_{1B}-AR account for its agonist-binding selectivity as compared to the α_{1A}-AR. The approach used to identify these two residues, at positions 5.39 (α_{1B} = A, α_{1A} = V) and 6.55 (α_{1B} = L, α_{1A} = M), is instructive. Based on the reasoning that the residues potentially involved in subtype selectivity should be distinct between the two receptor subtypes, only the 48 nonconserved residues forming the

TM segments were considered. Of these, candidate resides were selected based on the following criteria: (1) location in the ligand-binding extracellular half of the TM segments, and (2) orientation of side chains toward the putative ligand-binding pocket. Residues excluded were those on TM I because this helix was known not to be involved in ligand binding and those for which a lack of conservation was merely caused by interspecies differences given that α_1-subtype ligand-binding profiles are conserved across species. This allowed the initial set of 48 nonconserved residues to be reduced to only 7 that fulfilled all criteria, which were then subjected to mutational analysis. Mutation of A5.39 in the α_{1B}-AR to a valine, the residue found at this position in the α_{1A}-AR, resulted in an 80% conversion of agonist-selective binding from that of the α_{1B}- to that of the α_{1A}-subtype; the remaining 20% were accounted for by the additional substitution of L6.55 in the α_{1B}-AR to a methionine, the residue at this position in the α_{1A}-AR *(33)*. It was proposed that A5.39V-induced increase in the affinity for α_{1A}-AR-selective ligands was caused by an increased hydrophobic interaction between valine and the aromatic ring of agonist ligands; the additional 20% increase in affinity provided by L6.55M was caused by increased interactions resulting from the extended chain length of the ortho hydrophobic groups of synthetic ligands *(33)*, a postulate supported by the finding that the complementary substitutions of both V5.39A and M6.55V in the α_{1A}-AR converted its agonist selectivity entirely to that of the α_{1B}-AR.

Interestingly, neither the single mutations at the 5.39 or 6.55 positions nor the double mutations at both positions altered antagonist binding, demonstrating the agonist-specific nature of these interactions *(33)*. However, either single mutation (A5.39V or L6.55M in the α_{1B}-AR or V5.39A or M6.55L in the α_{1A}-AR) resulted in constitutive activity that could be rescued by additional substitution of the complimentary residue responsible for agonist selectivity *(33)*.

In contrast to the TM V and VI residues involved in subtype-selective agonist binding, residues in extracellular loop 2 (e_2) have been found to be responsible for the selective binding of antagonists by the α_{1A}- and α_{1B}-ARs. Thus, substitution of Gly[196], Val[197], and Thr[198] of the α_{1B}-AR to the corresponding residues (Gln, Ile, and Asn, respectively) in the α_{1A}-AR, or vice versa, leads to a change in the antagonist-binding profile to that of the other subtype *(34)* (Fig. 5). This finding, and those of several other studies, has provided evidence that α_1-selective antagonists bind at a site closer to the extracellular loops, which is above the plane of the binding site and skewed toward TM VII *(35,36)*. The binding of antagonists to e_2 also raises the question of the spatial arrangement of this loop with respect to the TM domains. In rhodopsin, e_2 covers the binding site like a lid. It is tethered by a disulfide bond (found in almost all G protein-coupled receptors [GPCRs]) connecting it to e_1 at the N-terminal end of TM III and forms multiple interactions with the chromophore ligand, 11-*cis* retinal *(37,38)*. It has been postulated that this structural arrangement traps the chromophore and prevents its extrusion into

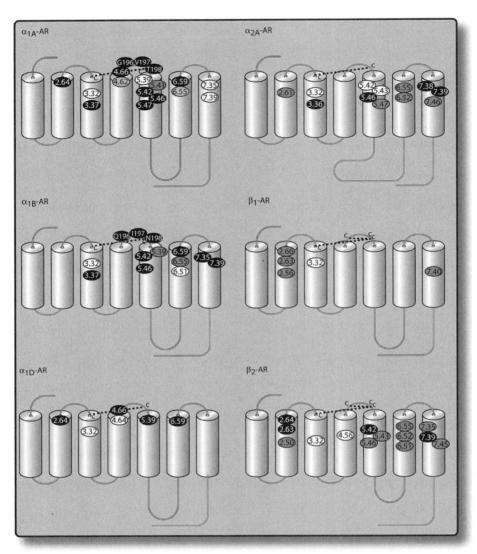

Fig. 5. Residues involved in determining subtype and ligand selectivity. Residues important for antagonist binding are shown in black, for agonist binding in grey, and for both in white. Residue numbers are indicated by the Ballesteros and Weinstein system (*see* the Appendix on page 65).

2.50 Mutation of D2.50 of the β_2-AR results in decreased affinity for agonists but not antagonists *(6)*

2.56 In the β_1-AR, L2.56 makes a major contribution to binding interactions for those agonists containing a dimethoxyphenyl group *(43,44)*

2.61 S2.61 is involved in the stereoselectivity of α_{2A}-AR for (−)-enantiomers of catecholamines; It has been proposed that this site represents an important point for attachment of the β-hydroxyl group of catecholamines *(287)*

2.63 In the β_1-AR, T2.63 constitutes a major binding interaction for those agonists containing a dimethoxyphenyl group *(43,44)*; in the β_2-AR, S2.63 interacts with *p*-aminobenzylcarazolol *(288)*

2.64	M2.64 of α_{1D}-AR imparts its selectivity for niguldipine vs α_{1A}-AR (F2.64) *(34,289,290)*; H2.64 of β_2-AR interacts with *p*-aminobenzylcarazolol *(291)*
2.66	V2.66 of the β_1-AR contributes to agonist binding *(43,44)*
3.32	D3.32 of the adrenergic receptors is important for binding of the amine moiety of ligands *(6,7,291)*
3.36	C3.36 of the α_{2A}-AR interacts with antagonist phenoxybenzamine; this position is important for binding of imidazoline derivatives *(292)*
3.37	T3.37 has been predicted to interact with the 2-methoxy group of the quinazoline ring of prazosin in the α_{1A}- and α_{1B}-AR *(36)*
4.56	The T4.56I mutation in the β_2-AR results in loss of affinity for agonists with a β-hydroxyl group *(27)*
4.62	F4.62 is involved in agonist binding to the α_{1A}-AR *(19)*
4.64	W4.64 of the α_{1D}-AR is involved in agonist and antagonist binding *(293)*
4.66	E4.66 of α_{1D}-AR imparts selectivity for KMD3213 vs α_{1A}-AR (Q4.66) *(36)*
e_2	The selectivity between α_{1A}-AR and α_{1B}-AR for the binding of the antagonists phentolamine and WB4101 is caused by differences in e_2; Q196 is predicted to hydrogen bond with the imidazoline nitrogen of phentolamine or the dioxan oxygen of WB4101; I197 is proposed to have hydrophobic interactions with the methyl of the phenyl ring or the ring itself of phentolamine and WB4101; N198 is thought to hydrogen bond with the nitrogen of the linker of these antagonists *(34)*
5.39	V5.39 of the human α_{1A}-AR imparts α_{1D} (A5.39) selectivity for oxazole antagonists and selectivity vs α_{1B} (A5.39) for agonists *(33,294)*
5.41	F5.41 is involved in agonist binding to the α_{1A}-AR *(19)*
5.42	S5.42 of the α_1-AR has been proposed to interact with the 1-nitrogen of the quinazoline of prazosin *(36)*; it has also been implicated in the binding of the *meta*-OH of phenethylamine ligands in the α_{2A}-AR *(295)*; removal of the hydroxyl moiety of S5.42 of the β_2-AR leads to loss of affinity of antagonists with nitrogen in their heterocyclic ring and isoproterenol; pindolol's heterocyclic ring has been predicted to hydrogen bond with S4.52, but this position has no effect on the affinity of β_2-AR for propranolol and alprenolol *(16)*
5.43	S5.43 of the α_{2A}-AR is responsible for the selectivity of UK14304 but not chlorpromazine and interspecies variation in yohimbine affinity *(296)*; in the β_2-AR, S5.43 is involved in isoproterenol binding *(297)*
5.46	S5.46 of the α-ARs has been predicted to interact with 2-methoxy of the quinazoline ring of prazosin *(36)*; in the β_2-AR S5.46 is involved in isoproterenol binding and binding of β-carbon hydroxyl of native ligands *(297)*
5.47	F5.47 of α_{1A}-AR has been demonstrated to interact with antagonists 5-methylurapidil, HEAT, and WB4101 but not niguldipine *(35)*
6.51	F6.51 has been shown to be an interaction site between agonists and antagonists and the α_{1B}-AR and has been suggested to be involved in ligand binding to the β_2-AR *(20,22)*
6.52	F6.52 of the α_{2A}-AR interacts with the catechol ring of agonists and has been suggested to be involved in ligand binding to the β_2-AR *(11,22)*
6.55	M6.55 of the α_{1A}-AR imparts selectivity vs α_{1B}-AR (L6.55) for agonists *(33)*; Y6.55 of the α_{2A}-AR interacts with catechol ring of agonists *(11)*; in the β_2-AR, N6.55 plays a role in the stereospecificity of agonists *(24)*
6.59	S6.59 of the α_1-ARs has been predicted to hydrogen bond with the carbonyl group between the piperazine and furan rings of prazosin *(36)*
7.35	F7.35 of α_{1A}- and α_{1B}-AR is a major contributor to the affinity of the antagonists prazosin, WB4101, niguldipine, and 5-methylurapidil; however, it is not involved in the binding of phenethylamine agonists (i.e., epinephrine) but is involved in the binding of imidazoline agonists such as oxymetazoline and cirazoline *(35)*; F7.35 is also responsible for high-affinity binding of TA-2005 to the β_2-AR *(45)* and is predicted to interact with the ether oxygen in side chain of salmeterol, formoterol, and procaterol and is important for β_2-AR selectivity *(46)*
7.38	F7.38 is important in the interaction of phenethylamines with α_{2A}-AR *(11)*
7.39	F7.39 of the α_1-ARs contributes to the interaction with antagonists and imidazoline agonists but not phenethylamine agonists *(35)*; F7.39 is also critical for the binding of yohimbine to the α_{2A}-AR *(48)*; in the β_2-AR, N7.39 is important for the binding of the antagonists propranolol and alprenolol; if this residue is substituted for Gln or Thr, an increase in affinity for the α-AR ligand yohimbine is seen *(47)*
7.40	W7.40 is proposed to play a role in agonist binding to the β_1-AR *(298)*
7.45	N7.45 of the β_2-AR is involved in agonist affinity *(6)*
7.46	S7.46 is involved in the affinity of the (–)-enantiomers of the catecholamines for the α_{2A}-AR but plays no role in the affinity of (+)-enantiomers *(23)*

the extracellular environment as rhodopsin undergoes the conformational rearrangement associated with its activation or may stabilize rhodopsin's active state. It is unlikely, however, that this structural rearrangement is entirely analogous in ARs because this would impede ligand entry from the extracellular milieu into the binding pocket. In the case of rhodopsin, the chromophore enters (and also exits after activation to be reisomerized back from the all-*trans* to the 11-*cis* conformation) from the cytoplasmic side *(39)*.

Other residues identified to be involved in antagonist binding by the α_{1A}-AR are two aromatics (F7.35 and F7.39) located at the extracellular end of TM VII *(35)*. Mutation of these residues, which are also conserved in other α_1-subtypes and in all α_2-ARs but not in β-ARs, markedly reduced the affinity of the receptor for all antagonists with no change in the affinity of phenethylamine-type agonists *(35)*. However, both residues were also shown to be involved in the binding of all imidazoline-type agonists *(35)*—a finding indicating that this class of agonists binds differently to phenethylamine agonists, as predicted by the Easson-Stedman hypothesis *(1)*. In this regard, imidazoline agonists are more antagonistlike, which may account for many of them being partial agonists *(40,41)*.

Phenylalanines (4.62 and 5.41) in TM IV and V of the α_{1A}-AR have also been identified as forming potentially novel contacts involved in agonist binding but not receptor activation. Interestingly, whereas substitution of both of these α_{1A}-residues with the corresponding Gln and Ala of the β_2-AR markedly reduced agonist affinity, the reverse substitutions in the β_2-AR increased agonist affinity *(19)*. Although antagonist binding was unaltered with these substitutions *(19)*, given that 4.62 is not conserved in other α_1-subtypes, it remains unclear if the affinity changes observed are caused by these residues forming direct ligand contacts or rather are indirect as a result of mutation-induced local conformational changes.

Macromolecular modeling studies have been undertaken to predict which receptor residues form critical interactions with the various moieties of α_1-antagonists, and contacts have been suggested with residues in TM III, IV, V, VI, and VII *(35,36,42)*. For the non-subtype-selective α_1-antagonist, prazosin (Fig. 4), for example, the 4-amino group and 1-nitrogen atom of its quinazoline ring have been suggested to interact with the carboxyl group of Asp 3.32 and hydroxyl group of Ser 5.42, respectively. Interaction of the two methoxy groups of its quinazoline ring with the hydroxyl groups of Thr 3.37 and Ser 5.46 and the carbonyl group between the piperazine and furan rings and Ser 6.59 have been identified for all α_1-AR subtypes *(36)*. For tamulosin, an α_{1D}-selective compound, more interactions were found for this subtype than for the other two α_1-subtypes, whereas for KMD-3213 (Fig. 4), an α_{1A}-selective compound, more interactions were found with the α_{1A}-AR *(36)*. However, these docking interactions have yet to be confirmed by formal structure–function studies.

Although TM V and VI are important for α_1-AR ligand discrimination, the selectivity of β-AR agonists is because of interactions with TM II and VII. β_1-AR selective agonists (e.g., denopamine; Fig. 4) interact with L2.56, T2.63, and V2.66, and it is these residues that have been demonstrated to impart selectivity *(43,44)*. Y7.35 at the extracellular end of TM VII has been demonstrated to be critical for the binding of several β_2-AR agonists *(43–46)*. The subtype selectivity of antagonist binding by the β_2-AR is also caused by an interaction with a TM VII residue, N7.39, which has been shown to be important for effective binding of β_2-AR antagonists, such as propranolol (Fig. 4) *(47)*. Interestingly, not only is the asparagine side chain required for the binding of β_2-antagonists, but also its substitution with Gln or Thr increases the affinity of the β_2-AR for the α_2-AR-selective antagonist yohimbine (Fig. 4) *(47)* despite the native residue at 7.39 in all α-AR being a phenylalanine. Conversely, if F7.39 of α_2-AR is replaced with Asn, the α_2-AR now displays decreased affinity for yohimbine and increases affinity for the β-antagonist alprenolol (Fig. 4) *(48)*.

2. Receptor Activation

2.1. Theory and Models

The concept of proteins as drug targets was proposed at the end of the 19th century. Ehrlich and Langley both contributed to the notion that compounds evoked biological activity by binding to cellular constituents (Ehrlich stated "corpora non agunt, nisi fixata," i.e., agents cannot act without binding; *[49]*) that were soon named *receptors* (Langley's "receptive substances"; *[50]*). Analogous to Fisher's lock-and-key theory of enzyme action *(51)*, these concepts led to a model of a receptor that is a rigid structure switched on by the turning of a key (ligand). A more dynamic picture of receptor activation evolved from about the middle of the twentieth century, with models failing to provide for more than one affinity state of the receptor (e.g., the collision coupling model of Tolkovsky et al. *[52]* and the random matrix hit model of Bergman et al. *[53]*) giving way to those that could because the existence of more than one affinity state was clearly evident experimentally. The last included the two noninterconvertible site model *(53)*; the cyclic (allosteric) model, initially proposed by Katz and Theleff *(54)* in 1957 and then used by Weiland and Taylor *(55)* to successfully model the binding of agonists and antagonists by cholinergic receptors; the divalent receptor model *(56)*; and eventually the ternary complex model *(57)*. The last was developed to explain the interaction of the agonist-bound receptor with its cognate G protein, with high agonist affinity observed when the receptor was complexed with its G protein, but low affinity when the receptor–G protein interaction was disrupted *(58)*.

This finding of modulation of affinity by a cognate interacting component, the G protein, was a major contravention of the accepted dogma of the time, which posited that receptor activation involved merely a binary interaction with ligand.

Nevertheless, intrinsic to all of these models, including the ternary complex model (Fig. 6), was the assumption that the binding of agonist is essential for receptor activation and signaling caused by a large energy barrier between the basal state R and the activated state R*. Accordingly, these models invoked an inductive step (ligand induction model) by which the free energy of agonist binding is required to allow the energy barrier between the inactive and active state to be surmounted.

The finding that receptors exhibit constitutive signaling, which is signaling in the absence of agonist (increased basal activity)—a property of GPCRs that was first revealed with the availability of cloned receptors that could be markedly overexpressed *(59)*—coupled also with the finding that mutations could render receptors constitutively active *(60–62)* led to proposal of an extended ternary complex (ETC) model (Fig. 6) *(63)*. Akin to the conformational selection model proposed by Koshland and Neet for enzymes *(64)*, central to this model is that receptors can spontaneously isomerize between R and R*, with the binding of agonist merely selecting or stabilizing the active state. In addition to explicitly allowing for spontaneous isomerization between R and R*, the ETC model also accounts for the G protein-independent high agonist (but not antagonist) affinity displayed by constitutively active mutant receptors and for the effects of different classes of drugs (full agonist, partial agonists, inverse agonist, neutral antagonists) *(65–67)*.

Although the ETC model explains most GPCR behavior, a more thermodynamically complete model, the cubic ternary complex (CTC) model (Fig. 6), was subsequently proposed *(68–70)*. This model is merely an extension of the ETC model (that is, the ETC model is one of the subsets making up the CTC model) that allows for the existence of an inactive ternary complex, ARG, although both models similarly predict GPCR behavior. However, at the time of development of the ETC and CTC models, neither specifically accommodated experimental

---

Fig. 6. *(Opposite page)* Evolution of receptor occupancy models. (i) The first models of receptor occupancy were based on the binding of an agonist A to the receptor R, leading to the generation of a response . However, this model could not account for experimental data showing high agonist affinity when the receptor was complexed with its G protein (G), but low affinity when the receptor–G protein interaction was disrupted *(58)*. (ii) This led to the development of the ternary complex model). (iii) The finding that receptors can exhibit constitutive signaling resulted in the extended ternary complex (ETC) model, which allows for spontaneous isomerization between inactive (R) and active (R*) receptor. However, the ETC assumes that only the active state of the receptor interacts with the G protein, and hence (iv) the cubic ternary complex model builds on the extended ternary complex model with the additional interaction of the inactive receptor with the G protein.   *(Figure caption continued on next page.)*

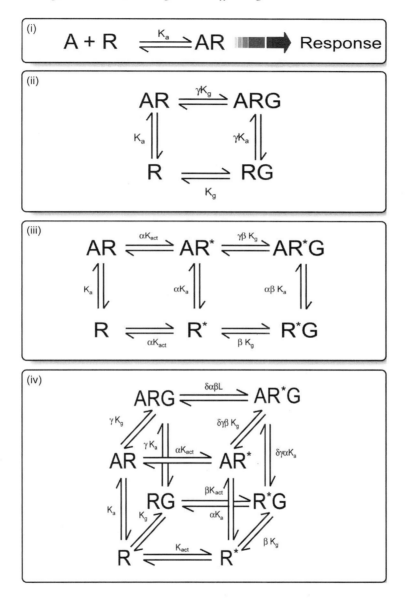

Fig. 6. *(Figure caption continued from previous page)* Modeling parameters: K_a, equilibrium constant for ligand binding; K_g, equilibrium constant for binding of G protein to inactive receptor; α, effect of ligand binding on receptor activation, effect of activation on ligand binding; β, effect of receptor activation on G protein binding, effect of G protein coupling on activation; γ, effect of ligand binding on G protein coupling; δ, measure of synergism between any two of receptor activation, G protein coupling, or ligand binding on the level of the third. (Based on a figure from ref. *299*.)

evidence predicting the formation of more than one active state (e.g., R_1^* and R_2^*), each of which can activate a distinct G protein and effector. Both the ETC and CTC models can accommodate agonist-specific receptor active conformations because the thermodynamic constants α and γ for ETC and α, γ, and δ for CTC allow for the microaffinity constant of the ligand-bound receptor to be specific to the ligand; that is, the affinity of ligand-bound receptor for G protein can vary *(71–73)*.

Intrinsic to all ternary complex models is the premise that agonists bind with higher affinity to the R^* state, and this is required to stabilize or select the active conformation. Kobilka and colleagues argued that this feature of the models does not accommodate the fact that agonists bind rapidly to R, whereas the kinetics of the agonist-induced conformational change in the absence of G protein is slow *(74)*. Moreover, both agonists, which supposedly stabilize the R^* state, and inverse agonists, which stabilize the basal state R, protect the receptor from thermal denaturation and from proteolytic degradation *(75)*. This implies that the conformations stabilized by both agonists and inverse agonists are distinct from that of the unliganded receptor. Accordingly, Gether and Kobilka *(76)* suggested that the unliganded receptor R represents a unique conformation that can undergo transition to either of at least two other states, R° and R^*, stabilized by inverse agonists and agonist, respectively. This model is consistent with findings from studies of various GPCR mutants, which can best be explained only by invoking the existence of conformations that are intermediate between R' and R^* *(20)*. Further, these studies suggest that whereas conformational selection can be invoked to account for a degree of basal activity—consistent with spontaneous isomerization from R to some intermediate R'—to get to the fully active R^* state requires an inductive step.

Of interest in this regard is a comparison of the transducin (the G protein coupled to rhodopsin) activation response resulting from photoactivation of rhodopsin vs that resulting from treatment of the protein opsin with the agonist all-*trans* retinal *(77)*. With the former, the chromophore 11-*cis* retinal is bound to opsin and functions as an inverse agonist that stabilizes the inactive state, even in the presence of mutations that would otherwise lead to constitutive activity *(78)*. Thus, photoactivation results in the complete transition from the inactive state (R° in the dark rhodopsin shows no appreciable binding to transducin) to the fully activated state (R^*). By contrast, all-*trans* retinal presumably only induces or stabilizes the transition of opsin from an intermediate state R (the unliganded state) to R^*. It is surprising, nonetheless, that the transducin response with all-*trans* retinal is a mere 14% of that observed with light activation *(77)*. Further, this extraordinarily low degree of activation by all-*trans* retinal occurs despite the fact that it binds much more rapidly to opsin than does 11-*cis* retinal *(77)*. Although rhodopsin is distinct from other GPCRs in having its basal state stabilized by a covalently bound inverse agonist, its activation mechanisms and the conformational changes that occur with activation are nonetheless very similar to those observed with other GPCRs, especially ARs. Thus, by analogy, activation of ARs by agonists, in which isomerization may be restricted only to a transition from R to R*, may only be realizing a fraction of the activation potential that might be possible with transition from R° to R*. These considerations also reinforce the notion that multiple conformations, R', R", and so on, probably exist between R° and R*. Such conformational intermediates are likely revealed by various mutations, which presumably lower the energy barrier required for the spontaneous adoption of a partially activated conformation (cf. refs. *20* and *79*).

It is evident that each successive model of receptor activation has been formulated to account parsimoniously for new experimental findings as they have been advanced. All, however, are based on two concepts. First, receptor activation involves a conformational change in the receptor protein that is imparted to its coupled intracellular machinery rather than some other mode of activation, such as relay of redox changes, as is operative, for example, with *Rhodopseudomonas viridis*, the first membrane protein receptor system yielding to high-resolution X-ray crystallographic structural analysis *(80)*. Evidence that activation of GPCRs indeed involves a conformational change in the receptor protein is now overwhelming, as exemplified, for example, by the spectroscopic identification of conformational intermediates with activation of rhodopsin *(81,82)* and, more recently, with activation of the β-AR *(83)*. In addition, direct evidence for helical movements with activation, initially obtained from studies of photocycle intermediates of the archaebacterial proton pump bacteriorhodopsin *(84)* and from site-directed spin-labeling studies of both bacteriorhodopsin and rhodopsin, have given rise to the helix movement model of GPCR activation *(85–87)*.

The second concept underlying receptor activation theory is the notion that it involves a single quiescent species that is activated by agonist; that is, there exist but two receptor states, R and R*. As indicated above, this notion has been challenged by evidence that receptors can isomerize to more than one active state (e.g., R*[1], R*[2], etc.), and that the output of receptor activation is not only limited to G protein and effector activation, but also involves a spectrum of effects: internalization, phosphorylation, and interaction with other membrane and cytosolic components, such as receptor activity-modifying proteins, arrestins, and the like, that can alter ligand-binding characteristics, relative potency, and thus the final receptor-mediated response. In other words, as indicated by Kenakin *(88)*, receptors can no longer be regarded as simple on/off switches, but must be considered more three-dimensionally as bipolar (or better still multipolar) recognition (or transduction) units. Accordingly, the binding of ligand at one recognition site governs its interaction with a variety of cognate "effectors" (used here broadly to cover not only the enzymes or channels activated by their cognate receptors, but also GPCR kinases (GRKs), arrestins, receptor activity-modifying proteins, etc.) at other recognition sites, and thus that ligand efficacy not only is a quantitative parameter, but also has a qualitative dimension.

This concept of a bipolar recognition unit can perhaps be best understood by consideration of Sakmar's elegant exposé of rhodopsin activation at the molecular level (89). He proposed that activation involves conformational changes at a variety of distinct topological receptor locations, such that those, for example, involved in forming the ligand-binding pocket may be in the "on" state (in other GPCRs, this would be evidenced by high-affinity agonist binding) without necessarily locking the G protein-activating domain into its active conformation and vice versa. Thus, he argued, a concerted transition of individual amino acid subsets may generate the overall active conformation but not all transitions may actually be essential for activation of the downstream effector (here used in the restrictive sense to designate the cognate enzyme or channel activated by a receptor). For example, a minimal subset of amino acids (in Kenakin's parlance, this would constitute a "recognition unit") may allow either high-affinity agonist binding, interaction with arrestins, receptor phosphorylation, and so on irrespective of the binary states (on/off) of all possible subsets constituting the active conformation. Further, the functional hierarchy of individual group transitions can be revealed by mutations in which the side chain of an individual amino acid within a particular recognition unit is influenced or locked into the on or off state. This simple binary model of group transitions allows one to reconcile the fact that mutations can result in constitutive activity without causing an increase in agonist affinity (90–92) or vice versa; can result in the binding but not the activation of the cognate G protein (93); can result in constitutive activation for one but not another receptor-coupled effector pathway (94); or can result in the dissociation of internalization, desensitization, phosphorylation, or dimerization from activation of the G protein-coupled response (72,95). Similarly, it provides an understanding of the identification of ligands that are seemingly antagonists (do not cause activation), and yet promote internalization (96,97), for ligands that result in dissociation of agonist efficacy vs phosphorylation (98) or even for series of ligands able to activate a single receptor but with different kinetics (99).

2.2. Agonist Trafficking

As indicated in Section 2.1, a growing body of experimental data supports the notion of more than two distinct receptor conformations. Further, it has been suggested that agonists can stabilize different receptor active states, which then selectively activate specific G protein signaling pathways. This phenomenon of promiscuous G protein coupling by distinct agonist-specific active states has been termed *agonist trafficking (100)*; a process that extends beyond G protein activation and includes functional outcomes such as receptor phosphorylation and internalization. For the β_2-AR, it has been demonstrated not only that different ligands induce different conformations *(74,101,102)*, but also that on agonist binding the receptor undergoes a temporal change in conformation *(83)*. Also, consistent with the notion of agonist trafficking is the finding of differences in ligand potency/efficacy-order for the activation of different signaling pathways by a single receptor *(71)*.

2.2.1. Multiple Activation States

In detailed studies of detergent-solubilized, purified β_2-AR, Kobilka and colleagues used several spectroscopic techniques to demonstrate not only that receptors exist in multiple conformations, but also that ligands induce conformational changes that vary depending on the ligand type, that is, agonists, partial agonists, or antagonists *(83,102–105)*. By derivitization of cysteine residues with *N,N'*-dimethyl-*N*-(iodoacetyl)-*N'*-(7-nitrobenz-2-oxa-1,3-diazol-4-yl)ethylenediamine, a fluorescent probe sensitive to its solvent environment, they demonstrated that agonists and partial agonists caused decreases in fluorescence that were proportional in magnitude to ligand efficacy, whereas antagonists increased fluorescence *(102)*. Using the technique of single-molecule spectroscopy, they further showed that, in the absence of ligand, the β_2-AR exists in multiple substates, suggesting that the receptor is spontaneously oscillating (or "breathing") between different conformations, and that on application of the agonist isoproterenol, a different subset of conformations was apparent *(105)*.

Using another environmentally sensitive probe (i.e., fluoresceine maleimide) in lifetime spectroscopy studies, discrete conformational states were evident within a population of receptors *(104)*. Moreover, whereas the unliganded receptor existed in a single flexible state and neutral antagonist, alprenolol, reduced conformational flexibility; agonists and partial agonists promoted the formation of two separate species with different fluorescence lifetimes *(104)*. The last two species are indicative of at least two distinct conformations, with the agonist-bound one representing the active conformation. Because the fluorescence lifetime (and thus the microenvironment around the fluorophore) differed with each of the agonists, it is likely that these species represent distinct agonist-specific active states *(104)*.

In additional studies, it was demonstrated that norepinephrine can induce at least two conformational states in the β_2-AR: one capable of activating G_s and another required for interaction of the receptor with G protein-receptor kinase (GRK) or arrestin and hence agonist-induced internalization *(83)*. In contrast, dopamine, which can stimulate G_s activation of the β_2-AR but not internalization, induced only one of the conformational states observed with norepinephrine *(83)*.

Further evidence of conformational variance in the ligand-bound β_2-AR has been provided by plasmon-waveguide resonance studies. These studies evaluated changes in mass density and mass distribution of receptors incorporated into a preformed (artificial) lipid bilayer, with changes in mass distribution caused by changes in structural anisotropy. Again, evidence for agonist-specific conformational states was apparent with the plasmon-waveguide resonance studies, and changes in resonance differed for agonists compared to antagonists *(103)*. However, shifts in resonance were detected for all ligand classes, with those for agonists and partial agonists multiphasic and those for antagonists monophasic *(103)*. This finding is consistent with receptor activation occurring through discrete conformational intermediates.

2.2.2. Pathway-Selective Mutants

Mutation of C3.35 in the α_{1B}-AR to phenylalanine results in a receptor that is constitutively active for the G_q/inositol-1,4,5-triphosphate (IP_3) pathway, but not for the G_i/arachidonic acid-coupled pathway *(94)*. Given that C3.35 is directed toward TM II and is immediately below D3.32, which is critically involved in stabilizing the inactive state via an interaction with K7.36 (cf., Sections 1.1. and 2.3.2), pathway-specific activation observed with the C3.35F mutation is likely because of the bulky phenylalanine side chain sterically altering the correct juxtapositioning of TM III with TM II; a conformational perturbation that presumably resembles the activated state for G_q- but not for G_i-signaling. Interestingly, this mutation also leads to increased affinity of the receptor for the endogenous catecholamines and other phenethylamines, but not for imidazoline agonists or for antagonists *(94)*.

Mutation of N6.55 of β_2-AR, a residue located at the extracellular end of TM VI that has been implicated in determining stereoselectivity of catechol agonist binding to an aspartate, results in a receptor that cannot respond to agonist activation of G_s/adenyl cyclase or to agonist stimulation of receptor phosphorylation, but nonetheless it continues to display wild-type-like basal activation *(106)*. Again, in keeping with distinct activated intermediates between R and R*, this suggests that the active-state conformation generated by spontaneous isomerization from the basal state is distinct from that achieved with agonist stimulation of the receptor *(106)*.

Like the C3.35F α_{1B}-AR mutant, an α_2-AR D2.50N mutant shows pathway-specific signaling. Thus, this mutant displays loss of G_q and G_s coupling but can still couple to G_i, albeit with reduced potency and despite retaining the same affinity for the agonist UK14304 (Fig. 4) as wild type α_2-AR *(107)* This mutant is unable to activate K^+ channels but shows unimpaired inhibition of cyclic adenosine 5'-monophosphate (cAMP) production or voltage-sensitive Ca^{2+} currents *(108,109)*.

2.2.3. Ligand-Specific Signaling

For both α_{1A}- and α_{1B}-ARs, *meta-* and *para-*octopamine have been shown to maximally stimulate one G protein-coupled pathway (pertussis toxin-sensitive PLA_2 activation) but are only partial agonists for another (G_q-mediated IP_3 production) *(110)*. In terms of PLA_2 activation, *para-*octopamine is a full agonist at the α_{1A}-AR but a partial agonist for the α_{1B}-AR, whereas *meta-*octopamine is a partial agonist at α_{1A}- and a full agonist at the α_{1B}-AR. However, norepinephrine is a full agonist for both pathways with both receptor subtypes *(110)*. Stimulation of the α_{1A}-AR by epinephrine also leads to activation of the IP_3 signaling pathway but, in contrast to α_{1B}-AR, does not cause receptor phosphorylation or internalization. However, the α_{1A}-AR is internalized by the imidazoline agonist oxymetazoline (Fig. 4). This suggests that a distinct conformation is required for receptor internalization, and that the generation of this conformation is ligand specific *(111)*.

Many examples of ligand-specific signaling have been documented for α_2-ARs. Thus, although α_{2B}-AR couples to both G_s and G_i, some agonists (e.g., UK14,304) show preference for coupling to G_i over G_s *(112–115)*. Also, despite a dissociation constant (K_d) of 670 nM for UK14,304 binding at the α_{2A}-AR, its EC_{50} varies widely: 0.09 nM for G_i signaling, 50 nM for G_q signaling, and 70 nM for G_s signaling *(107)*. *meta-*Octopamine selectively activates α_{2A}-AR coupling to G_i but promotes coupling of α_{2B}-AR and α_{2C}-AR to both G_i and G_s *(115)*. Further, at the α_{2C}-AR, *meta-*octopamine is one order of magnitude less potent than norepinephrine with respect to G_s coupling but is equipotent to norepinephrine for coupling to G_i and displays increased efficacy at stimulating this G protein when compared to norepinephrine *(115)*.

For all three α_2-ARs, the efficacy of G_s coupling is dependent on the structure of the agonists. Thus, compounds that act as full agonists with respect to G_i coupling do not necessarily display full efficacy for G_s coupling *(114)*. This is especially the case for the α_{2C}-AR, for which it has been suggested that oxymetazoline, BHT-920, and BHT-933 (Fig. 4) activate G_i but not G_s signaling *(114)*. However, this differential signaling activity of agonists acting on the α_{2C}-AR was not observed by others and has been attributed to the presence of spare receptors *(116)*.

It has also been shown that some ligands function as antagonists with respect to one receptor-coupled pathway but as partial agonists at the same receptor for another signaling pathway *(117)*. For example, for the α_{2A}-AR the imidazoline derivative dexefaroxan is a neutral antagonist for Ca^{2+} signaling via $G_{\alpha15}$, an inverse agonist for $G_{\alpha o}$ signaling by the mutant Cys[351]Ile, and a partial agonist for signaling by a constitutively active mutant α_{2A}-AR that couples via $G_{\alpha15}$ *(117)*.

Ligand-specific signaling is also evident with β-ARs. For example, at the β_2-AR, ICI118551 and propranolol (Fig. 4) have been found to act as inverse agonists for G_s-stimulated adenylyl cyclase but as partial agonists for $G_{s/l}$-independent extracellularly responsive kinase 1/2 (ERK1/2) activation. Because these two ligands promote β-arrestin recruitment to the $β_2$-AR, this receptor-coupled response is not an exclusive property of agonists, and ligands normally classified as inverse agonists have been shown to require β-arrestin for their signaling activity *(118)*.

2.3. Molecular Determinants of Activation

2.3.1. Helical Movements and Disruption of Helical Interactions

Experimental data and consideration of the crystal structure of rhodopsin suggest that intramolecular interactions stabilize the inactive conformation of GPCRs. Removal or rearrangement of these constraining interactions results in receptor activation as a result of movements of the TM helices, which are then relayed to the G protein-interacting intracellular loops. In the activated conformation, receptors display structural instability and enhanced conformational flexibility, as evidenced by the thermolability of constitutively active mutants *(75)*.

Of the GPCRs, the activation mechanism of rhodopsin has been most extensively studied using a variety of biophysical approaches, including tryptophan ultraviolet absorbance spectroscopy, Fourier transform infrared resonance spectroscopy, and site-directed spin-labeling studies. With the last, electron paramagnetic spin of pairs of cysteine-substituted residues labeled with sulfhydryl spin probes is monitored *(119–121)*. These studies have provided evidence that activation involves a small movement of TM III coupled with significant rigid body movement and counterclockwise (when viewed from the extracellular surface of the receptor) rotation of TM VI, leading to movement of the cytoplasmic end of TM VI away from TM III *(86)*. This finding was also supported by mutagenesis studies in which either an engineered disulfide bond *(122)* or the binding of zinc to a site engineered between two histidine-substituted residues *(87)*, one in TM III and one in TM VI, has been used to lock rhodopsin into the inactive state.

Studies of TM residue accessibility to water-soluble sulfhydryl-reactive compounds has allowed Javitch and coworkers to gain evidence that $β_2$-AR activation also involves a conformational rearrangement of TM VI *(123)*, whereas detailed fluorescence spectroscopy studies by Kobilka and coworkers indicated that the helical movements occurring with $β_2$-AR activation are almost identical to those for rhodopsin, that is, a counterclockwise rotation (when viewed from the extracellular surface of the receptor) of both TM III and TM VI, with a tilting of the cytoplasmic end of the latter toward TM V *(74,124)*. The importance of the orientation of TM VI, which is stabilized by interhelical interactions with TM V, comes from studies of the $α_1$-ARs, which showed that mutation of either the residue at 5.39 in TM V or 6.55 in TM VI of the α_{1B}-AR to that of the α_{1A}-AR or vice versa results in constitution activation, and further that the basal state could be restored by mutation of both residues in one subtype to those of the other subtype (double reciprocal mutation) *(125)*. Evidence for involvement of TM VI in α_{1B}-AR activation also comes from the delineation of F6.51 as a key switch residue involved in both agonist binding and receptor activation by this receptor, albeit that this residue appears only to be involved in the isomerization from R′ to R* and not from the basal state to R′ *(20)*. In other GPCRs, such as the NK-1 substance P receptor, interhelical stabilization of TM VI by TM V has been demonstrated from studies showing that an engineered zinc-binding site linking the extracellular ends of these two helices prevents activation *(126)*. Activation may also involve movement of other helices, such as TM VII, as demonstrated in studies of rhodopsin *(127)* and other GPCRs, such as the thyroid-stimulating hormone receptor *(128)*.

2.3.2. Molecular Basis for Helical Movements and G Protein Activation

In the case of rhodopsin, the ground state is stabilized by a salt bridge linking E3.28 in TM III with the protonated Schiff base formed by the covalent binding of the chromophore 11-*cis* retinal with K7.43 in TM VII *(129–131)*. Photoisomerization of the chromophore to the all-*trans* conformation disrupts the salt bridge as a result of deprotonation of the Schiff base *(132)*. Thus, movement of TM III is likely the first step in the rhodopsin activation process. Similarly, studies by Perez and coworkers *(5,133,134)* have provided evidence that a salt bridge between D3.32 and K7.36 stabilizes the ground state of the α_{1B}-AR, and that its disruption also is essential and probably the proximate step in activation. Thus, mutagenesis of either D3.32 or K7.36 to an alanine results in constitutive activation that can be rescued by reciprocal mutation of these residues, and activation can be induced even with triethylamine, a compound that mimics the protonated amine moiety of catecholamines *(5,133,134)*. However, other ARs, including the α_{2A}-, α_{2B}-, and all β-AR subtypes, lack a lysine at the 7.36 position and are thus unable to form a salt bridge with D3.32. Indeed, lack of such a strong bonding interaction to stabilize the basal state may explain why some receptors, such as the β_2-AR, are more likely to demonstrate constitutive activity because the energy barrier for spontaneous isomerization from R to R* would be lower.

Based on detailed fluorescence spectroscopy studies of the β_2-AR, it has been suggested that binding of the various moieties of catecholamine agonists is sequential *(83)*, and although interactions between the receptor and the catechol ring and amine group are rapid, whereas that with the chiral hydroxyl is slow, formation of the catechol ring interactions with TM VI and TM V precedes that between the amine and D3.32 in TM III, with the latter required only to stabilize the interactions with the catechol ring *(83)*. These findings could be interpreted to imply that, for the β_2-AR, movement of TM III may occur after that of TM VI, and thus that movement of TM VI, rather than TM III, is the initial step in receptor activation.

Another interhelical interaction that is disrupted, and likely plays a role in the activation process, is that between a glutamic acid at the cytoplasmic end of TM VI and residues of the (D/E)RY motif in TM III. This interaction is discussed in Section 2.3.3.

Movement of TM III and TM VI, which are contiguous with the G protein-interacting second and third intracellular loops (i_2 and i_3 loops), is consistent with their central involvement in the activation process. However, it remains unclear exactly how the binding of agonist to a site in the outer third of the TM domain is transmitted to the G protein-interacting loops on the cytoplasmic surface of the receptor—a distance of some 30–40 Å (135). The crystal structure of rhodopsin revealed that TM VI is kinked because of the presence of a proline (6.50) located approximately at the junction of the outer and middle thirds of the helix (135). This proline is highly conserved in GPCRs, including all ARs. In addition, the six residues N-terminal to 6.50 are highly homologous between ARs and rhodopsin. Given that the residues N-terminal of proline have been shown to be the determinants of proline-induced kinks, as well as other nonhelical elements in TM proteins (136), it is likely that a kink in TM VI is a conserved architectural feature of most GPCRs. The putative Pro-kink in ARs is surrounded by a cluster of aromatic residues (F6.44, W6.48, F6.51, F6.52). Because computational simulation studies indicated that Pro-kinks form flexible molecular hinges that can act as conformational switches in TM α-helices (137), it has been suggested that the aromatic residues of the β_2-AR that are clustered about 6.50 act as a toggle switch that modulates the TM VI kink (123). Specifically, based on both mutagenesis data and computer simulations of activation-induced structural changes in TM VI, Shi et al. (123) proposed that activation results in a switch in the rotamer conformations of C6.47, W6.48, and to a lesser degree F6.52, which result in a sweeping movement of the cytoplasmic end of TM VI away from TM III.

Although of interest, further experimental studies will be required to validate or refute this rotameric switch model, which runs contrary to data indicating that activation of rhodopsin involves rigid body movement of TM VI (86). In addition, in the study of Shi et al. (123), the molecular simulations of TM VI were performed with the helix isolated from the likely constraining influences of other TM helices; the rotamers assigned to the TM VI residue were those determined from studies of α-helices in soluble proteins, which may not pertain for residues in membrane-embedded helices. In agreement with the rhodopsin studies, site-directed fluorescence-labeling studies of the β_2-AR are entirely consistent with TM VI moving as a rigid body (124).

Based on engineered cysteine sensor studies of the β_2-AR, which provided evidence for movement not only of the cytoplasmic end of TM VI below the Pro-kink, but also of the extracellular end of the helix above P6.50, Chen et al. *(20)* suggested that rather than adding flexibility to TM VI, P6.50 rigidifies the helix into a stiff, kinked helical rod, a proposal supported by studies of other proteins showing increased thermostability with the substitution of an alanine by a kink-inducing proline *(138)*. As a result, the Pro-kink acts as a fulcrum to allow TM VI to pivot and thus amplify the conformational change associated with agonist binding. This results in productive propagation of the agonist signal from the agonist binding site to the G protein-binding site on the cytoplasmic face of the receptor.

Coupled with the findings of modeling studies of the β_2-AR, Chen et al. *(20)* further proposed mechanical momentum transfer as a plausible mechanism for the propagation of activation-induced movements over a distance of 30–40 Å, a mechanism suggested not only by the presence of a cluster of aromatic residues, but also by their interaction in a typical herringbone arrangement interspersed by strongly dipolar side chains (Asn 6.55, 7.39, 7.44, 7.49). Because buried amide side chains, or even charged ones, form thermodynamically stable dipolar/aromatic clusters as a result of π-cation interactions with aromatic Trp, Phe, and Tyr residues *(139)*, any local changes to such interactions resulting from ligand-induced residue rearrangements are likely to affect the stability of the whole cluster. This would explain how large-scale movements of side-chain clusters might be propagated along the length of the TM helices.

2.3.3. Extracellular Disulfide Bond Disruption

Even before the structure of any GPCR was known from molecular cloning, it was demonstrated that the β-AR was stabilized by a disulfide bond(s) *(140)*. Indeed, based on an analysis of β-AR disulfide bonding, Pedersen and Ross *(141)* suggested that its structure would be more akin to that of rhodopsin than to that of other types of TM receptors—an astonishingly prescient prediction. In that study, it was shown that treatment of the β-AR with thiol-reducing agents to disrupt disulfide linkages resulted in its activation *(141,142)*. Subsequently, with the cloning of the β_2-AR, the presence of a disulfide bond connecting extracellular loops 1 and 2 (e_1 and e_2, respectively) was suggested by the presence of cysteine residues in e_1 and e_2, which are also conserved in all ARs and most other GPCRs, and by structure–function studies *(143,144)*. However, it was not until some years later that the extracellular loop disulfide bond connectivity of the β_2-AR was confirmed and shown to be atypical in that it involved not one bond, as in other ARs, but two disulfide bonds connecting Cys[106] in e_1 and Cys[184] in e_2 with vicinal cysteines (Cys[191] and Cys[190], respectively) in e_2 *(145)*, both of which stabilize receptor structure, whereas only the Cys[106]–Cys[191] linkage is involved in activation *(145)*. Further, it was shown that formation of these disulfide bonds likely involves disulfide exchange during biogenesis of the nascent receptor, with initial bonding between Cys^{106} and Cys^{184}, the cysteine pair conserved in most other GPCRs *(145)*.

In contrast to the solvent accessibility of the β_2-AR disulfide bonds, that of the α_{1B}-AR *(146)*, like rhodopsin *(147)*, is solvent inaccessible, a finding consistent with their extracellular loop structures being different from that of the β_2-AR. Because the disulfide bond is masked in α_1-ARs, one cannot test if its reduction by thiols would also lead to activation. Nevertheless, because catecholamine agonists are reducing agents *(148)* and are inactive in their oxidized form *(149)*, whereas antagonists are redox inactive *(148)*, it has been suggested that receptor activation involves an essential reductive step, a postulate initially made for the α_2-AR *(150)* and later extended to β-AR *(148,151)* and dopamine receptors *(152)*. Further, it has been suggested that, because G proteins and adenylyl cyclase contain active sulfhydryl groups *(153)*, their activation by β_2-ARs may involve TM redox chemistry. Direct evidence, however, is lacking, and given the reducing environment of the cytoplasm *(154)*, one has to postulate that critical sulfhydryls of intracellular receptor link proteins must be masked in their inactive conformation if they are to react on receptor activation because otherwise they would already be reduced.

2.3.4. Involvement of the E/DRY Motif

It has long been known that photoactivation of rhodopsin is not only associated with deprotonation of the Schiff base linking the retinal chromophore to Lys^{296}, but also with proton uptake from the aqueous milieu *(155)*. Careful biophysical studies of wild-type rhodopsin and mutants indicated that it is E3.49 of the E/DRY motif at the cytoplasmic end of TM III that becomes protonated with photoactivation, that protonation occurs with significantly slower kinetics than retinal isomerization, and that two spectroscopically indistinguishable activated forms of rhodopsin (*isochromic* species known as metarhodopsin IIa and IIb) are generated by photoactivation. The first (MIIa), which is generated rapidly, is unable to activate transducin but results in E3.49 becoming available for protonation, and the second (MIIb), generated by proton uptake by E3.49, is able to activate signaling. In addition, mutation of E3.49 to an uncharged glutamine results in constitutively active opsin. Thus, E3.49 is involved in stabilizing the inactive state of rhodopsin.

As in rhodopsin, the residue at position 3.49 in adrenergic and other class A GPCRs, an aspartate, has been proposed as an important modulator of the transition from the inactive (R) to the active (R*) state, and not surprisingly, charge-neutralizing mutations of D3.49 in several such receptors have been shown to result in constitutive activity *(66,156–159)*. With the α_{1B}-AR, mutagenesis studies have suggested that, as with rhodopsin, activation involves protonation of D3.49. Further, based on computer simulations, Scheer et al. *(159)* proposed that, in the inactive state, R3.50 is constrained in a "polar pocket" formed by residues in TM I, II, and VII, with the counterion for R3.50 being D2.50 in TM II. However, for the β_2-AR, Ballesteros et al. *(160)* predicted the counterion to be the adjacent D3.49 of the DRY motif, with D3.49 protonated in the active state and R3.50 interacting with D2.50. In other studies of the β_2-AR, Ghanouni et al. *(161)* provided evidence that protonation increased basal activity by destabilizing the inactive state of the receptor.

Based on additional mutagenesis studies, cysteine accessibility data, and computer simulations, Ballesteros et al. *(160)* indicated that R3.50 forms ionic interactions with both the adjacent D3.49 and E6.30 in TM VI. Further, they suggested that disruption of this "ionic" lock might constitute a common switch governing the activation of many class A GPCRs. Although an attractive hypothesis, given the rhodopsin data showing that isomerization to MIIa precedes protonation and the generation of MIIb, it is unlikely that disruption of the putative D3.49/R3.50/E6.30 ionic lock is a primary step in receptor activation. Moreover, direct evidence for proton uptake from the aqueous milieu by receptors other than rhodopsin has yet to be provided. It is also of interest that the increased basal activity of the β_2-AR observed with reductions in pH could not be abrogated with alanine substitutions of D3.49 or E6.30. This suggests that the residue(s) mediating protonation-induced activation has yet to be identified, albeit that it would be interesting to test if the activating effect of pH reduction could be prevented with charge-neutralizing mutations of more than one residue forming the putative D3.49/R3.50/E6.30 interaction.

It has been suggested that, unlike rhodopsin or the α_{1B}- and β_2-ARs, the α_{2A}-AR does not follow the conventional GPCR mechanistic paradigm with respect to the function of the DRY motif; that is, D3.49 is involved in receptor activation, and R3.50 is involved in activation of the cognate G protein. Regarding the lack of involvement of D3.49 in receptor activation, this conclusion is based on the finding that D3.49I and D3.49N mutant α_{2A}-ARs did not display constitutive activity *(15,162)*. Although the same substitutions of D3.49 in the α_{1B}-AR do result in constitutive activity *(163)*, this conclusion should be interpreted with caution because the D3.49N mutation of the α_{1B}-AR induces the weakest constitutive activity of all 19 substitutions at this residue *(163)*. In addition, although the isoleucine substitution of D3.49 resulted in robust constitutive activation of the α_{1B}-AR, it is possible that its long hydrophobic side chain may interact with residues in other regions of the α_{2A}-AR receptor that are not conserved in the α_{1B}-AR and by so doing may prevent expression of an activated phenotype. Thus, additional data are required before it can be confidently concluded that the role of the DRY motif in the α_{2A}-AR is distinct from that in other class A GPCRs,

albeit that such a proposal has also been made for the M_1 and M_5 mAch receptors
(164,165). With both of these muscarinic receptors, however, involvement of
D3.49 in receptor folding and expression may have limited the analysis of its
contribution to signaling.

2.3.5. Role of TM V Serines

Based on studies of the α_{1A}-AR, it has been demonstrated that the *meta*-
hydroxyl of the endogenous agonists preferentially binds to S5.42, and it is this
hydrogen bond interaction, and not that between the *para*-hydroxyl and S5.46,
that allows receptor activation *(12)*.

In early studies of the β_2-AR, a critical interaction was demonstrated between
S5.42 and S5.46 and the *meta*- and *para*-hydroxyls of catecholamine agonists
(17). Using thermodynamic analyses of double mutant cycles in which wild-type
and mutant receptors with alanine substitutions of S5.42 and 5.46 were evaluated
for their ability to bind agonists with differing hydroxyl moieties on the 3,4
positions of the catechol ring, Ambrosia et al. *(166)* provided evidence that S5.42
and S5.46 not only provide agonist docking interactions, but also control the
equilibrium between the inactive (R) and active (R*) states or the receptor. Thus,
alanine substitution of both S5.42 and S5.46 in the wild-type β_2-AR and a constitutively active mutant inhibited basal signaling. In a similar analysis, Liapakis
et al. *(16)* also showed that the catechol *meta*-hydroxyl interacts not only with
S5.42, but also perhaps (through a bifurcated H-bond) with S5.43, and that the
interaction with the latter may play a role in partial agonism. Given that S5.43 is
not conserved in other ARs such as α_1- and α_2-ARs and in some cases is replaced
by an alanine that lacks H-bonding potential, catechol binding and the orientation
of the catechol ring clearly differ significantly between ARs.

3. Interaction of Adrenergic Receptors With Signaling Proteins

3.1. G Protein and Receptor Coupling

Like other GPCRs, ARs interact with heterotrimeric guanine nucleotide binding regulatory proteins or G proteins. The heterotrimeric nature of these proteins
is evident from their α-, β-, and γ-subunit composition, each subunit is encoded
by a distinct gene. The nucleotide-binding signature G_α subunit is structurally
related to small molecular weight G proteins and, like the latter, possesses intrinsic, but catalytically inefficient, GTPase activity *(167)*. The G_β- and G_γ-subunits
form a tightly interacting dimer that is bound to the plasma membrane via an
isoprenyl moiety covalently attached to the C-terminus of G_γ.

In the guanosine 5′-diphosphate (GDP)-bound state, G_α associates with $G_{\beta\gamma}$.
On activation by the cognate GPCR, GDP dissociation (the rate-limiting step) is
facilitated and allows G protein activation as a result of guanosine 5′-triphos-
phate (GTP) binding. The mechanisms by which receptors bind their cognate G

protein and catalyze GDP/GTP exchange are not well understood but involve interaction with the i_2 and i_3 receptor regions *(168)*. One possibility could be that GTP binding by G_α instigates a conformational change that may lower its affinity for $G_{\beta\gamma}$ and thereby leads to dissociation of G_α-GTP from $G_{\beta\gamma}$ (although some have suggested that, rather than dissociation, the trimeric complex merely undergoes a conformational rearrangement) *(169)*. Both G_α-GTP and $G_{\beta\gamma}$ can activate downstream effectors *(170)*. In addition to effector activation, G_α complexes have numerous signaling functions, including a role in membrane localization and activation of certain GRKs.

In mammals, there are at least 27 G_α-, 5 G_β-, and 13 G_γ-subtypes *(171)*; hence, the intracellular propagation of GPCR signaling is orchestrated by myriad $G_{\alpha\beta\gamma}$ combinations. On the basis of the primary sequence of the G_α-subunits, G proteins can be divided into different major families, including G_s, G_i, G_q, and G_{12} *(172)*. Each G_α protein subtype couples to specific effectors. Originally, both the specificity and the selectivity of GPCR signaling were thought to be achieved by the coupling of a given receptor with a single class of G proteins. However, this paradigm was abandoned because several GPCRs, including the β_2-AR, have been shown to be capable of coupling to several different G_α-subunits, a phenomenon dependent on the specific agonist employed or its concentration, which is referred to, as indicated in Section 2.2, as *agonist trafficking (100)*.

As detailed in Sections 3.2–3.4, the G proteins involved in AR signaling (Fig. 7) include G_s, which couples β-ARs to adenylyl cyclase stimulation, and G_i, which mainly couples α_2-ARs to AC inhibition. α_2-ARs activation can also lead to Ca^{2+} channel activation via G_o coupling. For α_1-ARs, the $G_{q/11}$ family can mediate receptor coupling to phospholipase Cβ (PLC-β) activation. In addition, the atypical G protein G_h/TGase 2 can mediate PLC-γ1 activation by the α_{1B}- and α_{1D}-, but not α_{1A}-, AR.

3.2. α_1-AR G Protein and Effector Activation

Stimulation of α_1-ARs results in the activation of various effectors, including PLC, phospholipase D (PLD), and phospholipase A_2 (PLA$_2$), as well as activation of Ca^{2+} channels and the Na^+/H^+ exchangers, modulation of K^+ channels *(173)*, and activation of other signaling pathways, such as that involving activation of mitogen-activated protein kinases, or leading to transcriptional activation of early and late response genes.

The main signaling pathways activated by α_1-ARs are depicted in Fig. 8. All three α_1-AR subtypes can activate phosphoinositide turnover and calcium signaling. Indeed, although the Ca^{2+} influx *(174,175)* response was initially thought to be specific for the α_{1A}-AR, it was later found to be mediated also by the other subtypes. Both voltage-dependent and -independent Ca^{2+} channels have been implicated in these responses. Using antisense technology, Marcrez-Lepetre and

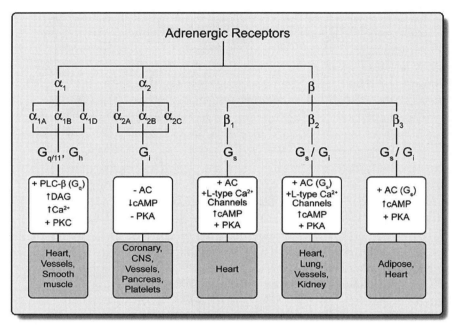

Fig. 7. Adrenergic receptor subtypes and their coupled G proteins and effectors. AC, adenylyl cyclase; c-AMP, cyclic adenosine-3′,5′-monophosphate; DAG, diacylglycerol; PKA, c-AMP-dependent protein kinase A; PKC, protein kinase C; PLC-β, phospholipase Cβ; +, activation; −, inhibition; ↑, increase; ↓, decrease.

coworkers have provided evidence that $G_{\alpha q}$ participates in α_1-AR-mediated phosphoinositide turnover and intracellular calcium mobilization, whereas $G_{\alpha 11}$ is involved in α_1-AR-mediated calcium influx *(176)*.

Like many other Ca^{2+}-mobilizing receptors, α_1-ARs mainly couple to the $G_{q/11}$ family of G proteins to increase intracellular free Ca^{2+} concentration. The $G_{q/11}$ family includes five α-subunits: α_q, α_{11}, α_{14}, α_{15}, and α_{16} *(177)*. Transient overexpression of both receptor and G protein α-subunit in COS-7 cells has shown that α_q and α_{11}, which are expressed in most cells, can mediate PLC activation by all α_1-AR subtypes *(178)*. This results predominantly from $G_{q/11}$-mediated activation of PLC-β *(173)*. In contrast, α_{14} and α_{16}, which are expressed in a limited subset of tissues but can also mediate PLC-β activation, couple differentially to α_1-AR subtypes. Thus, whereas the α_{1B}-AR signals efficiently via coupling to $G_{\alpha 14}$ or $G_{\alpha 16}$, the α_{1A}-AR signals via $G_{\alpha 14}$ but not $G_{\alpha 16}$, and the α_{1D}-AR poorly interacts with either *(178)*.

The activation of PLC-β by α_1-ARs results in the hydrolysis of a specific membrane lipid, phosphatidylinositol-4,5-bisphosphate, to release the diffusible

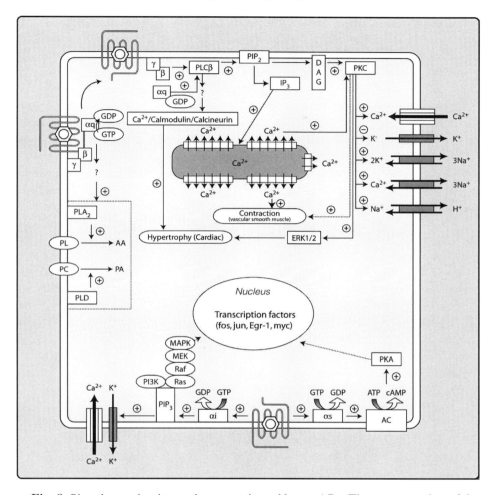

Fig. 8. Signal transduction pathways activated by α_1-ARs. The upper portion of the figure shows the classical receptor-linked phosphoinositide pathway and secondary effector activation. The lower portion shows additional α_1-AR-linked pathways, which include modulation of ion channels and activation of MAPK pathways via G_i-mediated PI3K stimulation. α_1-AR-mediated activation of adenylyl cyclase via $G_{\alpha s}$ has also been reported. AA, arachidonic acid; AC, adenylyl cyclase; ATP, adenosine 5-triphosphate; cAMP, cyclic adenosine 3',5'-monophosphate; DAG, diacylglycerol; ERK, extracellular signal-regulated kinase; GDP, guanosine diphosphate; GTP, guanosine triphosphate; IP_3, inositol-1,4,5-triphosphate; MAPK, mitogen-activated protein kinase; MEK, mitogen-activated protein kinase kinase; PA, phosphatidic acid; PC, phosphatidylcholine; PI3K, phosphatidylinositol-3 kinase; PIP_2, phosphatidyl inositol-4,5-bisphosphate; PIP_3, phosphatidylinositol 3,4,5-triphosphate; PKA, protein kinase A; PKC, protein kinase C; PL, phospholipids; PLA_2; phospholipase A_2; PLC-β, phospholipase Cβ; PLD, phospholipase D.

second messengers IP_3 and diacylglycerol (DAG) *(173)*. IP_3 then activates the release of Ca^{2+} from intracellular stores, such as the endoplasmic reticulum, resulting in a rapid increase in cytoplasmic Ca^{2+} concentration. The increased free Ca^{2+} binds to calcium-dependent regulatory proteins such as calmodulin. The complex formed with calmodulin regulates the activities of a variety of enzymes and other cellular proteins, which leads to a variety of physiological responses in different tissues. DAG, on the other hand, is an allosteric activator of PKC, which in turn phosphorylates seryl and threonyl residues on a variety of cellular protein substrates, including various ion channels (Ca^{2+} and K^+ channels), Na^+-H^+ exchanger, and Na^+-Ca^{2+} pump *(173)*. Regulation of these proteins by PKC results in a variety of cellular responses, including altered cardiac function.

There are at least 10 mammalian PLC isozymes, which can be divided into three types: β1-4, γ1-4, δ1-4 *(179)*. PLC-β can be activated by the α-subunits of all four members of the $G_{q/11}$ family. PLC-γ is mainly activated by receptor tyrosine kinases; the regulators of PLC-δ isoforms have not yet been clearly defined *(179)*. Feng et al. *(180)* have provided evidence that the α_{1B}-AR may couple to G_h to regulate PLC-δ activity, and that a G_h/PLC-δ1 complex is formed on α_{1B}-AR activation. Also, PLC-δ1 can be stimulated by activated G_h following reconstitution, suggesting that PLC-δ1 is a downstream effector of G_h *(181)*. However, Murthy et al *(182)* suggested that G_h may negatively regulate PLC-δ1 activity. They showed that the activity of PLC-δ1 is inhibited when it forms a complex with G_h in the empty or GDP-bound state, whereas dissociation of G_h from PLC-δ1 as a result of receptor-stimulated GTP/GDP exchange activates PLC-δ1. Both the α_{1B}- and the α_{1D}-ARs can utilize the atypical G protein G_h/TGase 2 to activate PLC-δ1 or maxi-K^+ channels *(180,183,184)*.

Stimulation of α_1-ARs has also been shown to induce arachidonic acid (AA) release in a variety of cells, including FRTL5 cells *(185)*, spinal cord neurons *(186)*, MDCK cells *(187)*, vascular smooth muscle cells *(186,188)*, striatal astrocytes *(189)*, and transfected COS-1 and CHO cells *(190)*. In most of these studies, evidence has been provided that activation of PLA_2, either directly or indirectly, was involved in AA release. PLA_2s are a family of enzymes that cleave the ester linkage in membrane glycerophospholipids at the *sn*-2 position of the glycerol moiety, producing a free fatty acid and a lysophospholipid *(191–193)*. There are three major types of PLA_2s: a 14-kDa secretory form, an 85-kDa cytosolic Ca^{2+}-dependent (cPLA_2) form, and an intracellular Ca^{2+}-independent PLA_2 (iPLA_2) form. Although all three PLA_2s mediate AA release, cPLA_2 possesses characteristics suggesting that it is the enzyme mainly involved in receptor-activated signaling *(194)*. The enzyme does not need Ca^{2+} for activation but is able to translocate to membranes in response to increases in intracellular Ca^{2+} to micromolar levels. It possesses a preference for AA-containing phospholipids as its substrate, and its activity is regulated by mitogen-activated protein kinase (MAPK)-mediated phosphorylation. α_1-ARs activate AA release through cPLA$_2$ *(195)*.

However, it is still unclear how the activity of PLA$_2$ is regulated. Studies of various cloned α_1-AR subtypes expressed in different eukaryotic expression systems suggested that their regulation of cPLA$_2$ activity is complicated and is probably cell type specific *(175)*. Some studies have shown that α_1-AR-mediated AA release as a result of PLA$_2$ activation secondary to stimulation of other signaling pathways, such as Ca^{2+} influx or PKC and MAPK activation. But, there is also evidence that α_1-ARs couple directly to PLA$_2$ activation. For example, Perez and coworkers *(190)* showed that stimulation of AA by either the α_{1B}- or α_{1D}-AR expressed in COS-1 cells is dependent on Ca^{2+} influx via dihydropyridine-sensitive L-type calcium channels, whereas in CHO cells, which lack a voltage-dependent calcium channel, α_1-AR-mediated AA release does not involve stimulation of PLC, Ca^{2+} influx, PKC, or DAG lipase or increase of intracellular Ca^{2+} but rather involves direct activation of PLA$_2$.

In addition to PLA$_2$-mediated mechanisms, it is worth noting that AA can also be generated from the activation of other pathways, including PLC, which forms DAG that could be cleaved to generate AA via the action of mono- or diglycerol lipase *(194)*. PLD-mediated cleavage of phosphatidylcholine may also generate phosphatidic acid (PA), which can be further metabolized by phosphatidic acid phosphohydrolase to DAG, and activation of AA release by α_1-ARs via the PLD pathway has been reported *(196)*.

As with other receptors, α_1-ARs may regulate PLA$_2$ activity via G proteins *(197,198)*. Thus, PLA$_2$ activity can be regulated by guanine nucleotides and in most cases is inhibited by pertussis toxin treatment—thus suggesting involvement of a G$_i$- or G$_o$-like G protein *(197,199,200)*. However, it is still unclear how activation of G proteins is linked to PLA$_2$ stimulation, although there is evidence that it may be by via a direct G$\beta\gamma$-mediated effect *(201)*.

The role of the released AA in cell functions is not completely understood, and AA itself can act as a second messenger to activate PKC *(202,203)* and PLCδ *(204)* and to influence membrane ion channel activity *(205,206)*. AA can also inhibit smooth muscle myosin light chain phosphatase activity *(207)* or can be converted through the lipoxygenase or cyclooxygenase pathways to a number of bioactive eicosanoids, including prostaglandins, thromboxanes, leukotrienes, epoxides, and hydroxyeicosatetraeinoic acids, which are involved in inflammation and cell proliferation *(194,208)*. Moreover, lysophospholipid, which is concomitantly released from phospholipid as a result of PLA$_2$ activation, can influence cell functions (e.g., proliferation) by acting on its receptor on the cell surface.

PLD mainly catalyzes the hydrolysis of phosphatidylcholine to PA and choline *(209)*. PA may act directly as a signaling molecule or can be converted by phosphohydrolase to the PKC activator DAG. Activation of PLD via α_1-ARs has been demonstrated in a variety of tissues and cell lines, including cerebral cortex *(210)*, artery *(211,212)*, parotid *(213)*, ventricular myocytes *(214)*, and MDCK cells *(215)*. Indeed, each of the three α_1-ARs subtypes, when expressed in rat-1 fibroblast cells, can activate PLD with the following order of efficiency: $\alpha_{1A} >$ $\alpha_{1B} > \alpha_{1D}$-AR *(196)*. However, the mechanisms involved in this activation are poorly understood. The activity of PLD can be regulated by multiple pathways, including by PKC or tyrosine kinases, as well as by small G proteins of the ADP-ribosylating factor and Rho families *(209)*. In a few studies that have examined the regulatory mechanisms, it was shown that extracellular Ca^{2+} but not PKC activation is required for stimulation of PLD via α_1-ARs *(215)*. In addition, there is evidence that α_1-AR-mediated PLD activation can be regulated by the cAMP–PKA (protein kinase A) signaling pathway *(196)*.

α_1-ARs can also signal via interaction with pertussis-sensitive G proteins. Thus, $G_{\alpha o}$ has been suggested to interact with α_1-ARs in mediating contraction and inositol phosphate generation in rat aorta *(216)*, a response that may involve effector activation by either the α- or $\beta\gamma$-complexes. Other α_1-AR-mediated actions, such as PLA_2 activation *(94,197)* and modulation of calcium influx *(217)*, are also mediated by pertussis toxin G proteins. Also, in rat aortic smooth muscle *(216)* or with overexpression of the α_{1B}-AR in oocytes *(218)*, PLC coupling involves interaction with G_o. Direct coupling of the α_{1B}-AR to G_s to stimulate adenylyl cyclase activity has also been reported in transfected CHO cells *(219)*. In addition to modulation of these classical effector pathways, α_1-ARs regulate growth responses via activation of the MAPK family, including ERK1/2, c-Jun N-terminal kinases (JNKs), and the p38 kinases. Thus, α_1-ARs can also activate the MAPK pathway *(175)*. MAPKs are a large family of widely expressed serine/threonine kinases *(220)*, involving three major subfamilies: the ERKs, the JNKs, and the p38 MAPKs. All three MAPKs can be activated α_1-ARs, albeit to variable extents *(175)*. In particular, their activation plays a critical role in the hypertrophic response of cardiac myocytes to α_1-AR stimulation *(221)*. The cellular pathways involved have not yet been completely elucidated, but activation of Ras, Rho, and their downstream kinases has been implicated *(175)*. The upstream signals probably involve various receptor-coupled second messengers, such as Ca^{2+} and PKC, as well as G proteins (both α- and $\beta\gamma$-subunits) *(220)*. In addition, they may involve tyrosine kinases (Pyk2, Src), adaptor proteins (Shc), and phosphoinositide-3 kinase (PI3K) *(175)*.

As with other GPCRs, the domains of the α_1-ARs involved in G protein coupling are the intracellular loops, particularly i_3 *(222)*. For example, substitution of a portion of i_3 of the α_{1B}-AR into the corresponding region of the β_2-AR results in a chimera that can now activate PI hydrolysis but not cAMP generation *(223)*. Moreover, overexpression of the i_3 segment of the α_{1B}-AR using a minigene construct inhibits coupling of this receptor to inositol phosphate turnover *(224)*. Finally, selective deletion of a portion of i_3 of the α_{1B}-AR impairs its ability to couple to $G_{q/11}$, G_{14}, and G_{16} *(225)*. The i_3 sequences involved in the activation of G proteins by the α_{1B}-AR subtype involve residues extending from Lys[240]-His[252] for activation via $G_{\alpha q}$ and $G_{\alpha 11}$ but not for activation via $G_{\alpha 14}$ or $G_{\alpha 16}$ *(225)*. Two segments in i_3—one at the amino terminus and another at the carboxy terminus— are required for $G_{\alpha i}$ activation and to some extent for coupling to $G_{\alpha 16}$ *(225)*. However, no consensus sequences have been defined that predict selective interaction of the various α_1-AR subtypes with specific G proteins *(222)*. This is not altogether surprising given that even when receptors belonging to the same family couple to similar G proteins, they share little or no amino acid identity within their G protein-interacting intracellular loops. As a corollary, in addition to primary amino acid sequence, the secondary and tertiary structures of the intracellular loops are likely critical for the specificity of receptor/G protein coupling.

3.3. α_2-ARs G Protein and Effector Activation

Signaling by α_2-ARs mainly involves coupling via G_i and hence leads to the inhibition of adenylyl cyclase *(107,226)*. Also, Eason and colleagues have demonstrated pertussis toxin-insensitive activation of cAMP in CHO cells expressing high levels of α_2-AR *(226)*. Moreover, they have also demonstrated a direct agonist-dependent physical coupling of the α_{2A}-AR to G_s. G_q coupling has been demonstrated in HEK293 cells transiently transfected with the porcine α_{2A}-AR and either murine $G_{\alpha q}$ or rat $G_{\alpha s}$ *(107)*. However, coupling of the α_{2A}-AR to endogenous G_i was approx 1000 times greater than that to G_s or G_q. Hence, α_2-ARs preferentially couple to the $G_{i/o}$ families of G proteins *(227)*, and different amino acids are responsible for the activation of G_i and G_s *(228,229)*.

Coupling of α_2-ARs to G_i leads to inhibition of adenylyl cyclase, which results in decreased cAMP generation. Coupling to several other signaling pathways has also been reported for the α_2-ARs, including activation of K^+ channels *(230)*; inhibition of calcium channels; activation of the Na^+/H^+ antiporter *(231)*; and mobilization of intracellular Ca^{2+} *(232)*.

The α_{2A}- and α_{2D}-ARs can couple to at least G_{i2}, G_{i3}, and G_{o1} *(233–237)*, whereas the α_{2C}-AR couples to G_{i1}, G_{o1}, or G_{o2} *(238,239)*. After reconstitution in phospholipid vesicles, both the α_{2A}- and α_{2C}-ARs have been shown to couple to members of the $G_{i/o}$ subfamily with the following potency: $G_{i3} > G_{i1} = G_{i2} > G_{o1}$ *(240)*.

In addition to inhibition of AC, stimulation of both the α_{2A}- and α_{2C}-ARs results in direct activation of PLC via a PTX-sensitive G protein *(241)*. Hence, as for many other receptor subtypes, α_2-ARs can couple to multiple effector systems, indicating heterogeneity of receptor–effector interactions. In addition, the effector pathway utilized is dependent on the specific ligand employed and its concentration.

3.4. β-AR G Protein and Effector Activation

All three β-AR subtypes activate effectors via coupling to G_s. In cardio-myocytes, stimulation of β-AR by nonselective agonists results in G_s-mediated adenylyl cyclase activation and enhanced c-AMP generation, which in turn causes activation of PKA. In some cells, enhanced cAMP generation also results in activation of cAMP-gated ion channels. As depicted in Fig. 9, PKA phospho-rylates several proteins that are involved in cardiac function, which results in activation of L-type calcium channels *(242,243)*; disinhibition of the sarcoendoplasmic reticular Ca^{2+}-ATPase as a result of phospholamban (PLB) phosphorylation *(244)*; and activation of troponin I *(245)*, ryanodine receptors *(246)*, and myosin-binding proteins *(247)*. In addition, PKA also phosphorylates and activates protein phosphatase inhibitor-1 *(248)*, which inhibits protein phos-phatase-1 and thus prevents dephosphorylation of PLB and other substrates. These β-AR-mediated effects enhance contractility by increasing Ca^{2+} influx (activation of L-type channels), increasing Ca^{2+} reuptake into the sarcoplasmic reticulum (PLB/SERCA), and modulating myofilament Ca^{2+} sensitivity (tropo-nin I, myosin binding protein C). Activation of β-ARs also results in enhanced cAMP-dependent gene transcription (Fig. 9, lower panel).

Although the cAMP pathway is activated by both β_1- and β_2-ARs in both cardiomyocytes *(249,250)* and transfected cells *(251,252)*, β_2-AR-mediated adenylyl cyclase activation is greater than that by β_1-ARs. These two β-AR subtypes also have opposing actions in regulating cardiomyocyte apoptosis: stimulation of the β_1-AR increases apoptosis, whereas stimulation of the β_2-AR inhibits it *(253)*. Such differences may be because, whereas the β_1-AR couples exclusively to $G_{\alpha s}$, the β_2-AR can also activate effectors via coupling to G_i *(254–256)*. For example, Daaka and colleagues *(254)* reported that, in HEK293 cells,

---

Fig. 9. *(Opposite page)* Classical and cardiomyocyte β-AR signaling pathways. Upper portion: Indicated in white rectangular boxes are the classical signaling path-ways mediated by the β-ARs, which mainly involve G_s-mediated PKA activation. The bold-lined boxes indicate the signaling molecules common to both β_1- and β_2-ARs signaling via G_s, whereas the thin-lined boxes indicate those activated solely by the β_2-AR. Indicated in oval boxes are the nonclassical signaling pathways. Of particular importance is the PKA-mediated switch in β_2-AR signaling from G_s to G_i coupling. Hence, both G_s- and G_i-mediated pathways lead to ERK activation by the β_2-AR. Signaling intermediates in gray are unique to either the G_s or the G_i pathway, whereas those without color are common to both pathways. Indicated in the dotted boxes are the two major mediators of β_2-AR desensitization: GPCR kinase (GRK) and β-arrestin (β-arr). Interaction of β-arrestin with the β_2-AR leads to its internalization and the activa-tion of new signaling pathways, which result in ERK activation. Lower portion: G protein and effector pathways involved in β_2-AR-mediated enhancement of cardiac inotropy via release of Ca^{2+} from the sarcoplasmic reticulum. *(Continued on next page)*

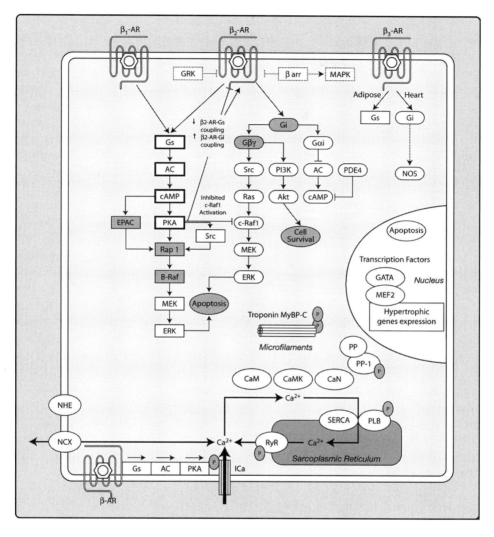

Fig. 9. *(Continued from opposite page)* AC, adenylyl cyclase; c-AMP, cyclic adenosine monophosphate; β-arr, β-arrestin; CaM, calmodulin; CaMK, calmodulin-dependent kinase; CaN, calcineurin; EPAC, exchange protein directly activated by cAMP; ERK, extracellular signal-regulated kinase; GRK, G protein coupled receptor kinase; MAPK, mitogen-activated protein kinase; MEK, mitogen-activated protein kinase kinase; MEF2, myocyte enhancing factor 2; NCX, sodium-calcium exchanger; NHE, sodium-hydrogen antiporter; NOS, nitric oxide synthase; P, a phosphate group that has modified the target protein as a result of phoshorylation; PDE, phosphodiesterase; PI3K, phosphatidylinositol-3 kinase; PKA, c-AMP-dependent protein kinase A; PLB, phospholamban; PP, protein phosphatase; RyR, ryanodine receptor; SERCA, sarcoendoplasmic reticular calcium ATPase. (This figure has been adapted from refs. *284* and *300*.)

activation of the β_2-AR results in initial PKA-mediated receptor phosphorylation. The resulting phosphorylated receptor is no longer able to activate adenylyl cyclase, but switches to activation of MAPK, a response mediated by a pathway involving stimulation of c-Src and Ras by the $G_{\beta\gamma}$-subunits of pertussis toxin-sensitive G_i.

This switch in the coupling of the β_2-AR from G_s to G_i signaling leads to the activation of not only ERKs *(254)*, but also Akt/protein kinase B *(257)*, phosphoinositide-3-kinase *(257)*, certain receptor tyrosine kinases *(258)* and inhibition of adenylyl cyclase *(259)*. In cardiomyocytes, G_i-mediated stimulation of the PI3K/Akt-dependent cell survival signaling pathway is thought to prevent cardiomyocytes from undergoing G_s-mediated apoptosis. This β_2-AR-coupled, G_i-mediated pathway may also result in the transactivation of the epidermal growth factor receptor *(254,257–262)* and has been demonstrated in a variety of different cell lines, including cultured rat cardiomyocytes *(261)*, HEK293 cells *(254)*, CHO cells *(262)*, and COS-7 cells *(258)*. Both the classical β_2-AR G_s-mediated ERK activation pathway and the G_s/G_i-mediated ERK activation pathway are depicted in Fig. 9.

In addition to PKA, the β_2-AR can be phosphorylated by PKC and GRKs as part of the desensitization response. GRKs phosphorylate the ligand-activated β_2-AR and thereby stimulate recruitment of arrestin, which targets the receptor for internalization. In addition, the receptor/β-arrestin complex recruits several proteins that initiate nonclassical signaling pathways. Because this GRK/β-arrestin targeting mechanism is more prominent with the β_2- than the β_1-AR, this could explain why the activation of these nonclassical signaling pathways is more evident with the former subtype. The differing behavior of the β-AR subtypes, in terms of β-arrestin binding and internalization, might also regulate some of their differential signaling properties. It has also been suggested that the receptors may initially be embedded into large signalosomes, which differ for the two subtypes. The hypothesis underlying this proposal is that spatial segregation of receptors allows their association with other sequestered proteins to form specific signaling complexes that mediate subtype-specific responses. In this context, it has been shown that, in neurons, a β_2-AR signalosome containing an entire signaling chain could be isolated *(263,264)*.

Although subtype-specific differences in receptor compartmentalization have been suggested, the mechanisms underlying such differential receptor segregation are not well understood. One possibility is that of differential plasma membrane localization of the two different receptors. Indeed, it has been shown that the β_2-AR could be copurified with caveolae from adult cardiomyocytes, whereas the β_1-AR was much more evenly distributed in these cells *(265)*. However, in rat neonatal cardiomyocytes, the β_1-AR is associated with caveolae *(250)*. cAMP signals might also be spatially regulated via their site of generation (receptor localization) and destruction (phosphodiesterases). In particular, activation of the β_2-AR leads to β-arrestin-mediated phosphodiesterase (PDE4) recruitment to the plasma membrane, which may regulate the switching from G_s- to G_i-mediated signaling *(266)*. Hence, it seems that although signals are usually measured as global changes in second messenger concentrations—which are therefore assumed to change in a uniform manner throughout the cell—compartmentalization of intracellular signaling might be essential, and both spatial and temporal regulation of receptor-induced signaling seems to be operative with both β_1- and β_2-ARs.

Finally, selective coupling of the β_1-AR only to G_s may not hold in all cell types because ERK activation via β_1-AR and G_i has been demonstrated in COS-7 cells, a response regulated by the PDZ domain-binding protein: GAIP-interacting protein, carboxy (C) terminus *(267)*. Indeed, both the β_1- and the β_2-AR contain carboxy-terminal PDZ-binding domains that can bind to PDZ domain-containing proteins *(268)*. In this context, the β_2-AR has been shown to interact with Na^+/H^+ exchanger regulatory factors in an agonist-dependent manner via its PDZ-binding domain *(268)*, and the β_1-AR interacts with MAGI-2 *(269)* and PSD-95 in a GRK5-dependent manner *(270)*. Expression of the β_3-AR subtype is mainly limited to the adipose tissue *(271)*, but several groups have reported β_3-AR effects and messenger ribonucleic acid (mRNA) in human, guinea pig, and canine heart and cardiomyocytes *(272–274)*. However, although it couples to G_s in fat cells, these reports suggest coupling to a nonclassical G_i/nitric oxide pathway that produces enhanced inotropic effects in human heart *(275, 276)*. β_1/β_2-Knockout mice have little or only very slight β_3-AR effects *(277–279)*, whereas with cardiac-specific overexpression of this receptor, enhanced cardiac contractility has been observed *(280)*. Thus, the physiological role of this subtype outside adipose tissue remains to be defined. A fourth receptor subtype, the β_4-AR, has also been postulated to mediate the cardiac effects of the agonist CGP12177, but studies with the β_1-AR and β_2-AR knockout mice revealed that these effects were actually mediated through the β_1-AR *(281)*.

3.5. Regulation of G Protein and Effector Coupling

To allow precise homeostatic regulation of cellular functions, signaling pathways that are turned on also need to be turned off, and to this end, agonist occupation of receptors has been shown to initiate a series of molecular processes that control temporal and spatial receptor input. Three such regulatory processes are desensitization, internalization, and downregulation. Desensitization—a phenomenon commonly described as the waning of the receptor response on continuous agonist exposure—is characterized by receptor/G protein uncoupling and occurs rapidly (within seconds to minutes). Two forms, homologous and heterologous, have been identified. The former refers to uncoupling that occurs with exposure of a receptor to its own agonist, the latter to uncoupling of a receptor as a result of continuous activation of a different receptor.

Although not fully understood, desensitization involves several mechanisms, including receptor phosphorylation and interactions with intracellular protein partners, especially arrestins, which by binding to the G protein recognition site, block the G protein/receptor interaction. Phosphorylation of GPCRs can be mediated by second messenger-dependent protein kinases (PKA or PKC), which phosphorylate receptors whether occupied by an agonist or not. Phosphorylation by these kinases thus is involved in heterologous desensitization. Receptor phosphorylation can also be mediated by GRKs, which selectively phosphorylate agonist-bound receptors and hence participate in homologous desensitization.

Downregulation, by contrast, occurs more slowly (over hours), and is caused by a decrease in the total number of receptor molecules in the cell, resulting from either a decrease in receptor synthesis, destabilization of receptor mRNA, or an increase in receptor degradation *(282,283)*. Recovery from downregulation therefore requires *de novo* protein synthesis. However, as downregulation is not necessarily coupled to receptor internalization, signals different from those involved in endocytosis are likely required.

Internalization or sequestration of receptors away from the cell surface also occurs more slowly (minutes to hours) than desensitization. Although it might be facilitated by receptor phosphorylation, it can also occur in the absence of phosphorylation. In many instances, internalization is dependent on an interaction with arrestin molecules, which then target receptors for endocytosis via clathrin-coated pits. Once internalized, receptors are either recycled to the cell surface (resensitization) or are degraded in lysosomes.

In addition to their roles in the desensitization and internalization of receptors, arrestins also initiate signals from receptors and have been shown to interact with different kinases and other regulatory proteins, such as Src-family tyrosine kinases, and act as receptor-regulated scaffolds for several ERKs, including JNKs and p38 MAPKs. ERKs are activated by a variety of diverse GPCRs (for review, *see* ref. *260*) via G_s, G_i, G_q, and G_o-mediated pathways. Thus, it is now well established that internalization, or at least the sequestration of GPCRs, plays a role in their signaling, and that interaction with arrestins is essential for activation of new signaling pathways. These new or nonclassical signaling pathways and paradigms are considered in the chapter "New Signal Transduction Paradigms" by KP Minneman.

Finally, there is increasing evidence for the specific intracellular localization of receptors with distinct signaling pathways, a process that allows spatial segregation of receptors and thus their association/interaction with other proteins to form signalosomes that may be responsible for subtype-specific responses *(284)*.

Appendix

Residue Identification

To allow residues to be readily compared between adrenergic receptor subtypes, the standardized numbering system of Ballesteros and Weinstein *(285)* is used throughout this chapter to identify residues in the TM helices. Each residue is designated by a three-digit number: The first digit (1 through 7) corresponds to the helix in which it is located; the second and third digits identify its position relative to the most-conserved residue in that helix, which is designated as ".50" (Table 2). Residues C-terminal to the conserved residue are designated by successively increasing numbers, whereas those N-terminal are identified by successively decreasing numbers. For example, residues of the "DRY" motif are designated as D3.49, R3.50, and Y3.51.

Table 2
Residue Designation [a]

Receptor	1.50	2.50	3.50	4.50	5.50	6.50	7.50
α_{1A}	N44	D72	R124	W151	P196	P287	P323
α_{1B}	N63	D91	R143	W170	P215	P309	P345
α_{1D}	N114	D142	R194	W221	P266	P363	P399
α_{2A}	N51	D79	R131	W158	P208	P351	P303
α_{2B}	N30	D58	R110	W137	P184	P386	P423
α_{2C}	N69	D97	R149	W176	P222	P396	P433
β_1	N76	D104	R156	W183	P236	P339	P374
β_2	N51	D79	R131	W158	P211	P288	P323
β_3	N55	D83	R135	W162	P216	P307	P343

[a] The numbers following the amino acids (identified using the single letter code) indicated below each Ballesteros and Weinstein position are those of the human adrenergic receptor sequences.

Glossary

The following definitions are based on those recommended by the International Union of Pharmacology, Committee on Receptor Nomenclature and Drug Classification *(286)*.

Affinity
  The equilibrium constant of the reversible reaction of a drug with a receptor to form a drug-receptor complex, dependent on the chemical natures of both the drug and the receptor.

Agonist
  A ligand that binds to a receptor and alters the receptor-state resulting in a biological response. Conventional agonists increase receptor activity, whereas *inverse agonists* reduce it.

Antagonist
   A ligand that inhibits receptor activation by another ligand, generally an agonist.

e_1, e_2, e_3
   Extracellular loop 1, extracellular loop 2, extracellular loop 3.

EC_{50}
   The molar concentration of an agonist that produces 50% of the maximal possible effect of that agonist.

Efficacy
   The degree to which different agonists produce a response, given the same proportion of occupied receptors. For example a *partial agonist* has a reduced efficacy compared to a *full agonist* for the same receptor

Full agonist
   An agonist which has the ability to produce the maximal response for a given system. The designation of full *vs* partial agonist is system-dependent.

i_1, i_2, i_3
   Intracellular loop 1, intracellular loop 2, intracellular loop 3.

Inverse agonist:
   A ligand that by binding to receptors reduces the fraction of receptors in the active conformation.

K_d
   The equilibrium dissociation constant of a ligand determined directly in a binding assay using a labeled form of the ligand.

Ligand
   A molecule that binds to a receptor.

Partial agonist
   An agonist that cannot elicit a maximal response (even when applied at high concentrations to ensure full receptor occupancy). The designation of full *vs* partial agonist is system-dependent.

Potency
   The activity of a drug, in terms of the concentration or amount needed to produce a defined effect.

References

1. Easson LH, Stedman E. CLXX. Studies on the relationship between chemical constitution and physiological action. V. Molecular dissymmetry and physiological activity. Biochem J 1933;27:1257–1266.
2. Dixon RA, Kobilka BK, Strader DJ, et al. Cloning of the gene and cDNA for mammalian β-adrenergic receptor and homology with rhodopsin. Nature 1986; 321:75–79.
3. Yarden Y, Rodriguez H, Wong SK, et al. The avian β-adrenergic receptor: primary structure and membrane topology. Proc Natl Acad Sci USA 1986;83:6795–6799.

4. Tota MR, Strader CD. Characterization of the binding domain of the β-adrenergic-receptor with the fluorescent antagonist carazolol—evidence for a buried ligand-binding site. J Biol Chem 1990;265:16,891–16,897.

5. Porter JE, Perez DM. Characteristics for a salt-bridge switch mutation of the α_{1B} adrenergic receptor—altered pharmacology and rescue of constitutive activity. J Biol Chem 1999;274:34,535–34,538.

6. Strader CD, Sigal IS, Register RB, Candelore MR, Rands E, Dixon RAF. Identification of residues required for ligand-binding to the β-adrenergic-receptor. Proc Natl Acad Sci USA 1987;84:4384–4388.

7. Strader CD, Sigal IS, Candelore MR, Rands E, Hill WS, Dixon RAF. Conserved aspartic-acid residue-79 and residue-113 of the β-adrenergic-receptor have different roles in receptor function. J Biol Chem 1988;263:10,267–10,271.

8. Gros J, Manning BS, Pietri-Rouxel F, Guillaume JL, Drumare MF, Strosberg AD. Site-directed mutagenesis of the human β_3-adrenoceptor—transmembrane residues involved in ligand binding and signal transduction. Eur J Biochem 1998;251:590–596.

9. Strader CD, Gaffney T, Sugg EE, et al. Allele-specific activation of genetically engineered receptors. J Biol Chem 1991;266:5–8.

10. Cavalli A, Fanelli F, Taddei C, DeBenedetti PG, Cotecchia S. Amino acids of the α_{1B}-adrenergic receptor involved in agonist binding: differences in docking catecholamines to receptor subtypes. FEBS Lett 1996;399:9–13.

11. Nyronen T, Pihlavisto M, Peltonen JM, et al. Molecular mechanism for agonist-promoted α_{2A}-adrenoceptor activation by norepinephrine and epinephrine. Mol Pharmacol 2001;59:1343–1354.

12. Hwa J, Perez DM. The unique nature of the serine interactions for α_1-adrenergic receptor agonist binding and activation. J Biol Chem 1996;271:6322–6327.

13. Wetzel JM, Salon JA, Tamm JA, et al. Modeling and mutagenesis of the human α_{1A}-adrenoceptor: orientation and function of transmembrane helix V sidechains. Receptors Channels 1996;4:165–177.

14. Peltonen JM, Nyronen M, Wurster S, et al. Molecular mechanisms of ligand-receptor interactions in transmembrane domain V of the α_{2A}-adrenoceptor. Br J Pharmacol 2003;140:347–358.

15. Wang CD, Buck MA, Fraser CM. Site-directed mutagenesis of α_{2A}-adrenergic receptors—identification of amino-acids involved in ligand-binding and receptor activation by agonists. Mol Pharmacol 1991;40:168–179.

16. Liapakis G, Ballesteros JA, Papachristou S, Chan WC, Chen X, Javitch JA. The forgotten serine—a critical role for Ser-203(5.42) in ligand binding to and activation of the β_2-adrenergic receptor. J Biol Chem 2000;275:37,779–37,788.

17. Strader CD, Candelore MR, Hill WS, Sigal IS, Dixon RAF. Identification of 2 serine residues involved in agonist activation of the β-adrenergic-receptor. J Biol Chem 1989;264:13,572–13,578.

18. Bilezikian JP, Dornfeld AM, Gammon DE. Structure-binding-activity analysis of β-adrenergic amines—I. Binding to the β receptor and activation of adenylate cyclase. Biochem Pharmacol 1978;27:1445–1454.

19. Waugh DJJ, Zhao MM, Zuscik MJ, Perez DM. Novel aromatic residues in transmembrane domains IV and V involved in agonist binding at α_{1A}-adrenergic receptors. J Biol Chem 2000;275:11,698–11,705.

20. Chen SH, Xu M, Lin F, Lee D, Riek P, Graham RM. Phe(310) in transmembrane VI of the α_{1B}-adrenergic receptor is a key switch residue involved in activation and catecholamine ring aromatic bonding. J Biol Chem 1999;274:16,320–16,330.

21. Strader CD, Sigal IS, Dixon RA. Structural basis of β-adrenergic receptor function. FASEB J 1989;3:1825–1832.

22. Dixon RA, Sigal IS, Strader CD. Structure-function analysis of the β-adrenergic receptor. Cold Spring Harb Symp Quant Biol 1988;53 Pt 1:487–497.

23. Hieble JP, Hehr A, Li YO, Ruffolo RR, Jr. Molecular basis for the stereoselective interactions of catecholamines with α-adrenoceptors. Proc West Pharmacol Soc 1998;41:225–228.

24. Wieland K, Zuurmond HM, Krasel C, Ijzerman AP, Lohse MJ. Involvement of Asn-293 in stereospecific agonist recognition and in activation of the β_2-adrenergic receptor. Proc Natl Acad Sci USA 1996;93:9276–9281.

25. MaloneyHuss K, Lybrand TP. Three-dimensional structure for the β_2 adrenergic receptor protein based on computer modeling studies. J Mol Biol 1992;225:859–871.

26. Trumpp-Kallmeyer S, Hoflack J, Bruinvels A, Hibert M. Modeling of G-protein-coupled receptors: application to dopamine, adrenaline, serotonin, acetylcholine, and mammalian opsin receptors. J Med Chem 1992;35:3448–3462.

27. Green SA, Cole G, Jacinto M, Innis M, Liggett SB. A Polymorphism of the Human β_2-Adrenergic Receptor within the fourth Transmembrane Domain Alters Ligand-Binding and Functional-Properties of the Receptor. J Biol Chem 1993;268:23,116–23,121.

28. Freddolino PL, Kalani MY, Vaidehi N, et al. Predicted 3D structure for the human β_2 adrenergic receptor and its binding site for agonists and antagonists. Proc Natl Acad Sci USA 2004;101:2736–2741.

29. Furse KE, Lybrand TP. Three-dimensional models for β-adrenergic receptor complexes with agonists and antagonists. J Med Chem 2003;46:4450–4462.

30. Salminen T, Varis M, Nyronen T, et al. Three-dimensional models of α_{2A}-adrenergic receptor complexes provide a structural explanation for ligand binding. J Biol Chem 1999;274:23,405–23,413.

31. Porter JE, Hwa J, Perez DM. Activation of the α_{1B}-adrenergic receptor is initiated by disruption of an interhelical salt bridge constraint. J Biol Chem 1996;271: 28,318–28,323.

32. Chen S, Finch AM, Graham RM. Unpublished observation. In 2001.

33. Hwa J, Reik RP, Graham RM, Perez DM. Effects of mutating specific amino-acids on the ligand-binding characteristics of α_1-adrenergic receptor subtypes. FASEB J 1995;9:A104–A104.

34. Zhao MM, Hwa J, Perez DM. Identification of critical extracellular loop residues involved in α_1-adrenergic receptor subtype-selective antagonist binding. Mol Pharmacol 1996;50:1118–1126.

35. Waugh DJJ, Gaivin RJ, Zuscik MJ, et al. Phe-308 and Phe-312 in transmembrane domain 7 are major sites of α_1-adrenergic receptor antagonist binding—imidazoline agonists bind like antagonists. J Biol Chem 2001;276:25,366–25,371.

36. Ishiguro M, Futabayashi Y, Ohnuki T, Ahmed M, Muramatsu I, Nagatomo T. Identification of binding sites of prazosin, tamsulosin and KMD-3213 with α_1-adrenergic receptor subtypes by molecular modeling. Life Sci 2002;71:2531–2541.

37. Sakmar TP, Menon ST, Marin EP, Awad ES. Rhodopsin: insights from recent structural studies. Annu Rev Biophys Biomol Struct 2002;31:443–484.

38. Yan EC, Kazmi MA, De S, et al. Function of extracellular loop 2 in rhodopsin: glutamic acid 181 modulates stability and absorption wavelength of metarhodopsin II. Biochemistry 2002;41:3620–3627.

39. Schadel SA, Heck M, Maretzki D, et al. Ligand channeling within a G-protein-coupled receptor. The entry and exit of retinals in native opsin. J Biol Chem 2003; 278:24,896–24,903.

40. Horie K, Obika K, Foglar R, Tsujimoto G. Selectivity of the imidazoline α-adrenoceptor agonists (oxymetazoline and cirazoline) for human cloned α_1-adrenoceptor subtypes. Br J Pharmacol 1995;116:1611–1618.

41. Kukkonen JP, Renvaktar A, Shariatmadari R, Akerman KE. Ligand- and subtype-selective coupling of human α_2 adrenoceptors to Ca++ elevation in Chinese hamster ovary cells. J Pharmacol Exp Ther 1998;287:667–671.

42. Hwa J, Graham RM, Perez DM. Identification of critical determinants of α_1-adrenergic receptor subtype selective agonist binding. J Biol Chem 1995;270: 23,189–23,195.

43. Kurose H, Isogaya M, Kikkawa H, Nagao T. Domains of β_1 and β_2 adrenergic receptors to bind subtype selective agonists. Life Sci 1998;62:1513–1517.

44. Isogaya M, Sugimoto Y, Tanimura R, et al. Binding pockets of the β_1- and β_2-adrenergic receptors for subtype-selective agonists. Mol Pharmacol 1999;56:875–885.

45. Kikkawa H, Isogaya M, Nagao T, Kurose H. The role of the seventh transmembrane region in high affinity binding of a β_2-selective agonist TA-2005. Mol Pharmacol 1998;53:128–134.

46. Isogaya M, Yamagiwa Y, Fujita S, Sugimoto Y, Nagao T, Kurose H. Identification of a key amino acid of the β_2-adrenergic receptor for high affinity binding of salmeterol. Mol Pharmacol 1998;54:616–622.

47. Suryanarayana S, Kobilka BK. Amino-acid substitutions at position 312 in the 7th hydrophobic segment of the β_2-adrenergic receptor modify ligand-binding specificity. Mol Pharmacol 1993;44:111–114.

48. Suryanarayana S, Daunt DA, Vonzastrow M, Kobilka BK. A point mutation in the 7th hydrophobic domain of the α_2 adrenergic-receptor increases its affinity for a family of β-receptor-antagonists. J Biol Chem 1991;266:15,488–15,492.

49. Ehrlich P. Chemotherapeutics: scientific principles, methods and results. Lancet 1913;2:445–451.

50. Langley J. On the contraction of muscle, chiefly in relation to the presence of 'receptive' substances. IV: The effect of curari and of some other substances on the nicotine response of the sartorius and gastrocnemius muscles of the frog. J Physiol (Lond) 1909;39:235–295.

51. Fisher E. Einfluss der configuration auf die wirkung der enzyme. Ber Dtsh Chem Ges 1894;27:2985–3005.

52. Tolkovsky AM, Levitzki A. Mode of coupling between the β-adrenergic receptor and adenylate cyclase in turkey erythrocytes. Biochemistry 1978;17:3795–3810.
53. Bergman RN, Hechter O. Neurohypophyseal hormone-responsive renal adenylate cyclase. IV. A random-hit matrix model for coupline in a hormone-sensitive adenylate cyclase system. J Biol Chem 1978;253:3238–3250.
54. Katz B, Thesleff S. A study of the desensitization produced by acetylcholine at the motor end-plate. J Physiol 1957;138:63–80.
55. Weiland G, Taylor P. Ligand specificity of state transitions in the cholinergic receptor: behavior of agonists and antagonists. Mol Pharmacol 1979;15:197–212.
56. De Lean A, Munson PJ, Rodbard D. Multi-subsite receptors for multivalent ligands. Application to drugs, hormones, and neurotransmitters. Mol Pharmacol 1979;15: 60–70.
57. De Lean A, Stadel JM, Lefkowitz RJ. A ternary complex model explains the agonist-specific binding properties of the adenylate cyclase-coupled β-adrenergic receptor. J Biol Chem 1980;255:7108–7117.
58. Lefkowitz RJ, Mullikin D, Williams LT. A desensitized state of the β adrenergic receptor not associated with high-affinity agonist occupancy. Mol Pharmacol 1978;14:376–380.
59. Chidiac P, Hebert TE, Valiquette M, Dennis M, Bouvier M. Inverse agonist activity of β-adrenergic antagonists. Mol Pharmacol 1994;45:490–499.
60. Allen LF, Lefkowitz RJ, Caron MG, Cotecchia S. G-protein-coupled receptor genes as protooncogenes - constitutively activating mutation of the α_{1B}-adrenergic receptor enhances mitogenesis and tumorigenicity. Proc Natl Acad Sci USA 1991; 88:11,354–11,358.
61. Javitch JA, Fu DY, Liapakis G, Chen JY. Constitutive activation of the β_2 adrenergic receptor alters the orientation of its sixth membrane-spanning segment. J Biol Chem 1997;272:18,546–18,549.
62. Lattion AL, Abuin L, Nenniger-Tosato M, Cotecchia S. Constitutively active mutants of the β_1-adrenergic receptor. FEBS Lett 1999;457:302–306.
63. Samama P, Cotecchia S, Costa T, Lefkowitz RJ. A mutation-induced activated state of the β_2-adrenergic receptor - extending the ternary complex model. J Biol Chem 1993;268:4625–4636.
64. Koshland DE, Jr., Neet KE. The catalytic and regulatory properties of enzymes. Annu Rev Biochem 1968;37:359–410.
65. Herrick-Davis K, Egan C, Teitler M. Activating mutations of the serotonin 5-HT$_{2C}$ receptor. J Neurochem 1997;69:1138–1144.
66. Morin D, Cotte N, Balestre MN, et al. The D136A mutation of the V2 vasopressin receptor induces a constitutive activity which permits discrimination between antagonists with partial agonist and inverse agonist activities. FEBS Lett 1998;441: 470–475.
67. Egan CT, Herrick-Davis K, Teitler M. Creation of a constitutively activated state of the 5-hydroxytryptamine$_{2A}$ receptor by site-directed mutagenesis: inverse agonist activity of antipsychotic drugs. J Pharmacol Exp Ther 1998;286:85–90.
68. Weiss JM, Morgan PH, Lutz MW, Kenakin TP. The cubic ternary complex receptor-occupancy model. III. Resurrecting efficacy. J Theor Biol 1996;181:381–397.

69. Weiss JM, Morgan PH, Lutz MW, Kenakin TP. The cubic ternary complex receptor-occupancy model .1. Model description. J Theor Biol 1996;178:151–167.

70. Weiss JM, Morgan PH, Lutz MW, Kenakin TP. The cubic ternary complex receptor-occupancy model .2. Understanding apparent affinity. J Theor Biol 1996;178: 169–182.

71. Watson C, Chen G, Irving P, Way J, Chen WJ, Kenakin T. The use of stimulus-biased assay systems to detect agonist-specific receptor active states: implications for the trafficking of receptor stimulus by agonists. Mol Pharmacol 2000;58: 1230–1238.

72. Kenakin T. Inverse, protean, and ligand-selective agonism: matters of receptor conformation. FASEB J 2001;15:598–611.

73. Kenakin T. Principles: Receptor theory in pharmacology. Trends Pharmacol Sci 2004;25:186–192.

74. Ghanouni P, Steenhuis JJ, Farrens DL, Kobilka BK. Agonist-induced conformational changes in the G-protein-coupling domain of the β_2 adrenergic receptor. Proc Natl Acad Sci USA2001;98:5997–6002.

75. Gether U, Ballesteros JA, Seifert R, SandersBush E, Weinstein H, Kobilka BK. Structural instability of a constitutively active G protein-coupled receptor—agonist-independent activation due to conformational flexibility. J Biol Chem 1997; 272:2587–2590.

76. Gether U, Kobilka BK. G protein-coupled receptors - II. Mechanism of agonist activation. J Biol Chem 1998;273:17,979–17,982.

77. Han M, Lin SW, Minkova M, Smith SO, Sakmar TP. Functional interaction of transmembrane helices 3 and 6 in rhodopsin. Replacement of phenylalanine 261 by alanine causes reversion of phenotype of a glycine 121 replacement mutant. J Biol Chem 1996;271:32,337–32,342.

78. Han M, Lin SW, Smith SO, Sakmar TP. The effects of amino acid replacements of glycine 121 on transmembrane helix 3 of rhodopsin. J Biol Chem 1996;271: 32,330–32,336.

79. Noda K, Feng YH, Liu XP, Saad Y, Husain A, Karnik SS. The active state of the AT1 angiotensin receptor is generated by angiotensin II induction. Biochemistry 1996;35:16,435–16,442.

80. Deisenhofer J, Epp O, Miki K, Huber R, Michel H. X-ray structure analysis of a membrane protein complex. Electron density map at 3 Å resolution and a model of the chromophores of the photosynthetic reaction center from Rhodopseudomonas viridis. J Mol Biol 1984;180:385–398.

81. Jager S, Lewis JW, Zvyaga TA, Szundi I, Sakmar TP, Kliger DS. Chromophore structural changes in rhodopsin from nanoseconds to microseconds following pigment photolysis. Proc Natl Acad Sci USA 1997;94:8557–8562.

82. Jager S, Lewis JW, Zvyaga TA, Szundi I, Sakmar TP, Kliger DS. Time-resolved spectroscopy of the early photolysis intermediates of rhodopsin Schiff base counterion mutants. Biochemistry 1997;36:1999–2009.

83. Swaminath G, Xiang Y, Lee TW, Steenhuis J, Parnot C, Kobilka BK. Sequential binding of agonists to the β_2 adrenoceptor: kinetic evidence for intermediate conformational states. J Biol Chem 2004;279:686–691.

84. Subramaniam S, Gerstein M, Oesterhelt D, Henderson R. Electron diffraction analysis of structural changes in the photocycle of bacteriorhodopsin. EMBO J 1993;12:1–8.
85. Lin SW, Sakmar TP. Specific tryptophan UV-absorbance changes are probes of the transition of rhodopsin to its active state. Biochemistry 1996;35:11,149–11,159.
86. Farrens DL, Altenbach C, Yang K, Hubbell WL, Khorana HG. Requirement of rigid-body motion of transmembrane helices for light activation of rhodopsin. Science 1996;274:768–770.
87. Sheikh SP, Zvyaga TA, Lichtarge O, Sakmar TP, Bourne HR. Rhodopsin activation blocked by metal-ion-binding sites linking transmembrane helices C and F. Nature 1996;383:347–350.
88. Kenakin T. Ligand-selective receptor conformations revisited: the promise and the problem. Trends in PharmacolSci 2003;24:346–354.
89. Sakmar TP. Rhodopsin: a prototypical G protein-coupled receptor. Prog Nucleic Acid Res Mol Biol 1998;59:1–34.
90. Beinborn M, Ren Y, Blaker M, Chen C, Kopin AS. Ligand function at constitutively active receptor mutants is affected by two distinct yet interacting mechanisms. Mol Pharmacol 2004;65:753–760.
91. Zhang WB, Navenot JM, Haribabu B, et al. A point mutation that confers constitutive activity to CXCR4 reveals that T140 is an inverse agonist and that AMD3100 and ALX40-4C are weak partial agonists. J Biol Chem 2002;277: 24,515–24,521.
92. Spalding TA, Burstein ES, Henderson SC, Ducote KR, Brann MR. Identification of a ligand-dependent switch within a muscarinic receptor. J Biol Chem 1998;273: 21,563–21,568.
93. Chen S, Lin F, Xu M, Hwa J, Graham RM. Dominant-negative activity of an α_{1B}-adrenergic receptor signal-inactivating point mutation. EMBO J 2000;19:4265–4271.
94. Perez DM, Hwa J, Gaivin R, Mathur M, Brown F, Graham RM. Constitutive activation of a single effector pathway: Evidence for multiple activation states of a G protein-coupled receptor. Mol Pharmacol 1996;49:112–122.
95. Kenakin T, Onaran O. The ligand paradox between affinity and efficacy: can you be there and not make a difference? Trends Pharmacol Sci 2002;23:275–280.
96. Roettger BF, Ghanekar D, Rao R, et al. Antagonist-stimulated internalization of the G protein-coupled cholecystokinin receptor. Mol Pharmacol 1997;51:357–362.
97. Willins DL, Alsayegh L, Berry SA, et al. Serotonergic antagonist effects on trafficking of serotonin 5-HT_{2A} receptors in vitro and in vivo. Ann N Y Acad Sci 1998; 861:121–127.
98. Yu Y, Zhang L, Yin X, Sun H, Uhl GR, Wang JB. Mu opioid receptor phosphorylation, desensitization, and ligand efficacy. J Biol Chem 1997;272:28,869–28,874.
99. Krumins AM, Barber R. The stability of the agonist β_2-adrenergic receptor-G_s complex: evidence for agonist-specific states. Mol Pharmacol 1997;52:144–154.
100. Kenakin T. Agonist-receptor efficacy. II. Agonist trafficking of receptor signals. Trends Pharmacol Sci 1995;16:232–238.

101. Kobilka B, Gether U, Seifert R, Lin SS, Ghanouni P. Examination of ligand-induced conformational changes in the β_2 adrenergic receptor. Life Sci 1998;62: 1509–1512.

102. Gether U, Lin SS, Kobilka BK. Fluorescent labeling of purified β_2 adrenergic-receptor—evidence for ligand-specific conformational-changes. J Biol Chem 1995;270:28,268–28,275.

103. Devanathan S, Yao Z, Salamon Z, Kobilka B, Tollin G. Plasmon-waveguide resonance studies of ligand binding to the human β_2-adrenergic receptor. Biochemistry 2004;43:3280–3288.

104. Ghanouni P, Gryczynski Z, Steenhuis JJ, et al. Functionally different agonists induce distinct conformations in the G protein coupling domain of the β_2 adrenergic receptor. J Biol Chem 2001;276:24,433–24,436.

105. Peleg G, Ghanouni P, Kobilka BK, Zare RN. Single-molecule spectroscopy of the β_2 adrenergic receptor: observation of conformational substates in a membrane protein. Proc Natl Acad Sci USA2001;98:8469–8474.

106. Hannawacker A, Krasel C, Lohse MJ. Mutation of Asn293 to Asp in transmembrane helix VI abolishes agonist-induced but not constitutive activity of the β_2-adrenergic receptor. Mol Pharmacol 2002;62:1431–1437.

107. Chabre O, Conklin BR, Brandon S, Bourne HR, Limbird LE. Coupling of the α_{2A}-adrenergic receptor to multiple G-proteins—a simple approach for estimating receptor-G-protein coupling efficiency in a transient expression system. J Biol Chem 1994;269:5730–5734.

108. Lakhlani PP, Lovinger DM, Limbird LE. Genetic evidence for involvement of multiple effector systems in α_{2A}-adrenergic receptor inhibition of stimulus-secretion coupling. Mol Pharmacol 1996;50:96–103.

109. Surprenant A, Horstman DA, Akbarali H, Limbird LE. A point mutation of the α_2-adrenoceptor that blocks coupling to potassium but not calcium currents. Science 1992;257:977–980.

110. Richardson J, Chatwin H, Hirasawa A, Tsujimoto G, Evans PD. Agonist-specific coupling of a cloned human α_{1A}-adrenoceptor to different second messenger pathways. Naunyn-Schmiedebergs Arch Pharmacol 2003;367:333–341.

111. Finch AM. unpublished observation. In 2004.

112. Nasman J, Kukkonen JP, Ammoun S, Akerman KE. Role of G-protein availability in differential signaling by α_2-adrenoceptors. Biochem Pharmacol 2001;62:913–922.

113. Airriess CN, Rudling JE, Midgley JM, Evans PD. Selective inhibition of adenylyl cyclase by octopamine via a human cloned α_{2A}-adrenoceptor. Br J Pharmacol 1997;122:191–198.

114. Eason MG, Jacinto MT, Liggett SB. Contribution of ligand structure to activation of α_2-adrenergic receptor subtype coupling to G_s. Mol Pharmacol 1994;45: 696–702.

115. Rudling JE, Richardson J, Evans PD. A comparison of agonist-specific coupling of cloned human α_2-adrenoceptor subtypes. Br J Pharmacol 2000;131:933–941.

116. Brink CB, Wade SM, Neubig RR. Agonist-directed trafficking of porcine α_{2A}-adrenergic receptor signaling in Chinese hamster ovary cells: l-isoproterenol selectively activates G_s. J Pharmacol Exp Ther 2000;294:539–547.

117. Pauwels PJ, Rauly I, Wurch T. Dissimilar pharmacological responses by a new series of imidazoline derivatives at precoupled and ligand-activated α_{2A}-adrenoceptor states: Evidence for effector pathway-dependent differential antagonism. J Pharmacol Exp Ther 2003;305:1015–1023.

118. Azzi M, Charest PG, Angers S, et al. β-Arrestin-mediated activation of MAPK by inverse agonists reveals distinct active conformations for G protein-coupled receptors. Proc Natl Acad Sci USA2003;100:11,406–11,411.

119. Ohkita YJ, Sasaki J, Maeda A, et al. Changes in structure of the chromophore in the photochemical process of bovine rhodopsin as revealed by FTIR spectroscopy for hydrogen out-of-plane vibrations. Biophys Chem 1995;56:71–78.

120. Farrens DL, Khorana HG. Structure and function in rhodopsin. Measurement of the rate of metarhodopsin II decay by fluorescence spectroscopy. J Biol Chem 1995;270:5073–5076.

121. Resek JF, Farahbakhsh ZT, Hubbell WL, Khorana HG. Formation of the meta II photointermediate is accompanied by conformational changes in the cytoplasmic surface of rhodopsin. Biochemistry 1993;32:12,025–12,032.

122. Struthers M, Yu H, Oprian DD. G protein-coupled receptor activation: analysis of a highly constrained, "straitjacketed" rhodopsin. Biochemistry 2000;39:7938–7942.

123. Lei S, Liapakis G, Xu R, Guarnieri F, Ballesteros JA, Javitch JA. β_2 adrenergic receptor activation—modulation of the proline kink in transmembrane 6 by a rotamer toggle switch. J Biol Chem 2002;277:40,989–40,996.

124. Gether U, Lin S, Ghanouni P, Ballesteros JA, Weinstein H, Kobilka BK. Agonists induce conformational changes in transmembrane domains III and VI of the β_2 adrenoceptor. EMBO J 1997;16:6737–6747.

125. Hwa J, Graham RM, Perez DM. Chimeras of α_1-adrenergic receptor subtypes identify critical residues that modulate active state isomerization. J Biol Chem 1996;271:7956–7964.

126. Elling CE, Schwartz TW. Connectivity and orientation of the seven helical bundle in the tachykinin NK-1 receptor probed by zinc site engineering. EMBO J 1996;15: 6213–6219.

127. Altenbach C, Cai K, Khorana HG, Hubbell WL. Structural features and light-dependent changes in the sequence 306-322 extending from helix VII to the palmitoylation sites in rhodopsin: a site-directed spin-labeling study. Biochemistry 1999;38:7931–7937.

128. Govaerts C, Lefort A, Costagliola S, et al. A conserved Asn in transmembrane helix 7 is an on/off switch in the activation of the thyrotropin receptor. J Biol Chem 2001;276:22,991–22,999.

129. Jager F, Fahmy K, Sakmar TP, Siebert F. Identification of glutamic acid 113 as the Schiff base proton acceptor in the metarhodopsin II photointermediate of rhodopsin. Biochemistry 1994;33:10,878–10,882.

130. Sakmar TP, Franke RR, Khorana HG. Glutamic acid-113 serves as the retinylidene Schiff base counterion in bovine rhodopsin. Proc Natl Acad Sci USA 1989;86: 8309–8313.

131. Nathans J. Determinants of visual pigment absorbance: identification of the retinylidene Schiff's base counterion in bovine rhodopsin. Biochemistry 1990;29: 9746–9752.

132. Longstaff C, Calhoon RD, Rando RR. Deprotonation of the Schiff base of rhodopsin is obligate in the activation of the G protein. Proc Natl Acad Sci USA 1986;83: 4209–4213.

133. Porter JE, Perez DM. Influence of a lysine 331 counterion on the pK_a of aspartic acid 125: Evidence for a salt-bridge interaction and role in α_{1B}-Adrenergic receptor activation. J Pharmacol Exp Ther2000;292:440–448.

134. Porter JE, Edelmann SE, Waugh DJ, Piascik MT, Perez DM. The agonism and synergistic potentiation of weak partial agonists by triethylamine in α_1-adrenergic receptor activation: Evidence for a salt bridge as the initiating process. Mol Pharmacol 1998;53:766–771.

135. Palczewski K, Kumasaka T, Hori T, et al. Crystal structure of rhodopsin: a G protein-coupled receptor. Science 2000;289:739–745.

136. Rigoutsos I, Riek P, Graham RM, Novotny J. Structural details (kinks and non-α conformations) in transmembrane helices are intrahelically determined and can be predicted by sequence pattern descriptors. Nucleic Acids Res 2003;31: 4625–4631.

137. Sansom MS, Weinstein H. Hinges, swivels and switches: the role of prolines in signalling via transmembrane α-helices. Trends Pharmacol Sci 2000;21:445–451.

138. Matthews BW, Nicholson H, Becktel WJ. Enhanced protein thermostability from site-directed mutations that decrease the entropy of unfolding. Proc Natl Acad Sci USA 1987;84:6663–6667.

139. Burley SK, Petsko GA. Aromatic-aromatic interaction: a mechanism of protein structure stabilization. Science 1985;229:23–28.

140. Vauquelin G, Bottari S, Kanarek L, Strosberg AD. Evidence for essential disulfide bonds in β_1-adrenergic receptors of turkey erythrocyte membranes. Inactivation by dithiothreitol. J Biol Chem 1979;254:4462–4469.

141. Pedersen SE, Ross EM. Functional activation of β-adrenergic receptors by thiols in the presence or absence of agonists. J Biol Chem 1985;260:4150–4157.

142. Lin SS, Gether U, Kobilka BK. Ligand stabilization of the β_2 adrenergic receptor: Effect of DTT on receptor conformation monitored by circular dichroism and fluorescence spectroscopy. Biochemistry 1996;35:14,445–14,451.

143. Strosberg AD. Molecular and functional properties of β-adrenergic receptors. Am J Cardiol 1987;59:3F–9F.

144. Fraser CM. Site-directed mutagenesis of β-adrenergic receptors—identification of conserved cysteine residues that independently affect ligand-binding and receptor activation. J Biol Chem 1989;264:9266–9270.

145. Noda K, Saad Y, Graham RM, Karnik SS. The high-affinity state of the β_2-adrenergic receptor requires unique interaction between conserved and nonconserved extracellular loop cysteines. J Biol Chem 1994;269:6743–6752.

146. Parini A, Homcy CJ, Graham RM. Structural properties of the α_1-adrenergic receptor: studies with membrane and purified receptor preparations. Circ Res 1987;61:I100–104.

147. Karnik SS, Khorana HG. Assembly of functional rhodopsin requires a disulfide bond between cysteine residues 110 and 187. J Biol Chem 1990;265:17,520–17,524.

148. Peterson DA, Gerrard JM. Reduction of a disulfide bond by β-adrenergic agonists: evidence in support of a general "reductive activation" hypothesis for the mechanism of action of adrenergic agents. Med Hypotheses 1987;22:45–49.

149. Wong A, Hwang SM, Cheng HY, Crooke ST. Structure-activity relationships of β-adrenergic receptor-coupled adenylate cyclase: implications of a redox mechanism for the action of agonists at β-adrenergic receptors. Mol Pharmacol 1987;31: 368–376.

150. Peterson DA, Gerrard JM, Glover SM, Rao GH, White JG. Epinephrine reduction of heme: implication for understanding the transmission of an agonist stimulus. Science 1982;215:71–73.

151. Peterson DA, Gerrard JM. Reduction of a metal or disulfide bond associated with the receptor: a general hypothesis for the mechanism of action of adrenergic agents. Med Hypotheses 1987;22:35–44.

152. Peterson DA, Butterfield J, Garrard JM. The dopaminergic D receptor: another example of reductive activation? Med Hypotheses 1988;26:73–75.

153. Korner M, Gilon C, Schramm M. Locking of hormone in the β-adrenergic receptor by attack on a sulfhydryl in an associated component. J Biol Chem 1982;257: 3389–3396.

154. Hwang C, Sinskey AJ, Lodish HF. Oxidized redox state of glutathione in the endoplasmic reticulum. Science 1992;257:1496–1502.

155. Radding CM, Wald G. Acid-base properties of rhodopsin and opsin. J Gen Physiol 1956;39:909–922.

156. Alewijnse AE, Timmerman H, Jacobs EH, et al. The effect of mutations in the DRY motif on the constitutive activity and structural instability of the histamine H_2 receptor. Mol Pharmacol 2000;57:890–898.

157. Ge HF, Scheinin M, Kallio J. Constitutive precoupling to G_i and increased agonist potency in the α_{2B}-adrenoceptor. Biochem Biophysl Res Commun 2003;306: 959–965.

158. Rasmussen SGF, Jensen AD, Liapakis G, Ghanouni P, Javitch JA, Gether U. Mutation of a highly conserved aspartic acid in the β_2 adrenergic receptor: constitutive activation, structural instability, and conformational rearrangement of transmembrane segment 6. Mol Pharmacol 1999;56:175–184.

159. Scheer A, Fanelli F, Costa T, DeBenedetti PG, Cotecchia S. Constitutively active mutants of the α_{1B}-adrenergic receptor: role of highly conserved polar amino acids in receptor activation. EMBO J 1996;15:3566–3578.

160. Ballesteros JA, Jensen AD, Liapakis G, et al. Activation of the β_2-adrenergic receptor involves disruption of an ionic lock between the cytoplasmic ends of transmembrane segments 3 and 6. J Biol Chem 2001;276:29,171–29,177.

161. Ghanouni P, Schambye H, Seifert R, et al. The effect of pH on β_2 adrenoceptor function—evidence for protonation-dependent activation. J Biol Chem 2000;275: 3121–3127.

162. Chung DA, Wade SM, Fowler CB, et al. Mutagenesis and peptide analysis of the DRY motif in the α_{2A} adrenergic receptor: evidence for alternate mechanisms in G protein-coupled receptors. Biochem Biophys Res Commun 2002;293:1233–1241.

163. Scheer A, Fanelli F, Costa T, DeBenedetti PG, Cotecchia S. The activation process of the α_{1B}-adrenergic receptor: potential role of protonation and hydrophobicity of a highly conserved aspartate. Proc Natl Acad Sci USA 1997;94:808–813.

164. Lu ZL, Curtis CA, Jones PG, Pavia J, Hulme EC. The role of the aspartate-arginine-tyrosine triad in the M_1 muscarinic receptor: mutations of aspartate 122 and tyrosine 124 decrease receptor expression but do not abolish signaling. Mol Pharmacol 1997;51:234–241.

165. Burstein ES, Spalding TA, Brann MR. The second intracellular loop of the M_5 muscarinic receptor is the switch which enables G-protein coupling. J Biol Chem 1998;273:24,322–24,327.

166. Ambrosio C, Molinari P, Cotecchia S, Costa T. Catechol-binding serines of β_2-adrenergic receptors control the equilibrium between active and inactive receptor states. Mol Pharmacol 2000;57:198–210.

167. Sprang SR. G protein mechanisms: Insights from structural analysis. Annu Rev Biochem 1997;66:639–678.

168. Bockaert J, Pin JP. Molecular tinkering of G protein-coupled receptors: an evolutionary success. EMBO J 1999;18:1723–1729.

169. Bunemann M, Frank M, Lohse MJ. G_i protein activation in intact cells involves subunit rearrangement rather than dissociation. Proc Natl Acad Sci USA 2003;100: 16,077–16,082.

170. Bourne HR. How receptors talk to trimeric G proteins. Curr OpinCell Biol 1997;9: 134–142.

171. Venter JC, Adams MD, Myers EW, et al. The sequence of the human genome. Science 2001;291:1304–1351. Erratum in Science 2001;292:1838.

172. Wilkie TM, Gilbert DJ, Olsen AS, et al. Evolution of the mammalian G-protein α-subunit multigene family. Nat Genet 1992;1:85–91.

173. Graham RM, Perez DM, Hwa J, Piascik MT. α_1-Adrenergic receptor subtypes. Molecular structure, function, and signaling. Circ Res 1996;78:737–749.

174. Lepretre N, Mironneau J, Arnaudeau S, et al. Activation of α_{-1A} adrenoceptors mobilizes calcium from the intracellular stores in myocytes from rat portal vein. J Pharmacol Exp Ther 1994;268:167–174.

175. Zhong HY, Minneman KP. α_1-Adrenoceptor subtypes. Eur J Pharmacol 1999;375: 261–276.

176. MacrezLepretre N, Kalkbrenner F, Schultz G, Mironneau J. Distinct functions of G_q and G_{11} proteins in coupling α_1-adrenoreceptors to Ca^{2+} release and Ca^{2+} entry in rat portal vein myocytes. J Biol Chem 1997;272:5261–5268.

177. Offermanns S, Simon MI. Genetic analysis of mammalian G-protein signalling. Oncogene 1998;17:1375–1381.

178. Wu DQ, Katz A, Lee CH, Simon MI. Activation of phospholipase-C by α_1-adrenergic receptors is mediated by the α-subunits of G_q family. J Biol Chem 1992; 267:25,798–25,802.

179. Rhee SG. Regulation of phosphoinositide-specific phospholipase C. Annu Rev Biochem 2001;70:281–312.

180. Feng JF, Rhee SG, Im MJ. Evidence that phospholipase delta 1 is the effector in the G_h (transglutaminase II)-mediated signaling. J Biol Chem 1996;271:16,451–16,454.

181. Im MJ, Riek RP, Graham RM. A novel guanine nucleotide-binding protein coupled to the α_1-adrenergic receptor. II. Purification, characterization, and reconstitution. J Biol Chem 1990;265:18,952–18,960.

182. Murthy SNP, Lomasney JW, Mak EC, Lorand L. Interactions of G_h/transglut-aminase with phospholipase C delta 1 and with GTP. Proc Natl Acad Sci USA 1999;96:11,815–11,819.

183. Chen S, Lin F, Iismaa S, Lee KN, Birckbichler PJ, Graham RM. α_1-adrenergic receptor signaling via G_h is subtype specific and independent of its transglut-aminase activity. J Biol Chem 1996;271:32,385–32,391.

184. Feng JF, Gray CD, Im MJ. α_{1B}-adrenoceptor interacts with multiple sites of transglutaminase II: Characteristics of the interaction in binding and activation. Biochemistry 1999;38:2224–2232.

185. Burch RM, Luini A, Mais DE, et al. α_1-Adrenergic stimulation of arachidonic-acid release and metabolism in a rat-thyroid cell-line—mediation of cell replication by prostaglandin-E2. J Biol Chem 1986;261:1236–1241.

186. Kanterman RY, Felder CC, Brenneman DE, Ma AL, Fitzgerald S, Axelrod J. α_1-Adrenergic receptor mediates arachidonic-acid release in spinal-cord neurons independent of inositol phospholipid turnover. J Neurochem 1990;54:1225–1232.

187. Insel PA, Weiss BA, Slivka SR, Howard MJ, Waite JJ, Godson CA. Regulation of phospholipase-A2 by receptors in MDCK-Di cells. Biochem Soc Trans 1991;19:329–333.

188. Nebigil C, Malik KU. Prostaglandin synthesis elicited by adrenergic stimuli is mediated via α_{2c} and α_{1A} adrenergic-receptors in cultured smooth-muscle cells of rabbit aorta. J Pharmacol Exp Ther1992;260:849–858.

189. Marin P, Stella N, Cordier J, Glowinski J, Premont J. Role of arachidonic-acid and glutamate in the formation of inositol phosphates induced by noradrenaline in striatal astrocytes. Mol Pharmacol 1993;44:1176–1184.

190. Perez DM, DeYoung MB, Graham RM. Coupling of expressed α_{1B}- and α_{1D}-adrenergic receptor to multiple signaling pathways is both G protein and cell type specific. Mol Pharmacol 1993;44:784–795.

191. Dennis EA. Diversity of group types, regulation, and function of phospholipase A_2. J Biol Chem 1994;269:13,057–13,060.

192. Dennis EA. Phospholipase-A_2 regulation and signal-transduction. J Cell Biochem 1994;Suppl 18D:67.

193. Mukherjee AB, Miele L, Pattabiraman N. Phospholipase A_2 enzymes - regulation and physiological-role. Biochem Pharmacol 1994;48:1–10.

194. Balsinde J, Balboa MA, Insel PA, Dennis EA. Regulation and inhibition of phospholipase A_2. Annu Rev Pharmacol Toxicol 1999;39:175–189.

195. Xing MB, Insel PA. Protein kinase C-dependent activation of cytosolic phospholipase A_2 and mitogen-activated protein kinase by α_1-adrenergic receptors in Madin-Darby canine kidney cells. J Clin Invest 1996;97:1302–1310.

196. Ruan Y, Kan H, Parmentier JH, Fatima S, Allen LF, Malik KU. α_{1A} adrenergic receptor stimulation with phenylephrine promotes arachidonic acid release by activation of phospholipase D in rat-1 fibroblasts: inhibition by protein kinase A. J Pharmacol Exp Ther1998;284:576–585.

197. Burch RM, Luini A, Axelrod J. Phospholipase-A_2 and phospholipase-C are activated by distinct GTP-binding proteins in response to α_1-adrenergic stimulation in Frtl5 thyroid-cells. Proc Natl Acad Sci USA 1986;83:7201–7205.

198. Cockcroft S. G-protein-regulated phospholipase-C, phospholipase-D and phospholipase-A_2-mediated signaling in neutrophils. Biochimica Et Biophysica Acta 1992;1113:135–160.
199. Cockcroft S, Nielson CP, Stutchfield J. Is phospholipase-A_2 activation regulated by G-proteins. Biochem Soc Trans 1991;19:333–336.
200. Perez DM, Deyoung MB, Graham RM. Coupling of expressed α_{1B}-adrenergic and α_{1D}-adrenergic receptors to multiple signaling pathways is both G-protein and cell-type-specific. Mol Pharmacol 1993;44:784–795.
201. Jelsema CL, Axelrod J. Stimulation of phospholipase-A_2 activity in bovine rod outer segments by the $\beta\gamma$-subunits of transducin and its inhibition by the α-subunit. Proc Natl Acad Sci USA 1987;84:3623–3627.
202. McPhail LC, Clayton CC, Snyderman R. A Potential 2nd messenger role for unsaturated fatty-acids—activation of Ca^{2+}-dependent protein-kinase. Science 1984; 224:622-625.
203. Sekiguchi K, Tsukuda M, Ogita K, Kikkawa U, Nishizuka Y. 3 Distinct Forms of rat-brain protein-kinase-C—differential response to unsaturated fatty-acids. Biochem Biophysl Res Commun 1987;145:797–802.
204. Hwang SC, Jhon DY, Bae YS, Kim JH, Rhee SG. Activation of phospholipase Cγ by the concerted action of tau proteins and arachidonic acid. J Biol Chem 1996;271: 18,342–18,349.
205. Vanderzee L, Nelemans A, Denhertog A. Arachidonic-Acid Is functioning as a 2nd-messenger in activating the Ca^{2+} entry process on H_1-histaminoceptor stimulation in Ddt1 Mf-2 cells. Biochem J 1995;305:859–864.
206. Ordway RW, Walsh JV, Singer JJ. Arachidonic-acid and other fatty-acids directly activate potassium channels in smooth-muscle cells. Science 1989;244:1176–1179.
207. Gong MC, Kinter MT, Somlyo AV, Somlyo AP. Arachidonic-acid and diacylglycerol release associated with inhibition of myosin light-chain dephosphorylation in rabbit smooth-muscle. J Physiol (Lond) 1995;486:113–122.
208. Leslie CC. Properties and regulation of cytosolic phospholipase A_2. J Biol Chem 1997;272:16,709–16,712.
209. Exton JH. New developments in phospholipase D. J Biol Chem 1997;272:15,579–15,582.
210. Llahi S, Fain JN. α_1-Adrenergic receptor-mediated activation of phospholipase-D in rat cerebral-cortex. J Biol Chem 1992;267:3679–3685.
211. Gu H, Trajkovic S, Labelle EF. Norepinephrine-induced phosphatidylcholine hydrolysis by phospholipase-D and phospholipase-C in rat tail artery. Am J Physiol 1992;262:C1376–C1383.
212. LaBelle EF, Fulbright RM, Barsotti RJ, Gu H, Polyak E. Phospholipase D is activated by G protein and not by calcium ions in vascular smooth muscle. Am J Physiol Heart Circ Physiol 1996;39:H1031–H1037.
213. Guillemain I, Rossignol B. Receptor-mediated and phorbol ester-mediated phospholipase-D activation in rat parotid involves 2 different pathways. Am J Physiol 1994;266:C692–C699.
214. Ye HP, Wolf RA, Kurz T, Corr PB. Phosphatidic-acid increases in response to noradrenaline and endothelin-1 in adult-rabbit ventricular myocytes. Cardiovasc Res 1994;28:1828–1834.

215. Balboa MA, Insel PA. Stimulation of phospholipase D via α_1-adrenergic receptors in Madin-Darby canine kidney cells is independent of PKC α and -epsilon activation. Mol Pharmacol 1998;53:221–227.

216. Gurdal H, Seasholtz TM, Wang HY, Brown RD, Johnson MD, Friedman E. Role of $G_{\alpha q}$ or $G_{\alpha o}$ proteins in α_1-adrenoceptor subtype mediated responses in Fischer 344 rat aorta. Mol Pharmacol 1997;52:1064–1070.

217. Butta N, Urcelay E, Gonzalezmanchon C, Parrilla R, Ayuso MS. Pertussis toxin inhibition of α_1-adrenergic or vasopressin-induced Ca^{2+} fluxes in rat-liver—selective-inhibition of the α_1-adrenergic receptor-coupled metabolic-acttvation. J Biol Chem 1993;268:6081–6089.

218. Blitzer RD, Omri G, Devivo M, et al. Coupling of the expressed α_{1B}-adrenergic receptor to the phospholipase-C pathway in Xenopus oocytes—the role of G_O. J Biol Chem 1993;268:7532–7537.

219. Horie K, Itoh H, Tsujimoto G. Hamster α_{1B}-adrenergic receptor directly activates G_S in the transfected Chinese-hamster ovary cells. Mol Pharmacol 1995;48: 392–400.

220. Gutkind JS. The pathways connecting G protein-coupled receptors to the nucleus through divergent mitogen-activated protein kinase cascades. J Biol Chem 1998; 273:1839–1842.

221. Lamorte VJ, Thorburn J, Absher D, et al. G_q-Dependent and Ras-dependent pathways mediate hypertrophy of neonatal rat ventricular myocytes following α_1-adrenergic stimulation. J Biol Chem 1994;269:13,490–13,496.

222. Wess J. Molecular basis of receptor/G-protein-coupling selectivity. Pharmacol Ther 1998;80:231–264.

223. Cotecchia S, Exum S, Caron MG, Lefkowitz RJ. Regions of the α_1-adrenergic receptor involved in coupling to phosphatidylinositol hydrolysis and enhanced sensitivity of biological function. Proc Natl Acad Sci USA 1990;87:2896–2900.

224. Luttrell LM, Ostrowski J, Cotecchia S, Kendall H, Lefkowitz RJ. Antagonism of catecholamine receptor signaling by expression of cytoplasmic domains of the receptors. Science 1993;259:1453–1457.

225. Wu DQ, Jiang HP, Simon MI. Different α_1-adrenergic receptor sequences required for activating different G_α subunits of G_q class of G-proteins. J Biol Chem 1995;270: 9828–9832.

226. Eason MG, Kurose H, Holt BD, Raymond JR, Liggett SB. Simultaneous coupling of α_2-adrenergic receptors to two G-proteins with opposing effects—subtype-selective coupling of α_{2c10}, α_{2c4}, and α_{-2c2} adrenergic-receptors to G_i and G_s. J Biol Chem 1992;267:15,795–15,801.

227. Limbird LE. Receptors linked to inhibition of adenylate-cyclase—additional signaling mechanisms. FASEB J 1988;2:2686–2695.

228. Eason MG, Liggett SB. Chimeric mutagenesis of putative G-protein coupling domains of the α_{2A}-adrenergic receptor - Localization of two redundant and fully competent G_i coupling domains. J Biol Chem 1996;271:12,826–12,832.

229. Wade SM, Lim WK, Lan KL, Chung DA, Nanamori M, Neubig RR. G_i activator region of α_{2A}-adrenergic receptors: distinct basic residues mediate G_i versus G_s activation. Mol Pharmacol 1999;56:1005–1013.

230. Aghajanian GK, Vandermaelen CP. α_2-Adrenoceptor-mediated hyperpolarization of locus coeruleus neurons—intracellular studies in vivo. Science 1982;215: 1394–1396.

231. Isom LL, Cragoe EJ, Limbird LE. α_2-Adrenergic receptors accelerate Na^+/H^+ exchange in neuroblastoma-X glioma-cells. J Biol Chem 1987;262:6750–6757.

232. Michel MC, Brass LF, Williams A, Bokoch GM, Lamorte VJ, Motulsky HJ. α_2-Adrenergic receptor stimulation mobilizes intracellular Ca^{2+} in human erythroleukemia-cells. J Biol Chem 1989;264:4986–4991.

233. Simonds WF, Goldsmith PK, Codina J, Unson CG, Spiegel AM. G_{i2} Mediates α_2-adrenergic inhibition of adenylyl cyclase in platelet membranes—*in situ* identification with G_α C-terminal antibodies. Proc Natl Acad Sci USA 1989;86: 7809–7813.

234. Gerhardt MA, Neubig RR. Multiple G_i protein subtypes regulate a single effector mechanism. Mol Pharmacol 1991;40:707–711.

235. Gerhardt MA, Neubig RR. α_{2A}-Adrenergic receptors (α_2-AR) efficiently inhibit adenylate-cyclase in transfected CHO-K1 cells. FASEB J 1991;5:A1594–A1594.

236. McClue SJ, Selzer E, Freissmuth M, Milligan G. G_{i3} Does Not Contribute to the Inhibition of adenylate-cyclase when stimulation of an α_2-adrenergic receptor causes activation of both G_{i2} and G_{i3}. Biochem J 1992;284:565–568.

237. Remaury A, Larrouy D, Daviaud D, Rouot B, Paris H. Coupling of the α_2-adrenergic receptor to the inhibitory G-protein G_i and adenylate-cyclase in HT29 cells. Biochem J 1993;292:283–288.

238. Duzic E, Lanier SM. Factors determining the specificity of signal transduction by guanine nucleotide-binding protein-coupled receptors. 3. Coupling of α_2-adrenergic receptor subtypes in a cell type-specific manner. J Biol Chem 1992;267:24,045–24,052.

239. Duzic E, Coupry I, Downing S, Lanier SM. Factors determining the specificity of signal transduction by guanine nucleotide-binding protein-coupled receptors. 1. Coupling of α_2-adrenergic receptor subtypes to distinct G-proteins. J Biol Chem 1992;267:9844–9851.

240. Kurose H, Regan JW, Caron MG, Lefkowitz RJ. Functional interactions of recombinant-α_2 adrenergic-receptor subtypes and G-proteins in reconstituted phospholipid-vesicles. Biochemistry 1991;30:3335–3341.

241. Cotecchia S, Kobilka BK, Daniel KW, et al. Multiple 2nd messenger pathways of α-adrenergic receptor subtypes expressed in eukaryotic cells. J Biol Chem 1990; 265:63–69.

242. Zhao XL, Gutierrez LM, Chang CF, Hosey MM. The α_1-subunit of skeletal-muscle L-type Ca channels is the key target for regulation by α-kinase and protein phosphatase-1c. Biochem Biophysl Res Commun 1994;198:166–173.

243. Gerhardstein BL, Puri TS, Chien AJ, Hosey MM. Identification of the sites phosphorylated by cyclic AMP-dependent protein kinase on the β_2 subunit of L-type voltage-dependent calcium channels. Biochemistry 1999;38:10,361–10,370.

244. Simmerman HKB, Jones LR. Phospholamban: protein structure, mechanism of action, and role in cardiac function. Physiol Rev 1998;78:921–947.

245. Sulakhe PV, Vo XT. Regulation of phospholamban and troponin-I phosphorylation in the intact rat cardiomyocytes by adrenergic and cholinergic roles of cyclic-

nucleotides, calcium, protein-kinases and phosphatases and depolarization. Mol Cell Biochem 1995;149:103–126.

246. Marx SO, Reiken S, Hisamatsu Y, et al. PKA phosphorylation dissociates FKBP 12.6 from the calcium release channel (ryanodine receptor): defective regulation in failing hearts. Cell 2000;101:365–376.

247. Kunst G, Kress KR, Gruen M, Uttenweiler D, Gautel M, Fink RHA. Myosin binding protein C, a phosphorylation-dependent force regulator in muscle that controls the attachment of myosin heads by its interaction with myosin S2. Circ Res 2000;86:51–58.

248. Zhang ZY, Zhou B, Xie LP. Modulation of protein kinase signaling by protein phosphatases and inhibitors. Pharmacol Ther 2002;93:307–317.

249. Bristow MR, Hershberger RE, Port JD, Minobe W, Rasmussen R. β_1-Adrenergic and β_2-adrenergic receptor-mediated adenylate-cyclase stimulation in non-failing and failing human ventricular myocardium. Mol Pharmacol 1989;35:295–303.

250. Ostrom RS, Gregorian C, Drenan RM, Xiang Y, Regan JW, Insel PA. Receptor number and caveolar co-localization determine receptor coupling efficiency to adenylyl cyclase. J Biol Chem 2001;276:42,063–42,069.

251. Green SA, Holt BD, Liggett SB. β_1-Adrenergic and β_2-adrenergic receptors display subtype-selective coupling to G_s. Mol Pharmacol 1992;41:889–893.

252. Levy FO, Zhu X, Kaumann AJ, Birnbaumer L. Efficacy of β_1-adrenergic receptors is lower than that of β_2-adrenergic receptors. Proc Natl Acad Sci USA 1993;90: 10,798–10,802.

253. Communal C, Singh K, Sawyer DB, Colucci WS. Opposing effects of β_1- and β_2-adrenergic receptors on cardiac myocyte apoptosis—role of a pertussis toxin-sensitive G proteins. Circulation 1999;100:2210–2212.

254. Daaka Y, Luttrell LM, Lefkowitz RJ. Switching of the coupling of the β_2-adrenergic receptor to different G proteins by protein kinase A. Nature 1997;390:88–91.

255. Kompa AR, Gu XH, Evans BA, Summers RJ. Desensitization of cardiac β-adrenoceptor signaling with heart failure produced by myocardial infarction in the rat. Evidence for the role of G_i but not G_s or phosphorylating proteins. J Mol Cell Cardiol 1999;31:1185–1201.

256. Xiao RP, Cheng HP, Zhou YY, Kuschel M, Lakatta EG. Recent advances in cardiac β_2-adrenergic signal transduction. Cir Res 1999;85:1092–1100.

257. Zhu WZ, Zheng M, Koch WJ, Lefkowitz RJ, Kobilka BK, Xiao RP. Dual modulation of cell survival and cell death by β_2-adrenergic signaling in adult mouse cardiac myocytes. Proc Natl Acad Sci USA2001;98:1607–1612.

258. Maudsley S, Pierce KL, Zamah AM, et al. The β_2-adrenergic receptor mediates extracellular signal-regulated kinase activation via assembly of a multi-receptor complex with the epidermal growth factor receptor. J Biol Chem 2000;275:9572–9580.

259. Lawler OA, Miggin SM, Kinsella BT. Protein kinase A-mediated phosphorylation of serine 357 of the mouse prostacyclin receptor regulates its coupling to G_s, to G_i, and to G_q-coupled effector signaling. J Biol Chem 2001;276:33,596–33,607.

260. Luttrell LM, Daaka Y, Lefkowitz RJ. Regulation of tyrosine kinase cascades by G-protein-coupled receptors. Curr Opin Cell Biol 1999;11:177–183.

261. Zou YZ, Komuro I, Yamazaki T, et al. Both G_s and G_i proteins are critically involved in isoproterenol-induced cardiomyocyte hypertrophy. J Biol Chem 1999; 274:9760–9770.

262. Zamah AM, Delahunty M, Luttrell LM, Lefkowitz RJ. Protein kinase A-mediated phosphorylation of the β_2-adrenergic receptor regulates its coupling to G_s and G_i - Demonstration in a reconstituted system. J Biol Chem 2002;277: 31,249–31,256.

263. Davare MA, Avdonin V, Hall DD, et al. A β_2 adrenergic receptor signaling complex assembled with the Ca^{2+} channel Ca(v)1.2. Science 2001;293:98–101.

264. Davare MA. *Correction*: A β_2 adrenergic receptor signaling complex assembled with the Ca^{2+} channel Ca(v)1.2 (2001;293:98). Science 2001;293:804–804.

265. Rybin VO, Xu XH, Lisanti MP, Steinberg SF. Differential targeting of β-adrenergic receptor subtypes and adenylyl cyclase to cardiomyocyte caveolae: a mechanism to functionally regulate the cAMP signaling pathway. J Biol Chem 2000;275: 41,447–41,457.

266. Baillie GS, Sood A, McPhee I, et al. β-Arrestin-mediated PDE4 cAMP phosphodiesterase recruitment regulates β-adrenoceptor switching from G_s to G_i. Proc Natl Acad Sci USA 2003;100:940–945.

267. Hu LYA, Chen W, Martin NP, Whalen EJ, Premont RT, Lefkowitz RJ. GIPC interacts with the β_1-adrenergic receptor and regulates β_1-adrenergic receptor-mediated ERK activation. J Biol Chem 2003;278:26,295–26,301.

268. Hall RA, Premont RT, Chow CW, et al. The β_2-adrenergic receptor interacts with the Na^+/H^+-exchanger regulatory factor to control Na^+/H^+ exchange. Nature 1998; 392:626–630.

269. Xu JG, Paquet M, Lau AG, Wood JD, Ross CA, Hall RA. β_1-Adrenergic receptor association with the synaptic scaffolding protein membrane-associated guanylate kinase inverted-2 (MAGI-2) - Differential regulation of receptor internalization by MAGI-2 and PSD-95. J Biol Chem 2001;276:41,310–41,317.

270. Hu LA, Chen W, Premont RT, Cong M, Lefkowitz RJ. G protein-coupled receptor kinase 5 regulates β_1-adrenergic receptor association with PSD-95. J Biol Chem 2002;277:1607–1613.

271. Krief S, Lonnqvist F, Raimbault S, et al. Tissue distribution of β_3-adrenergic receptor messenger-RNA in man. J Clin Invest 1993;91:344–349.

272. Cheng HJ, Zhang ZS, Onishi K, Ukai T, Sane DC, Cheng CP. Upregulation of functional β_3-adrenergic receptor in the failing canine myocardium. Cir Res 2001; 89:599–606.

273. Gauthier C, Langin D, Balligand JL. β_3-Adrenoceptors in the cardiovascular system. Trends Pharmacol Sci 2000;21:426–431.

274. Kitamura T, Onishi K, Dohi K, Okinaka T, Isaka N, Nakano T. The negative inotropic effect of β_3-adrenoceptor stimulation in the beating guinea pig heart. J Cardiovasc Pharmacol 2000;35:786–790.

275. Gauthier C, Tavernier G, Charpentier F, Langin D, LeMarec H. Functional β_3-adrenoceptor in the human heart. J Clin Invest 1996;98:556–562.

276. Gauthier C, Leblais V, Kobzik L, et al. The negative inotropic effect of β_3-adrenoceptor stimulation is mediated by activation of a nitric oxide synthase pathway in human ventricle. J Clin Invest 1998;102:1377–1384.

277. Heubach JF, Graf EM, Molenaar P, et al. Murine ventricular L-type Ca^{2+} current is enhanced by zinterol via β_1-adrenoceptors, and is reduced in TG4 mice overexpressing the human β_2-adrenoceptor. Br J Pharmacol 2001;133:73–82.

278. Tavernier G, Galitzky J, Bousquetmelou A, Montastruc JL, Berlan M. The positive chronotropic effect induced by BRL-37344 and CGP-12177, 2 β_3 adrenergic agonists, does not involve cardiac β-adrenoceptors but baroreflex mechanisms. J Pharmacol Exp Ther1992;263:1083–1090.

279. Devic E, Xiang Y, Gould D, Kobilka B. β-adrenergic receptor subtype-specific signaling in cardiac myocytes from β_1 and β_2 adrenoceptor knockout mice. Mol Pharmacol 2001;60:577–583.

280. Kohout TA, Lin FT, Perry SJ, Conner DA, Lefkowitz RJ. β-arrestin 1 and 2 differentially regulate heptahelical receptor signaling and trafficking. Proc Natl Acad Sci USA2001;98:1601–1606.

281. Konkar AA, Zhai Y, Granneman JG. β_1-adrenergic receptors mediate β_3-adrenergic-independent effects of CGP 12177 in brown adipose tissue. Mol Pharmacol 2000;57:252–258.

282. Lefkowitz RJ. G protein-coupled receptors III. New roles for receptor kinases and β-arrestins in receptor signaling and desensitization. J Biol Chem 1998;273: 18,677–18,680.

283. Pitcher JA, Freedman NJ, Lefkowitz RJ. G protein-coupled receptor kinases. Annu Rev Biochem 1998;67:653-692.

284. Lohse MJ, Engelhardt S, Eschenhagen T. What is the role of β-adrenergic signaling in heart failure? Cir Res 2003;93:896–906.

285. Ballesteros JA, Weinstein H. Integrated Methods for the construction of three dimensional models and computational probing of structure-function relations in G-protein coupled receptors. Methods in Neurosciences. Academic Press, Sand Diego, CA, 1995, pp. 366–428.

286. Neubig RR, Spedding M, Kenakin T, Christopoulos A. International Union of Pharmacology Committee on Receptor Nomenclature and Drug Classification. XXXVIII. Update on terms and symbols in quantitative pharmacology. Pharmacol Rev 2003;55:597–606.

287. Hehr A, Hieble JP, Li YO, et al. Ser(165) of transmembrane helix IV is not involved in the interaction of catecholamines with the α_{2A}-adrenoceptor. Pharmacology 1997;55:18–24.

288. Dohlman HG, Caron MG, Strader CD, Amlaiky N, Lefkowitz RJ. Identification and sequence of a binding site peptide of the β_2-adrenergic receptor. Biochemistry 1988;27:1813–1817.

289. Hamaguchi N, True TA, Saussy DL, Jeffs PW. Phenylalanine in the second membrane-spanning domain of α_{1A}-adrenergic receptor determines subtype selectivity of dihydropyridine antagonists. Biochemistry 1996;35:14,312–14317.

290. Zhao M, Hwa J, Perez DM. Identification of critical extracellular loop residues involved in α_1-adrenergic receptor subtype selective antagonist binding. FASEB J 1996;10:2411–2411.

291. Stadel JM, De Lean A, Lefkowitz RJ. Molecular mechanisms of coupling in hormone receptor-adenylate cyclase systems. Adv Enzymol Relat Areas Mol Biol 1982;53:1–43.

292. Frang H, Cockcroft V, Karskela T, Scheinin M, Marjamaki A. Phenoxybenzamine binding reveals the helical orientation of the third transmembrane domain of adrenergic receptors. J Biol Chem 2001;276:31,279–31,284.

293. Carrieri A, Centeno NB, Rodrigo J, Sanz F, Carotti A. Theoretical evidence of a salt bridge disruption as the initiating process for the α_{1D}-adrenergic receptor activation: a molecular dynamics and docking study. Proteins 2001;43:382–394.

294. Hamaguchi N, True TA, Goetz AS, Stouffer MJ, Lybrand TP, Jeffs PW. α_1-Adrenergic receptor subtype determinants for 4-piperidyl oxazole antagonists. Biochemistry 1998;37:5730–5737.

295. Marjamaki A, Pihlavisto M, Cockcroft V, Heinonen P, Savola JM, Scheinin M. Chloroethylclonidine binds irreversibly to exposed cysteines in the fifth membrane-spanning domain of the human α_{2A}-adrenergic receptor. Mol Pharmacol 1998;53:370–376.

296. Cockcroft V, Frang H, Pihlavisto M, Marjamaki A, Scheinin M. Ligand recognition of serine-cysteine amino acid exchanges in transmembrane domain 5 of α_2-adrenergic receptors by UK 14,304. J Neurochem 2000;74:1705–1710.

297. Sato T, Kobayashi H, Nagao T, Kurose H. Ser(203) as well as Ser(204) and Ser(207) in fifth transmembrane domain of the human β_2-adrenoceptor contributes to agonist binding and receptor activation. Br J Pharmacol 1999;128: 272–274.

298. Wong SKF, Slaughter C, Ruoho AE, Ross EM. The catecholamine binding-site of the β-adrenergic-receptor is formed by juxtaposed membrane-spanning domains. J Biol Chem 1988;263:7925–7928.

299. Christopoulos A, Kenakin T. G protein-coupled receptor allosterism and complexing. Pharmacol Rev 2002;54:323–374.

300. Lefkowitz RJ, Pierce KL, Luttrell LM. Dancing with different partners: protein kinase A phosphorylation of seven membrane-spanning receptors regulates their G protein-coupling specificity. Mol Pharmacol 2002;62:971–974.

3

New Signal Transduction Paradigms

Kenneth P. Minneman

Summary

All adrenergic receptors (ARs) are members of the G protein-coupled receptor superfamily and have been assumed to initiate signals primarily by activation of heterotrimeric G proteins. The three major AR families (α_1, α_2, β) each contain three subtypes, with all receptors within a subfamily acting through the same G proteins to initiate the same signals. α_1-ARs activate $G_{q/11}$ to increase Ca^{2+}, α_2-ARs activate $G_{i/o}$ to decrease cyclic adenosine 5'-monophosphate, and β-ARs activate G_s to increase cyclic adenosine 5'-monophosphate. This raises questions regarding how apparently redundant receptor subtypes have survived evolutionarily and continue to mediate distinct functions in all known higher organisms. Although the primary importance of G proteins in signaling is not in doubt, it is increasingly clear that understanding AR signaling requires additional complexity. ARs have now been shown also to interact directly with other proteins, which may be important in signaling. One class includes other G protein-coupled receptors, and increasing reports of receptor heterodimerization are transforming our view of these receptors as solitary cellular sentinels for detecting incoming signals. Another class is adaptor or scaffolding proteins responsible for local organization of specific signaling complexes, for which proximity of effector molecules may result in increased or unexpected responses. Other proteins, such as regulators of G protein signaling, may affect the specificity or extent of G protein activation. Finally, internalization of receptors may be required for certain responses, which may be independent of G protein signaling. Thus, the traditional view of a linear signaling cascade of ligand/receptor/G protein/second messenger activation is turning into a much more complex, combinatorial, and context-dependent view of AR signaling.

From: *The Receptors: The Adrenergic Receptors: In the 21st Century*
Edited by: D. Perez © Humana Press Inc., Totowa, NJ

Key Words: Dimerization; internalization; mitogen-activated protein kinase; PDZ domains; phosphorylation; RGS proteins; scaffolding; tyrosine kinase.

1. Introduction

All adrenergic receptors (ARs) are members of the large G protein-coupled receptor (GPCR) superfamily, which comprises one of the largest family of proteins encoded by the human genome, with several hundred distinct genes *(1)*. These receptors share a common structure, predicted to have seven transmembrane-spanning helices, an extracellular N-terminus, an intracellular C-terminus, and extracellular and intracellular loops of varying lengths *(2)*. It has long been assumed that ligand-induced activation of these receptors initiates signals by interaction of their intracellular domains with heterotrimeric G proteins, stimulating these G proteins to dissociate into α- and $\beta\gamma$-subunits *(3)*. These G protein subunits then act on effector molecules, particularly enzymes and channels, to increase or decrease their activity. This increases the concentration of second messenger molecules such as cyclic adenosine 5′-monophosphate (cAMP), diacylglycerol, inositol 1,4,5-trisphosphate, or calcium or changes in membrane voltage or capacitance *(4)*. These ultimately result in alterations in protein phosphorylation, activation or inhibition of particular enzymes, and eventually specific cellular responses to receptor activation. Until recently, this relatively linear cascade of ligand activation of receptor, receptor activation of G protein, G protein activation of effector, and effector-induced changes in cellular physiology has been the standard paradigm for understanding signaling by this important receptor superfamily.

Increasingly, however, this relatively straightforward signaling cascade has been challenged by new observations suggesting much more complex and context-dependent signaling mechanisms for many GPCRs *(1,4)*. It is now increasingly clear that many GPCRs form heterodimers, which have a great impact on their trafficking, pharmacology, signaling, and internalization. In addition, a variety of adaptor or scaffolding proteins have now been found to interact directly with GPCRs and may serve as effector molecules themselves, independent of G protein activation. Regulators of G protein signaling proteins have been found to associate directly with GPCRs to regulate their interactions with G proteins *(5)*, and some responses have been found to require agonist-induced translocation of the receptor in the absence of G protein activation. Thus, the relatively small intracellular surface of GPCRs appears to have become a hotbed of interacting proteins, some affecting G protein signaling and some of which may initiate independent signals. These new findings have stimulated tremendous interest in the possibility of alternative signaling pathways for GPCRs.

ARs have served as prototypes for GPCRs for decades *(6)*. ARs were among the first to be recognized as having molecularly and pharmacologically distinct subtypes; to have their signaling pathways elucidated; to be specifically labeled with radioligand-binding assays; and to be purified, sequenced, and cloned *(4)*. With such a distinguished history, it is not surprising that they have also been prototypes for our increased understanding of alternative signaling pathways used by GPCRs. In this chapter, I provide an overview of some of this new information and how it has an impact on our understanding of the biological function of these important signaling molecules.

2. Signals Activated by AR Subtypes

In most cases, it has been found that each member of an AR subfamily couples faithfully to a single G protein type. The α_1-ARs (α_{1A}, α_{1B}, α_{1D}) act through $G_{q/11}$ to increase intracellular Ca^{2+}, α_2-ARs (α_{2A}, α_{2B}, α_{2C}) act through G_i to decrease cAMP, and β-ARs (β_1, β_2, β_3) act through G_s to increase cAMP. The dual G protein specificity observed with other GPCRs, such as angiotensin II receptors (which activate both $G_{q/11}$ and G_i families) *(7)*, has not generally been observed with AR subtypes.

2.1. Multiple Effects Caused by Multiple Subtypes

The multiplicity of AR subtypes suggests that they may activate many different, redundant, or potentially conflicting signaling pathways, resulting in a multitude of different functional responses. This is in fact the case because AR activation causes effects ranging from contraction or relaxation of vascular smooth muscle; contraction of cardiac muscle; decreased motility of intestinal smooth muscle; release of energy stores from liver, fat, and skeletal muscle; and many others. Many of these different effects are simply caused by the presence or absence of particular AR subtypes in a particular tissue and are thus to be expected. For example, bronchial smooth muscle contains primarily β_2-ARs, which cause relaxation; most vascular smooth muscles contain primarily α_1-ARs, which cause contraction.

2.2. Unexpected Responses to Individual Subtypes

On the other hand, there are cases for which well-defined AR subtypes have been found to activate signaling pathways that would not normally be expected to be activated by that receptor. For example, although mitogen-activated protein kinase (MAPK) pathways were primarily thought to be activated by growth factor receptors with intrinisic tyrosine kinase activity *(8)*, it quickly became clear that many GPCRs could also activate these pathways *(9)*. Subsequently, it has been found that α_1- *(10)*, α_2- *(11)*, and β- *(12)* ARs all activate MAPKs in a variety of systems despite their specificity in coupling to different G proteins (α_1/$G_{q/11}$, α_2/G_i, β/G_S), some of which stimulate opposing signals (G_i, G_S). Part of this may be explained by independent effects of common $\beta\gamma$-subunits (11), but this does not entirely explain the results because not all ARs activate MAPK in a single cell type (13), although they all undoubtedly release $\beta\gamma$-subunits when activated. In addition, all three AR subfamilies have been reported to activate tyrosine kinase pathways (14,15), again possibly involving release of $\beta\gamma$-subunits.

The α_1-ARs have also been reported to activate the Jak/Stat signaling pathway normally associated with cytokine receptors (16), similar to that observed with angiotensin II receptors, which have been much more extensively studied (17). Also, α_1-ARs increase inositol phosphate formation in primary brain cell cultures through a pertussis toxin-sensitive G protein (18), despite the fact that none of the $G_{q/11}$ proteins are inactivated by pertussis toxin. Finally, a large array of transcriptional reporters were activated by stimulation of α_1-ARs expressed in various cells (19,20) that were often insensitive to drugs thought to block downstream second messenger responses. Similar unexpected responses have been observed with β-ARs, for which coupling of β_3-ARs to both G_S and G_i has been suggested (21). Similarly, coupling of the β_2-AR to G_i proteins appears to be important under some circumstances (22), and it has been suggested that activation of cAMP-dependent protein kinase switches the signaling specificity of this receptor from G_S to G_i (23). Thus, it is clear that specific signaling pathways for ARs are still not completely understood.

3. Identification of Novel Protein-Binding Partners

ARs have been known for many years to interact directly with heterotrimeric G proteins, as well as with a variety of kinases and phosphatases that result in reversible phosphorylation of the receptors on specific serine, threonine, or tyrosine residues. However, until recently only slight attention was paid to the possibility that ARs might form oligomeric signaling complexes with other proteins, which might be critical for their function. Many reports now suggest that multiple proteins interact directly with particular AR families. To date, most of the specific protein–protein interactions have been identified for β-ARs, although some have also been reported for α_1- and α_2-AR subtypes. The specific functions of each of the protein–protein interactions that have been identified are in many cases still poorly understood. However, a few models have been proposed that may illustrate their potential importance in alternative signaling pathways.

3.1. β-AR Interacting Proteins

The β-ARs are the most widely studied of the AR subtypes, with the widely expressed β_2-AR subtype among the most heavily examined GPCR to date (4).

Thus, it is perhaps not surprising that the most interacting proteins have been identified for this subfamily.

3.1.1. β-Arrestins

The first protein other than G proteins or enzymes that was found to bind directly to β_2-ARs was an analog of arrestin, a protein involved in enhancing the inactivating effect of rhodopsin phosphorylation by rhodopsin kinase *(24)*. Purification and cloning of this protein showed that it had a high degree of similarity to retinal arrestin but was specific for β_2-ARs compared to rhodopsin *(25)*; it was therefore named β-arrestin. It is now clear that β-arrestin binds directly to β_2-ARs following phosphorylation by a specific GPCR kinase (GRK2 or β-ARK) and has a central coordinating role in processes involved in receptor internalization *(4)*. There are two β-arrestin isoforms (1 and 2) outside the visual system, which are widely expressed and have been reported to differentially regulate phosphorylation and internalization of a variety of GPCRs *(4)*. Although attention was first focused primarily on the role of β-arrestins in regulating receptor phosphorylation *(24)*, it has recently become clear that this protein plays several critical roles in receptor signaling and desensitization, including acting as a scaffolding protein for local assembly of particular signaling molecules *(4)*. This is discussed more extensively in Section 5.

3.1.2. Na^+/H^+ Exchange Regulatory Factor

The Na^+/H^+ exchange regulatory factor/ezrin-radixin-moesin-binding phosphoprotein-50 (NHERF/EBP50) originally was identified as a cofactor required for cAMP-dependent protein kinase-mediated inhibition of the Na^+/H^+ exchanger (NHE3 isoform) in renal and gastrointestinal epithelial cells. NHERF contains two N-terminal PDZ domains and an ezrin-radixin-moesin (ERM)-binding domain at its C-terminus, allowing it to interact with multiple proteins. In 1998, Hall and coworkers *(26)* identified NHERF as a protein that binds specifically to the C-terminal tail of β_2-ARs in an agonist-dependent manner. NHERF binds to the β_2-AR by means of an interaction between the first PDZ domain of NHERF and the last four amino acid residues of the receptor C-terminus *(27)*. PDZ domains were first recognized as conserved elements in the PSD–95 (postsynaptic density), Dgl (Discs–large), and ZO (zonula occludans) proteins. Mutation of the final C-terminal amino acid abolished the ability of the β_2-AR to bind to NHERF, as well as β_2-AR regulation of NHE3 in cells, however without altering stimulation of adenylyl cyclase. These observations suggest that agonist-dependent β_2-AR binding of NHERF plays a role in regulation of Na^+/H^+ exchange.

Interestingly, the same interaction was identified independently in a search for proteins regulating sorting of β_2-ARs between endosomes and lysosomes *(28)*.

Agonist-mediated endocytosis of β_2-ARs promotes dephosphorylation and resensitization, and recycling to the cell surface makes them ready for further agonist stimulation. Disrupting the interaction of NHERF/EBP50 with either the PDZ or ERM domain or drug-induced depolymerization of the actin cytoskeleton itself caused missorting of endocytosed β_2-ARs. Such disruptions did not affect the recycling of transferrin receptors, suggesting it is specific to GPCRs. Thus, it appears that NHERF/EBP50 plays multiple functions in regulating both signaling (Na^+/H^+ exchange) and recycling. The relationship between these multiple functions and their interaction with the traditional signaling G_S/cAMP signaling pathway have not yet been clarified.

The functional importance of the PDZ-binding motif at the C-terminus of β_2-ARs has been elegantly clarified in cardiac myocytes from β_1- and β_2-AR knock-out mice *(29)*. Mutation of the three C-terminal amino acids in the mouse β_2-AR disrupted recycling of the receptor after agonist-induced internalization in cardiac myocytes. Nevertheless, stimulation of this mutated β_2-AR produced a greater contraction rate increase than caused by the wild-type β_2-AR. This enhanced stimulation of contraction was attributed in part to the failure of the mutated β_2-AR to couple to G_i. These studies showed clearly that association of the PDZ ligand domain of the C-terminus of the β_2-AR with other proteins dictates signaling specificity and trafficking in cardiac myocytes.

3.1.3. A Kinase Anchoring Proteins (AKAPs)

The β-ARs increase cAMP, thus activating protein kinase A (PKA, or A kinase). A kinase anchoring proteins (AKAPs) localize PKA to its substrates by interacting with its regulatory subunit *(30)*, as well as phosphatases and possibly other proteins. This creates a spatially organized system for rapid control of receptor phosphorylation, contributing to desensitization and internalization *(4)*. One particular AKAP (gravin, AKAP250) has been found to form a dynamic complex with β_2-ARs in cells, showing a phosphorylation-dependent association of a multiprotein complex with the receptor, including both PKA and protein phosphatases *(31)*. This interaction occurs in the C-terminal tail *(32)*, and gravin-mediated signaling complexes appear to be essential in agonist-induced internalization and resensitization of β_2-ARs *(33)*.

Another AKAP, AKAP150, coimmunoprecipitates with the β_2-AR from various tissue extracts, resulting in a signaling complex including PKA, protein kinase C (PKC), and protein phosphatase 2B *(34)*. AKAP150 was reported to directly and constitutively interact with β_2-ARs and promote receptor phosphorylation following agonist stimulation. Functional studies showed that PKA anchoring enhanced β_2-AR phosphorylation and facilitated downstream activation of MAPK, suggesting a role for AKAP150 in recruitment of second messenger-regulated signaling enzymes to β_2-ARs.

3.1.4. Postsynaptic Density-95

Postsynaptic density 95 (PSD-95), a multiple PDZ domain-containing scaffolding protein, was identified by as a specific binding partner of the β_1-AR-C-terminus using a yeast two hybrid approach *(35)*. The interaction was confirmed with in vitro fusion proteins, which showed a specific interaction with the third PDZ domain of PSD-95. In addition, the full-length β_1-AR was found to associate with PSD-95 in cells by coimmunoprecipitation experiments and co-localization. This interaction was mediated by the last few amino acids of the β_1-AR because mutation of the C-terminus eliminated the binding and disrupted co-localization. Agonist-induced internalization of β_1-ARs in HEK293 cells was markedly attenuated by PSD-95 coexpression, whereas coexpression of PSD-95 did not affect either β_1-AR desensitization or cAMP accumulation. PSD-95 also facilitated formation of a complex between β_1-ARs and *N*-methyl-D-aspartate receptors as assessed by coimmunoprecipitation *(35)*. These data suggest that PSD-95 is a specific β_1-AR-binding partner that modulates its function and facilitates physical association with synaptic proteins.

3.1.5. Membrane-Associated Guanylate Kinase Inverted-2/Synaptic Scaffolding Molecule

Overlay and pull-down techniques were used to show that the β_1-AR C-terminus also associates with membrane-associated guanylate kinase inverted-2 (MAGI-2), a protein also known as synaptic scaffolding molecule (S-SCAM) *(36)*. MAGI-2 is a multidomain scaffolding protein that contains nine potential protein–protein interaction modules, including six PDZ domains, two WW domains, and a guanylate kinase-like domain. The β_1-AR C-terminus is bound with high affinity to the first PDZ domain of MAGI-2, with the last few amino acids of the β_1-AR C-terminus the key determinants. Association of full-length β_1-ARs with MAGI-2 in cells occurred constitutively and was enhanced by agonist stimulation. Agonist-induced internalization of β_1-ARs was markedly increased by coexpression with MAGI-2, in contrast to the effect of coexpression with PSD-95 described in Section 3.1.4. MAGI-2 also promoted association of β_1-ARs with the cytoplasmic signaling protein β-catenin, a known MAGI-2 binding partner. Thus, MAGI-2 appears to be a specific β_1-AR binding partner that modulates its function and may facilitate its association with intracellular proteins involved in signal transduction and synaptic regulation, possibly acting as a molecular scaffold.

3.1.6. CNrasGEF

Pak et al. *(37)* reported that β_1-ARs binds to the PDZ domain of the cAMP-dependent Ras exchange factor, CNrasGEF, via its C-terminal SKV motif. When cells were cotransfected with β_1-ARs and CNrasGEF, Ras was found to be activated by isoproterenol, suggesting an agonist-dependent association. This activation was abolished in β_1-AR mutants that could not bind CNrasGEF or in CNrasGEF mutants lacking the catalytic CDC25 domain or cAMP-binding domain, suggesting it depended on direct interactions. In addition, the activation required $G_S\alpha$ and not $G\beta\gamma$. In contrast, β_2-ARs could neither bind CNrasGEF nor activate it after agonist stimulation. These results suggest that a physical interaction between β_1-ARs and CNrasGEF facilitates $G_S\alpha$-mediated cyclic AMP production into Ras activation.

3.1.7. c-Src

The nonreceptor tyrosine kinase c-Src has been implicated in the pathways by which β_2-ARs activate MAPK. Fan et al. *(38)* showed that agonist stimulation triggered tyrosine phosphorylation of β_2-ARs and recruitment and activation of c-Src. Phosphorylation of tyrosine 350 in the β_2-AR C-terminus created a canonical Src homology 2 (SH2) binding site and appeared to be obligatory for agonist-induced desensitization, suggesting a role for this nonreceptor tyrosine kinase in this phenomenon.

c-Src was also shown to be required for extracellular signal regulated kinase (ERK) activation by β_2-ARs and be recruited to activated receptor through binding of the Src homology 3 (SH3) domain to proline-rich regions of the adapter protein β-arrestin-1. In this manner, it appears to terminate receptor–G protein coupling and initiate a second wave of signal transduction in which the "desensitized" receptor functions as a critical structural component of a mitogenic signaling complex *(39)* (*see also* Section 5).

Although β_3-ARs lack sites for phosphorylation and β-arrestin binding, MAPK activation by β_3-ARs still requires c-Src. Cao and coworkers *(40)* showed that ERK activation and Src coimmunoprecipitation with β_3-ARs occurs in adipocytes in an agonist-dependent and pertussis toxin-sensitive manner. Protein interaction studies showed that β_3-ARs interact directly with the SH3 domain of Src through proline-rich motifs (PXXP) in the third intracellular loop and the C-terminus. ERK activation and Src coimmunoprecipitation were abolished in cells expressing point mutations in these PXXP motifs, suggesting a novel mechanism for activation of MAPK by β_3-ARs, in which the intracellular domains directly recruit c-Src.

3.1.8. Endophilins

The β_1-ARs contain polyproline motifs within their intracellular domains, which in other proteins are known to mediate interactions with SH3 domains. Using the proline-rich third intracellular loop of the β_1-AR as bait, Tang et al. *(41)* identified SH3p4/p8/p13 (also referred to as endophilin 1/2/3), a SH3 domain-containing protein family, as binding partners for β_1-ARs. Both in vitro and in

HEK293 cells, SH3p4 specifically bound to the third intracellular loop of β_1-ARs but not β_2-ARs. The interaction appeared to be mediated by the C-terminal SH3 domain of SH3p4, and it was found that overexpression of SH3p4 promoted agonist-induced internalization and caused a small decrease in coupling to Gs. These results suggest a role for the SH3p4/p8/p13 protein family in β_1-AR signaling through an interaction with the third intracellular loop.

3.1.9. Eukaryotic Initiation Factor 2B

The α-subunit of eukaryotic initiation factor 2B (eIF-2B), a guanine nucleotide exchange factor that helps regulate translation, was found to associate with the C-terminal domains of α_{2A}- and α_{2B}-ARs in a yeast two-hybrid screen *(42)*. This interaction was shown to be specific for a subset of GPCRs, including the α_{2A}-, α_{2B}-, α_{2C}, and β_2-ARs. eIF-2Bα specifically coimmunoprecipitated with full-length β_2-ARs and was co-localized by fluorescence microscopy in intact cells. This co-localization appeared exclusively in plasma membrane regions in contact with the extracellular medium but not in membranes making cell–cell contacts. Overexpression of eIF-2Bα in 293 cells caused a small (~15%) but specific enhancement of β_2-AR-mediated activation of adenylyl cyclase, suggesting that this guanine nucleotide exchange factor may influence AR signaling.

3.2. α_1-AR Interacting Proteins

Less attention has been focused on α_1-AR interacting proteins, although some binding partners have been identified. Because of their relatively long C-terminal tails, most attention has been focused on finding proteins interacting with this domain.

3.2.1. Transglutaminase II

The α_1-ARs have been shown to copurify with and activate a high molecular weight G protein, G_h, which is structurally unrelated to heterotrimeric G proteins and has been shown to be the enzyme transglutaminase II *(43)*. This response has been shown to be activated by the α_{1B}- and α_{1D}-, but not the α_{1A}-, subtypes *(44)*. However, the functional significance of this pathway remains unclear because G_h knockout mice show no overt phenotype with respect to α_1-AR signaling *(45)*.

3.2.2. gC1qR

A yeast two-hybrid screen of a complementary deoxyribonucleic acid (cDNA) library from rat liver with the C-tail of the hamster α_{1B}-AR identified gC1qR as a potential protein-binding partner *(46)*. gC1qR was initially described as a receptor for the globular heads of the complement factor C1q and is also known as p32 or p33. gC1qR has been found to recognize multiple ligands, is present in different cellular compartments, and has been implicated in several different functions *(47)*. Interestingly, α_{1B}-ARs expressed alone were exclusively found on the plasma membrane, gC1qR was localized in the cytoplasm when expressed alone; however, cells coexpressing α_{1B}-ARs and gC1qR showed that most of the α_{1B}-ARs were co-localized with gC1qR in intracellular compartments. In addition, a remarkable downregulation of receptor expression was observed, suggesting a possible role for gC1qR in expression and localization of this receptor subtype (48). The interaction appears to occur through an arginine-rich motif located shortly after the seventh transmembrane-spanning domain. Because a similar domain is found in α_{1D}-, but not α_{1A}-, ARs, not surprisingly further studies suggested that gC1qR interacts specifically with α_{1B}- and α_{1D}-, but not α_{1A}-, ARs, and this interaction depends on the presence of an intact C-tail (49).

3.2.3. Neuronal Nitric Oxide Synthase

The C-terminal four amino acids (GEEV) of human α_{1A}-ARs were reported to interact with the PDZ domain of neuronal nitric oxide synthase (nNOS) in a yeast two-hybrid system (50). The other two α_1-AR subtypes have no sequence homology in this region, suggesting that this might be an example of subtype-specific interactions. Using coimmunoprecipitation and functional approaches with epitope-tagged α_1-ARs, it was found that cotransfection of α_{1A}-ARs and nNOS resulted in the expected interaction (51). However, the interaction between α_{1A}-ARs and nNOS did not appear to be subtype specific, and nNOS also coimmunoprecipitated with α_{1B}- and α_{1D}-ARs, with each of the three α_1-AR subtypes that had been C-terminally truncated, epitope-tagged β_1- and β_2-ARs. Thus, despite the apparent specificity in the yeast two hybrid screen (50), it appears that nNOS does interact with full-length α_{1A}-ARs, but that this interaction is not subtype-specific and does not require the C-terminal tail, raising questions about its functional significance (51).

3.2.4. AP2

A yeast two-hybrid screen identified the μ 2 subunit of the clathrin adaptor complex 2 as a protein interacting with the C-tail of the α_{1B}-AR (52). Direct association between α_{1B}-ARs and μ 2 was also demonstrated using an overlay assay. The α_{1B}-AR/μ 2 interaction also appeared to occur in intact cells because they could be coimmunoprecipitated following cotransfection. Mutational analysis of α_{1B}-ARs revealed that the μ 2 binding site involved the same highly charged arginine-rich stretch in the receptor C-tail as gC1qR (48). Binding of μ 2 involved both its N-terminus and subdomain B of its C-terminal portion (52). The α_{1B}-AR specifically interacted with μ 2, but not with μ 1, μ 3, or μ 4 subunits belonging to other AP complexes. Deletion of the μ 2 binding site in the C-tail markedly decreased agonist-induced receptor internalization, and thus it was suggested that this interaction might be involved in clathrin-mediated receptor endocytosis.

3.3. α_2-AR Interacting Proteins

Similarly, only a few interacting proteins have been identified for α_2-AR subtypes. Compared to α_1-ARs, α_2-ARs have shorter C-terminal tails and much longer third intracellular loops, so most attention has been given to the third intracellular loops of these receptors.

3.3.1. Spinophilin

Spinophilin is a PDZ domain-containing protein that appears to interact with α_2-ARs via a novel, non-PDZ domain-mediated mechanism involving the third intracellular loops of the receptors *(53)*. Spinophilin is ubiquitously expressed, but its localization in dendritic spines led to its name. Spinophilin was found to interact with all three α_2-AR subtypes in an agonist-regulated fashion and was suggested to contribute to both α_2-AR localization and signaling in polarized epithelial cells, particularly by stabilizing surface expression of α_{2B}-ARs *(54)*.

3.3.2. 14-3-3 ζ

Gel overlay assays were used to demonstrate that the third intracellular loop of α_2-ARs interact with the ζ isoform of the ubiquitously expressed, predominantly cytosolic, 14-3-3 proteins. These proteins exist as dimers with a conserved ligand-binding surface and regulate many cellular effectors, including protein kinases, members of the ras signaling pathway, RGS proteins, and cell cycle components *(55)*. α_2-AR third intracellular loops bound 14-3-3 ζ in a subtype-dependent manner ($\alpha_{2B} \geq \alpha_{2C} >> \alpha_{2A}$). The 14-3-3 ζ also interacted with all three native α_2-AR subtypes with different affinities through their third intracellular loops. Subsequent studies suggested that sequential or competitive interactions among spinophilin, arrestin, or 14-3-3 ζ may play a role in α_{2A}-AR function *(56)*.

3.3.3. β-Arrestins

Wu et al. *(57)* first showed that β-arrestins bind to the third intracellular loop of α_2-ARs. The role of these proteins in trafficking of α_2-ARs was examined subsequently *(58)*, and it was shown that internalization of α_{2B}-, α_{2C}-, and to a lesser extent α_{2A}-ARs is both arrestin and dynamin dependent, although arrestin did not appear to play a role in MAPK activation by these receptors. Later studies showed that arrestin-3 (β-arrestin 2) binds to two discrete regions within the α_{2B}-AR third intracellular loop *(59)*, and that disruption of arrestin binding selectively blocked agonist-promoted receptor internalization.

3.3.4. eIF2Bα

As mentioned in Section 3.1.9., elongation factor 2Bα, appears to interact with each of the three known α_2-AR subtypes, although the functional consequences of this interaction are still unclear *(54)*.

4. Dimerization of ARs

Dimerization of growth factor and cytokine receptors is essential for their signaling *(60)*. However, GPCRs have traditionally been thought to function as monomers, with a single receptor binding ligand and activating G proteins. Although early studies showed that two binding-deficient muscarinic/adrenergic chimeras could form a receptor capable of ligand binding and signaling on coexpression *(61)*, little attention was paid to the likelihood of receptor dimerization until 1999. In that year, it was shown by several groups that $GABA_B$ receptors required heteroligomerization of two different GPCRs to form a single functional receptor *(1,4)*. Since that time, reports of GPCR homo- and heterodimerization have appeared with increasing frequency *(62)*, and it is now clear that dimerization plays important roles in GPCR function, although except in isolated instances the specifics are not yet well understood.

4.1. Homodimerization

The first evidence for AR homodimerization came from Hebert et al. *(63)*, using β_2-ARs. Coimmunoprecipitation using β_2-ARs with different epitope tags provided direct biochemical evidence for β_2-AR homodimers *(63)*. An interesting feature of these dimers was their relative resistance to sodium dodecyl sulfate (SDS) denaturation on SDS polyacrylamide gel electrophoresis. They often migrated as mixtures of molecular species corresponding to monomers, dimers, or higher order oligomers based on the predicted monomeric mass. This resistance to SDS is also commonly observed with other highly hydrophobic proteins forming dimers in cells *(64)*, such as glycophorin A. The functional importance of β_2-AR dimerization was supported by the observation that a peptide-derived transmembrane domain VI, thought to be involved in homodimer formation, inhibited β_2-AR stimulation of adenylyl cyclase *(63)*. Similar results were obtained with other receptor types *(62)*, including epitope-tagged α_1-ARs, for which it was found that all three subtypes exist as monomers, dimers, and higher order oligomers on Western blots *(65)*.

In an effort to determine whether GPCR dimers exist in living cells, several groups took advantage of biophysical assays based on light resonance energy transfer. Using GPCRs fused via their C-tails to bioluminescent (luciferase) or fluorescent (green fluorescent) proteins, bioluminescence resonance energy transfer (BRET) or fluorescence resonance energy transfer (FRET) were used to show homodimerization of human β_2-ARs *(66)*. Subsequent studies showed similar results for a variety of GPCRs *(62)*, including α_{1A} and α_{1B}-ARs *(67,68)*. These results suggest that many GPCRs form constitutive homodimers in intact cells and raise the question of the role of this phenomenon in receptor activation because most of these homodimers appear essentially independent of agonist stimulation *(62)*.

4.2. Heterodimerization With Other ARs

Heterodimerization between ARs of different subtypes is observed with increasing frequency *(67,69–72)*. These include β_1/β_2 *(73)*, β_1/α_{2A} *(69)*, α_{1A}/α_{1B} *(67,70)*, and α_{1B}/α_{1D} *(70)*.

Heterodimerization between members of the α_1-AR subfamily has now been reported by two separate groups *(67,70)* and appears to be of particular interest. Uberti et al. *(70)* reported that α_1-AR heterodimerization is subtype specific, with α_{1B}-ARs interacting with α_{1A}- or α_{1D}-ARs, but with no detectable interactions between α_{1A}- and α_{1D}-ARs. Interestingly, heterodimerization did not alter apparent ligand-binding properties, but rather resulted in increased receptor expression. In particular, α_{1B}/α_{1D}-AR heterodimerization increased cell surface expression of α_{1D}-ARs as monitored by a luminometer assay. Because α_{1D}-ARs are almost always exclusively intracellular following heterologous expression in various cell types *(74,75)*, this was quite intriguing.

Further studies using green fluorescent protein or cyan fluorescent protein tagged receptors showed that α_{1B}/α_{1D}-AR heterodimerization appeared to completely control the surface expression and functional coupling of α_{1D}-ARs on the plasma membrane *(76)*. Coexpression of α_{1B}, but not α_{1A}-, ARs resulted in almost exclusively surface localization of the normally intracellular α_{1D}-ARs, consistent with the specificity observed in previous coimmunoprecipitation studies. Further studies showed that the hydrophobic core of the α_{1B}-AR is the major structural determinant of this interaction, and that G protein coupling was not required *(76)*. These studies suggest that subtype-specific heterodimerization of ARs may control surface expression, and that these observations may be relevant to many other class I G protein-coupled receptors, for which the functional consequences of this phenomenon are still poorly understood.

4.3. Heterodimerization With Other Receptor Types

Jordan et al. *(77)* observed coimmunoprecipitation of β_2-AR and δ-opioid receptors and found that β_2-AR agonists promoted δ-opioid internalization, suggesting a functional heterodimer was expressed at the cell surface. However, some caution in interpreting these results was provided by McVey and colleagues *(78)*. These authors showed that homodimerization of β_2-ARs and δ-opioid receptors could be detected by coimmunoprecipitation, BRET, and FRET. However, heterodimerization was detected only after coimmunoprecipitation, and no significant BRET or FRET signals were observed with coexpression. The authors concluded that heterodimerization might represent a biochemical artifact of aggregation of hydrophobic proteins during coimmunoprecipitation *(78)*. Such conflicting results are not unexpected in an emerging field but emphasize the care that must be used in data extrapolation. Heterodimerization between α_{1B}-ARs and histamine H1 receptors has also been proposed *(68)*, and use of inactive mutants and G protein fusion proteins resulted in the conclusion that dimerization resulted in transactivation of the associated G proteins. This surprising result will clearly need further corroboration before it is likely to be widely adopted.

5. Role of Receptor Internalization in Signaling

Agonist treatment of ARs leads not only to activation of receptor signaling and desensitization, but also to internalization of the receptor from the cell surface *(4)*. This was first thought to be only part of the process of desensitization; however, internalization is now also known to positively regulate receptor signalling *(4)*. Multiple pathways of internalization have been described, some of which involve clathrin-coated pits, cavolae, or even uncoated vesicles. However, the best-characterized mechanism for β_2-AR internalization is β-arrestin dependent through clathrin-coated vesicles. β-Arrestins bind to agonist-occupied, phosphorylated receptors as described above and with clathrin and the β2-adaptin subunit of the clathrin adaptor protein AP-2 *(4)*, targeting the ARs to clathrin-coated pits. These pits are pinched off by the actions of the large GTPase dynamin, and the receptors are rapidly recycled, targeted to larger endosomes and recycled more slowly, or degraded in lysosomes *(4)*.

It is now clear that β-arrestins also function as adaptor/scaffolds that bind proteins such as c-Src. Interaction of β-arrestin with c-Src regulates β_2-AR internalization by promoting tyrosine phosphorylation of dynamin. β-Arrestins also lead to activation and subcellular targeting of two different MAPK cascades (ERK and c-Jun N-terminal kinase 3 [JNK3]) by interacting with the last three kinases in each cascade. β-Arrestins bring these kinases into proximity, facilitating phosphorylation and activation. Surprisingly, this scaffolding leads to cytosolic retention of the active kinases, thereby promoting receptor internalization and co-localization of the receptor, β-arrestin, and the components of the MAPK cascade in large endocytic vesicles *(4)*. This enhances overall MAPK activation but inhibits their traditional nuclear signaling. It should be noted that these β-arrestin-scaffolded pathways are only one of many ways by which ARs can activate MAPK cascades, and cellular context is critical for determining which MAPK pathways are used. However, it now seems clear that direct interactions with such scaffold/adaptor proteins is important not only in internalization and subcellular localization, but also in particular signaling pathways.

6. Summary and Models
for New Signal Transduction Paradigms

It is now abundantly clear that the relatively linear signaling pathways activated by ARs, widely accepted for decades, are much more complex than previously realized. Individual ARs can interact with each other directly to form homo- or heterodimers, possibly creating pharmacologically and functionally

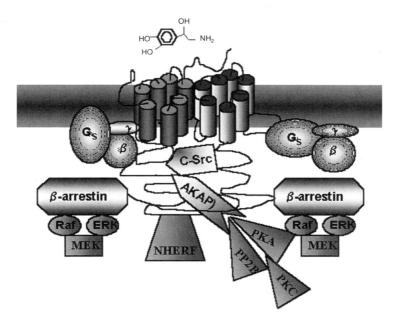

Fig. 1. Potential complexity of signaling involving adrenergic receptor dimers, G proteins, and scaffolding/adaptor proteins. As an illustration, dimers of two β_2-ARs are shown in a contact dimer formation *(62)* with *some* of the large variety of proteins suggested to bind to their intracellular surfaces, illustrating the potential complexity of intracellular signaling that may be initiated by receptor activation. Transmembrane helices are indicated by the barrel-like structures and intracellular and extracellular domains as lines. Interacting proteins are shown as various shapes in the approximate localization where they are thought to bind. Abbreviations are defined in the text. MEK, MAPK/ERK kinase.

distinct receptor species. ARs can interact with multiple G proteins, depending on cellular context and prior signaling history, and appear to be able to switch their G protein preferences under particular conditions. Most strikingly, ARs are now known to interact directly with a large variety of scaffold and adaptor proteins in addition to their specific G proteins, sometimes in a regulated, phosphorylation-dependent mechanism. The startling large number and variety of such proteins that have been identified suggest that the intracellular surface of ARs must be a very busy place indeed, with multiple large proteins competing for interacting sites (Fig. 1).

The structural effects of these scaffolding proteins, their participation in novel signaling pathways, and their competitive/interactive natures remain largely to be determined. Although a few examples of functional consequences of such interactions are now clear, many more are likely to appear in the near future.

Finally, the role of internalization in receptor signaling, particularly through intracellular pathways such as the MAPK pathways, has been made abundantly clear. Thus, the complexity of the system extends to receptor compartmentation and subcellular localization within cells, resulting in even more potentially complex scenarios. In the age of proteomics, these complexities are likely to expand exponentially until the underlying organizing principles are clearly elucidated. Until then, we are likely to see more and more examples of such signaling complexity and will have our hands full trying to understand its meaning.

References

1. Bockaert J, Marin P, Dumuis A, Fagni L. The "magic tail" of G protein-coupled receptors: an anchorage for functional protein networks. FEBS Lett 2003;546: 65–72.
2. Otaki JM, Firestein S. Length analyses of mammalian G-protein-coupled receptors. J Theor Biol 2001;211:77–100.
3. Gilman AG. Nobel Lecture. G proteins and regulation of adenylyl cyclase. Biosci Rep 1995;15:65–97.
4. Pierce KL, Premont RT, Lefkowitz RJ. Seven-transmembrane receptors. Nat Rev Mol Cell Biol 2002;3:639-650.
5. Chen JG, Willard FS, Huang J, et al. A seven-transmembrane RGS protein that modulates plant cell proliferation. Science 2003;301:1728–1731.
6. Furchgott RF. Pharmacological characterization of receptors: its relation to radioligand-binding studies. Fed Proc 1978;37:115–120.
7. Guo DF, Sun YL, Hamet P, Inagami T. The angiotensin II type 1 receptor and receptor-associated proteins. Cell Res 2001;11:165–180.
8. Schlessinger J. Cell signaling by receptor tyrosine kinases. Cell 2000;103: 211–225.
9. Crespo P, Xu N, Simonds WF, Gutkind JS. Ras-dependent activation of MAP kinase pathway mediated by G-protein $\beta\gamma$ subunits. Nature 1994;369:418–420.
10. Zhong H, Minneman KP. Differential activation of mitogen-activated protein kinase pathways in PC12 cells by closely related α_1-adrenergic receptor subtypes. J Neurochem 1999;72:2388–2396.
11. Koch WJ, Hawes BE, Allen LF, Lefkowitz RJ. Direct evidence that G_i-coupled receptor stimulation of mitogen-activated protein kinase is mediated by G $\beta\gamma$ activation of p21ras. Proc Natl Acad Sci USA 1994;91:12,706--12,710.
12. Crespo P, Cachero TG, Xu N, Gutkind JS. Dual effect of β-adrenergic receptors on mitogen-activated protein kinase. Evidence for a $\beta\gamma$-dependent activation and a G α s- cAMP-mediated inhibition. J Biol Chem 1995;270:25,259–25,265.
13. Williams NG, Zhong H, Minneman KP. Differential coupling of α_1-, α_2-, and β-adrenergic receptors to mitogen-activated protein kinase pathways and differentiation in transfected PC12 cells. J Biol Chem 1998;273:24,624–24,632.
14. Della Rocca GJ, van Biesen T, Daaka Y, Luttrell DK, Luttrell LM, Lefkowitz RJ. Ras-dependent mitogen-activated protein kinase activation by G protein-coupled receptors. Convergence of G_i- and G_q-mediated pathways on calcium/calmodulin, Pyk2, and Src kinase. J Biol Chem 1997;272:19,125–19,132.

15. Zhong H, Minneman KP. Activation of tyrosine kinases by α_{1A}-adrenergic and growth factor receptors in transfected PC12 cells. Biochem J 1999;344:889–894.
16. Zhong H, Murphy TJ, Minneman KP. Activation of signal transducers and activators of transcription by α_{1a}-adrenergic receptor stimulation in PC12 cells. Mol Pharmacol 2000;57:961–967.
17. Ali MS, Sayeski PP, Bernstein KE. Jak2 acts as both a STAT1 kinase and as a molecular bridge linking STAT1 to the angiotensin II AT1 receptor. J Biol Chem 2000;275:15,586–15,593.
18. Wilson KM, Minneman KP. Pertussis toxin inhibits norepinephrine-stimulated inositol phosphate formation in primary brain cell cultures. Mol Pharmacol 1990;38:274–281.
19. Minneman KP, Lee D, Zhong H, Berts A, Abbott KL, Murphy TJ. Transcriptional responses to growth factor and G protein-coupled receptors in PC12 cells: comparison of α_1-adrenergic receptor subtypes. J Neurochem 2000;74:2392–2400.
20. Gonzalez-Cabrera PJ, Gaivin RJ, Yun J, et al. Genetic profiling of α_1-adrenergic receptor subtypes by oligonucleotide microarrays: coupling to interleukin-6 secretion but differences in STAT3 phosphorylation and gp-130. Mol Pharmacol 2003;63:1104–1116.
21. Chaudhry A, MacKenzie RG, Georgic LM, Granneman JG. Differential interaction of β_1- and β_3-adrenergic receptors with G_i in rat adipocytes. Cell Signal 1994;6: 457–465.
22. Xiao RP, Avdonin P, Zhou YY, et al. Coupling of β_2-adrenoceptor to G_i proteins and its physiological relevance in murine cardiac myocytes. Circ Res 1999;84:43–52.
23. Daaka Y, Luttrell LM, Lefkowitz RJ. Switching of the coupling of the β_2-adrenergic receptor to different G proteins by protein kinase A. Nature 1997;390:88–91.
24. Benovic JL, Kuhn H, Weyand I, Codina J, Caron MG, Lefkowitz RJ. Functional desensitization of the isolated β-adrenergic receptor by the β-adrenergic receptor kinase: potential role of an analog of the retinal protein arrestin (48-kDa protein). Proc Natl Acad Sci USA 1987;84:8879–8882.
25. Lohse MJ, Benovic JL, Codina J, Caron MG, Lefkowitz RJ. β-Arrestin: a protein that regulates β-adrenergic receptor function. Science 1990;248:1547–1550.
26. Hall RA, Premont RT, Chow CW, et al. The β_2-adrenergic receptor interacts with the Na^+/H^+-exchanger regulatory factor to control Na^+/H^+ exchange. Nature 1998; 392:626–630.
27. Hall RA, Ostedgaard LS, Premont RT, et al. A C-terminal motif found in the β_2-adrenergic receptor, P2Y1 receptor and cystic fibrosis transmembrane conductance regulator determines binding to the Na^+/H^+ exchanger regulatory factor family of PDZ proteins. Proc Natl Acad Sci USA 1998;95:8496–8501.
28. Cao TT, Deacon HW, Reczek D, Bretscher A, von Zastrow M. A kinase-regulated PDZ-domain interaction controls endocytic sorting of the β_2-adrenergic receptor. Nature 1999;401:286–290.
29. Xiang Y, Kobilka B. The PDZ-binding motif of the β_2-adrenoceptor is essential for physiologic signaling and trafficking in cardiac myocytes. Proc Natl Acad Sci USA 2003;100:10,776–10,781.
30. Scott JD. A-kinase-anchoring proteins and cytoskeletal signalling events. Biochem Soc Trans 2003;31:87–89.

31. Shih M, Lin F, Scott JD, Wang HY, Malbon CC. Dynamic complexes of β_2-adrenergic receptors with protein kinases and phosphatases and the role of gravin. J Biol Chem 1999;274:1588–1595.
32. Fan G, Shumay E, Wang H, Malbon CC. The scaffold protein gravin (cAMP-dependent protein kinase-anchoring protein 250) binds the β_2-adrenergic receptor via the receptor cytoplasmic Arg-329 to Leu-413 domain and provides a mobile scaffold during desensitization. J Biol Chem 2001;276:24,005–24,014.
33. Lin F, Wang H, Malbon CC. Gravin-mediated formation of signaling complexes in β_2-adrenergic receptor desensitization and resensitization. J Biol Chem 2000;275:19,025–19,034.
34. Fraser ID, Cong M, Kim J, et al. Assembly of an A kinase-anchoring protein-β_2-adrenergic receptor complex facilitates receptor phosphorylation and signaling. Curr Biol 2000;10:409–412.
35. Hu LA, Tang Y, Miller WE, et al. β_1-Adrenergic receptor association with PSD-95. Inhibition of receptor internalization and facilitation of β_1-adrenergic receptor interaction with N-methyl-D-aspartate receptors. J Biol Chem 2000;275:38,659–38,666.
36. Xu J, Paquet M, Lau AG, Wood JD, Ross CA, Hall RA. β_1-Adrenergic receptor association with the synaptic scaffolding protein membrane-associated guanylate kinase inverted-2 (MAGI-2). Differential regulation of receptor internalization by MAGI-2 and PSD-95. J Biol Chem 2001;276:41,310–41,317.
37. Pak Y, Pham N, Rotin D. Direct binding of the β_1 adrenergic receptor to the cyclic AMP-dependent guanine nucleotide exchange factor CNrasGEF leads to Ras activation. Mol Cell Biol 2002;22:7942–7952.
38. Fan G, Shumay E, Malbon CC, Wang H. c-Src tyrosine kinase binds the β_2-adrenergic receptor via phospho-Tyr-350, phosphorylates G-protein-linked receptor kinase 2, and mediates agonist-induced receptor desensitization. J Biol Chem 2001;276:13,240–13,247.
39. Luttrell LM, Ferguson SS, Daaka Y, et al. β-Arrestin-dependent formation of β_2 adrenergic receptor-Src protein kinase complexes. Science 1999;283:655–661.
40. Cao W, Luttrell LM, Medvedev AV, et al. Direct binding of activated c-Src to the β_3-adrenergic receptor is required for MAP kinase activation. J Biol Chem 2000;275:38,131–38,134.
41. Tang Y, Hu LA, Miller WE, et al. Identification of the endophilins (SH3p4/p8/p13) as novel binding partners for the β_1-adrenergic receptor. Proc Natl Acad Sci USA 1999;96:12,559–12,564.
42. Klein U, Ramirez MT, Kobilka BK, von Zastrow M. A novel interaction between adrenergic receptors and the α-subunit of eukaryotic initiation factor 2B. J Biol Chem 1997;272:19,099–19,102.
43. Nakaoka H, Perez DM, Baek KJ, et al. Gh: a GTP-binding protein with transglutaminase activity and receptor signaling function. Science 1994;264:1593–1596.
44. Chen S, Lin F, Iismaa S, Lee KN, Birckbichler PJ, Graham RM. α_1-Adrenergic receptor signaling via Gh is subtype specific and independent of its transglutaminase activity. J Biol Chem 1996;271:32,385–391.
45. Nanda N, Iismaa SE, Owens WA, Husain A, Mackay F, Graham RM. Targeted inactivation of Gh/tissue transglutaminase II. J Biol Chem 2001;276:20,673–20,678.

46. Xu Z, Hirasawa A, Shinoura H, Tsujimoto G. Interaction of the α_{1B}-adrenergic receptor with gC1q-R, a multifunctional protein. J Biol Chem 1999;274:21,149–21,154.
47. Ghebrehiwet B, Lim BL, Kumar R, Feng X, Peerschke EI. gC1q-R/p33, a member of a new class of multifunctional and multicompartmental cellular proteins, is involved in inflammation and infection. Immunol Rev 2001;180:65–77.
48. Xu Z, Hirasawa A, Shinoura H, Tsujimoto G. Interaction of the α_{1B}-adrenergic receptor with gC1q-R, a multifunctional protein. J Biol Chem 1999;274:21,149–21,154.
49. Pupo AS, Minneman KP. Specific interactions between gC1qR and α_1-adrenoceptor subtypes. J Recept Signal Transduct Res 2003;23:185–195.
50. Schepens J, Cuppen E, Wieringa B, Hendriks W. The neuronal nitric oxide synthase PDZ motif binds to -G(D,E)XV* carboxyterminal sequences. FEBS Lett 1997;409:53–56.
51. Pupo AS, Minneman KP. Interaction of neuronal nitric oxide synthase with α_1-adrenergic receptor subtypes in transfected HEK-293 cells. BMC Pharmacol 2002; 2:17.
52. Diviani D, Lattion AL, Abuin L, Staub O, Cotecchia S. The adaptor complex 2 directly interacts with the α_{1b}-adrenergic receptor and plays a role in receptor endocytosis. J Biol Chem 2003;278:19,331–19,340.
53. Richman JG, Brady AE, Wang Q, Hensel JL, Colbran RJ, Limbird LE. Agonist-regulated interaction between α_2-adrenergic receptors and spinophilin. J Biol Chem 2001;276:15,003–15,008.
54. Brady AE, Limbird LE. G protein-coupled receptor interacting proteins: emerging roles in localization and signal transduction. Cell Signal 2002;14:297–309.
55. Fu H, Subramanian RR, Masters SC. 14-3-3 proteins: structure, function, and regulation. Annu Rev Pharmacol Toxicol 2000;40:617–647.
56. Wang Q, Limbird LE. Regulated interactions of the α_{2A} adrenergic receptor with spinophilin, 14-3-3 zeta, and arrestin 3. J Biol Chem 2002;277:50,589–50,596.
57. Wu G, Krupnick JG, Benovic JL, Lanier SM. Interaction of arrestins with intracellular domains of muscarinic and α_2-adrenergic receptors. J Biol Chem 1997;272: 17,836–17,842.
58. DeGraff JL, Gagnon AW, Benovic JL, Orsini MJ. Role of arrestins in endocytosis and signaling of α_2-adrenergic receptor subtypes. J Biol Chem 1999;274:11,253–11,259.
59. DeGraff JL, Gurevich VV, Benovic JL. The third intracellular loop of α_2-adrenergic receptors determines subtype specificity of arrestin interaction. J Biol Chem 2002;277:43,247–43,252.
60. Heldin CH. Dimerization of cell surface receptors in signal transduction. Cell 1995;80:213–223.
61. Maggio R, Vogel Z, Wess J. Coexpression studies with mutant muscarinic/adrenergic receptors provide evidence for intermolecular "cross-talk" between G-protein- linked receptors. Proc Natl Acad Sci USA 1993;90:3103–3107.
62. Bouvier M. Oligomerization of G-protein-coupled transmitter receptors. Nat Rev Neurosci 2001;2:274–286.
63. Hebert TE, Moffett S, Morello JP, et al. A peptide derived from a β_2-adrenergic receptor transmembrane domain inhibits both receptor dimerization and activation. J Biol Chem 1996;271:16,384–16,392.

64. Furthmayr H, Marchesi VT. Subunit structure of human erythrocyte glycophorin A. Biochemistry 1976;15:1137–1144.
65. Vicentic A, Robeva A, Rogge G, Uberti M, Minneman KP. Biochemistry and pharmacology of epitope-tagged α_1-adrenergic receptor subtypes. J Pharmacol Exp Ther 2002;302:58–65.
66. Angers S, Salahpour A, Joly E, et al. Detection of β_2-adrenergic receptor dimerization in living cells using bioluminescence resonance energy transfer (BRET). Proc Natl Acad Sci USA 2000;97:3684–3689.
67. Stanasila L, Perez JB, Vogel H, Cotecchia S. Oligomerization of the α_{1a}- and α_{1b}-adrenergic receptor subtypes. Potential implications in receptor internalization. J Biol Chem 2003;278:40,239–40,251.
68. Carrillo JJ, Pediani J, Milligan G. Dimers of class A G protein-coupled receptors function via agonist-mediated trans-activation of associated G proteins. J Biol Chem 2003;278:42,578–42,587.
69. Xu J, He J, Castleberry AM, Balasubramanian S, Lau AG, Hall RA. Heterodimerization of α_{2A}- and β_1-adrenergic receptors. J Biol Chem 2003;278:10,770–10,777.
70. Uberti MA, Hall RA, Minneman KP. Subtype-specific dimerization of α_1-adrenoceptors: effects on receptor expression and pharmacological properties. Mol Pharmacol 2003;64:1379–1390.
71. Lavoie C, Mercier JF, Salahpour A, et al. β_1/β_2-Adrenergic receptor heterodimerization regulates β_2-adrenergic receptor internalization and ERK signaling efficacy. J Biol Chem 2002;277:35,402–35,410.
72. Lavoie C, Hebert TE. Pharmacological characterization of putative β_1-β_2-adrenergic receptor heterodimers. Can J Physiol Pharmacol 2003;81:186–195.
73. Mercier JF, Salahpour A, Angers S, Breit A, Bouvier M. Quantitative assessment of β_1- and β_2-adrenergic receptor homo- and heterodimerization by bioluminescence resonance energy transfer. J Biol Chem 2002;277:44,925–44,931.
74. Hague C, Chen Z, Pupo AS, Schulte N, Toews ML, Minneman KP. The N-terminus of the human α_{1D}-adrenergic receptor prevents cell surface expression. J Pharm Exp Ther 2004; 309: 388–397.
75. Chalothorn D, McCune DF, Edelmann SE, Garcia-Cazarin ML, Tsujimoto G, Piascik MT. Differences in the cellular localization and agonist-mediated internalization properties of the α_1-adrenoceptor subtypes. Mol Pharmacol 2002;61:1008–1016.
76. Hague C, Uberti M, Chen Z, Hall RA, Minneman KP. Cell surface expression of α_{1D}-ARs is controlled by heterodimerization with α_{1B}-adrenergic receptors. J Biol Chem 2004; 279:15,541–15,549.
77. Jordan BA, Trapaidze N, Gomes I, Nivarthi R, Devi LA. Oligomerization of opioid receptors with β_2-adrenergic receptors: a role in trafficking and mitogen-activated protein kinase activation. Proc Natl Acad Sci USA 2001;98:343–348.
78. McVey M, Ramsay D, Kellett E, et al. Monitoring receptor oligomerization using time-resolved fluorescence resonance energy transfer and bioluminescence resonance energy transfer. The human δ-opioid receptor displays constitutive oligomerization at the cell surface, which is not regulated by receptor occupancy. J Biol Chem 2001;276:14,092–14,099.

4

Regulation of the Cellular Localization and Trafficking of the Adrenergic Receptors

Michael T. Piascik, Mary Lolis García-Cazarin, and Steven R. Post

Summary

The family of adrenergic receptors (ARs; the α_1-, α_2-, and β-ARs) are key regulators of the sympathetic division of the autonomic nervous system, involved in both central and peripheral cardiovascular function. Here, we review our current understanding of the cellular localization and trafficking properties of the α_1-, α_2-, and β-ARs. We then examine recent evidence indicating that the cellular localization of these receptors and their excursion into intracellular compartments play an underappreciated role in the activation of both G protein and novel non-G protein-dependent cellular signaling.

Key Words: Adrenergic receptors; cellular localization or receptors; cellular trafficking of receptors; receptor subtypes; signaling from intracellular receptor complexes.

1. Introduction

The regulation of cellular signaling by the adrenergic receptors (ARs) is a complex and multifaceted process. Indeed, as our knowledge of these processes increases, so does an appreciation of the breadth of this complexity. As depicted in Fig. 1, cellular signaling was viewed as a linear process with a G protein-coupled receptor (GPCR) envisioned to couple to a single, or small subset, of G protein(s), which in turn activated a discrete set of second messenger systems common to all GPCRs. This signaling paradigm has been found to be entirely too simplistic and inadequate to account for recent observations.

From: *The Receptors: The Adrenergic Receptors: In the 21st Century*
Edited by: D. Perez © Humana Press Inc., Totowa, NJ

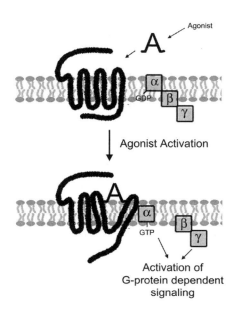

Fig. 1. Linear relationship among a GPCR, G proteins, and the activation of cellular signaling.

To illustrate, we know that subtypes of the β-ARs, the α_1 and α_2-ARs, can be expressed in intracellular compartments. Furthermore, despite having similar sequences and the fact that the α- and β-AR subtypes can couple to similar signaling pathways in heterologous expression systems, these receptors exhibit a high degree of signaling fidelity in vivo. For example, the α_{1B}-AR and α_{1D}-ARs can couple to inositol phosphate formation, increasing intracellular calcium and mitogen-activated protein kinases (MAPKs) when expressed in Chinese hamster ovary (CHO) cells or Rat1 fibroblast cells *(1,2)*. However, these receptors differ significantly in the ability to contract vascular smooth muscle and regulate systemic arterial blood pressure, cardiac contraction, and hypertrophic responses. This is but one example.

It is not completely understood how the specificity of coupling for GPCRs is achieved. An emerging concept is that the different sequences within the receptor control novel interactions with modulators of cellular signaling and target the receptor to discrete signaling packages within the cell. These signaling packages would contain different G proteins and other signaling molecules. Thus, the formation of the signaling complexes offers a degree of complexity and specificity not possible by cell surface receptors dependent on random interactions with G proteins to trigger changes in cellular activity.

In this review, we consider the regulation of cellular localization and trafficking of the family of ARs. Because cellular trafficking appears to be inexorably linked to the activation of novel signaling pathways and the formation of signaling packages within the cell, we also include a discussion of these processes.

2. The β-Adrenergic Receptors

There are three known β-ARs: β_1, β_2, and β_3. Pharmacological evidence of a β_4-AR has been suggested; however, it now appears that the β_4-AR may actually be an ortholog of the β_1-AR *(3)*. Our knowledge of the cellular trafficking of the family of the β-ARs has been extensively reviewed in a number of excellent articles and thus is only briefly summarized here *(4–8)*. We then delve into the more recent and provocative findings regarding the regulation of cellular trafficking and signaling for the β-ARs.

2.1. Overview of β-AR Phosphorylation, Internalization, and Downregulation

Figure 2 is a diagrammatic representation of our understanding of the trafficking of the β-ARs and was adapted from similar figures *(4,6–8)*. Agonist activation of the β-AR results in breaking of intramolecular bonds within the receptor, allowing surfaces in the third intracellular loop and C-terminal tail to interact with the G protein heterotrimer promoting the exchange of guanosine 5′-diphosphate for guanosine 5′-triphosphage and the initiation of G protein-mediated cellular signaling. Also activated are a series of incompletely understood reactions and protein interactions that significantly affect receptor function as well as receptor cellular localization and signaling. Receptor desensitization and downregulation occur as a consequence of activating these regulatory pathways. *Receptor desensitization* refers to the phenomenon by which the receptor is less efficiently coupled to its cognate G protein(s). Receptor downregulation occurs when there is a decrease in the number of cell surface receptors.

β-AR activation results in the activation of specific protein kinases, which can in turn regulate receptor function *(4–8)*. For example, protein kinase A (PKA) phosphorylation reduces β-AR interactions with G_s proteins. Because PKA-mediated phosphorylation of the receptor is not occupancy dependent and can occur following activation of other GPCRs coupled to increases in cyclic adenosine 5′-monophosphate, this type of cross regulation is referred to as *heterologous desensitization*. The β-ARs are also phosphorylated by a unique family of protein kinases, the G protein-coupled receptor kinases (GRKs) *(4–6)*. Originally referred to as βARK (β-adrenergic receptor kinase), at least seven GRK family members have been identified. In contrast to PKA, GRK phosphorylation of receptors occurs only when the receptor is occupied with agonist. Thus, GRK-dependent phosphorylation allows for a much more specific form of desensitization, referred to as *homologous desensitization*.

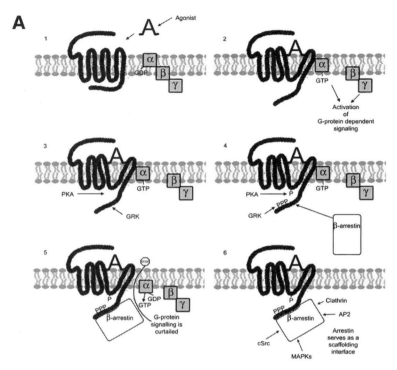

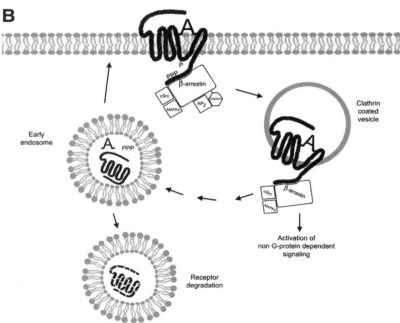

GRK-mediated phosphorylation of the β-AR promotes the binding of an arrestin molecule to the receptor. Arrestins are a family of regulatory proteins that bind to GPCRs following GRK-dependent phosphorylation *(4–6)*. Four arrestin family members have been identified *(5)*. Arrestin binding inhibits receptor–G protein interaction, further curtails G protein-mediated signaling, and initiates receptor internalization. Arrestins bind to clathrin and to the β-subunit of the clathrin adaptor protein AP2. This begins the assembly of clathrin-coated vesicles *(4–9)*. The nascent vesicles containing the ligand–receptor complex is pinched from the cell surface by the actions of dynamin. The internalized receptor–ligand complex is then transported to early endosomes, in which the low pH of the endosome causes the ligand to dissociate from the receptor. The acidic environment stimulates the dephosphorylation of the receptor by endosomal-associated phosphatases. Ligand dissociation and receptor dephosphorylation cause arrestins to dissociate from the receptor. Subsequently, the receptor can be recycled to the cell membrane, where it can be reinserted as a signaling competent receptor or be transported to late endosomes and then degraded in lysosomes.

2.2. Arrestin Scaffolds as Signaling Complexes

In addition to binding to the phosphorylated β-AR and restricting further G protein signaling, arrestins serve an intracellular scaffolding function. Engagement of the internalization/endocytotic machinery positions the β_2-AR–arrestin complex in discrete cellular locations in association with a diverse array of signaling proteins *(4–9)*. This localization is envisioned to allow for activation of a series of signals not based on G proteins. For example, it was recently shown that GRK forms a cytosolic complex with phosphoinositide-3 kinase (PI3K), and that activation of the β-AR recruits the GRK–PI3K complex to the cell membrane *(10)*. This results in both receptor phosphorylation by GRK and the phosphorylation of phosphoinositides by PI3K. PI3K-mediated phosphorylation of membrane phospholipids is involved in the recruitment of multiple endocytic proteins and may serve to enhance β-AR internalization.

Other data demonstrated that activation of the MAPK extracellular signal-regulated kinase 1/2 (ERK1/2) by the β_2-AR occurs as a result of engaging the endocytotic machinery *(11,12)*. These studies also showed that treatment of HEK-293 cells with isoproterenol induced an interaction between the tyrosine kinase Src and β-arrestin. The β-arrestin–Src complex is localized with AP2 and the nascent clathrin-coated pit. Using β-arrestin mutants unable to bind to clathrin inhibited β_2-AR-mediated activation of ERK1/2, indicating that arrestin-medi-

---

Fig. 2. *(Opposite page)* Agonist-mediated internalization, desensitization, and down-regulation of the β_2-AR.

ated formation of β_2-AR complexes is important for activation of certain signaling pathways. Further, Fan and associates *(13)* demonstrated that GRK-dependent phosphorylation of the β_2-AR is enhanced by Src. These authors postulated that association of Scr with β_2-AR promotes GRK activation and β_2-AR desensitization. Together, these data indicate that the formation of multiprotein complexes regulates receptor internalization and desensitization as well as the activation of specific signaling pathways.

2.3. β-AR Regulatory Activities
Resulting From Novel Protein Interactions

As discussed in Sections 2.1. and 2.2., β_2-AR interactions with novel binding proteins could have profound effects on β-AR signaling (*see also* Chapter 3). Of particular interest are PDZ proteins that interact with C-terminus of the β_2-AR and the localization of β_2-AR to cell surface microdomains, such as caveolae.

2.3.1. β-AR–PDZ Protein Interaction

PDZ-binding domains are binding cassettes contained within a discrete set of regulatory proteins thought to be vital in the targeting and assembly of protein complexes *(14)*. The interaction between a PDZ protein and the target interacting protein is thought to result in the anchoring of proteins to a particular cellular domain as well as the construction of signaling scaffolds. Both the β_1-AR and β_2-AR contain PDZ domains in the last several amino acids in the C-terminal tail. The PDZ-binding sequence in the β_2-AR is SDSLL; in the β_1-AR, the sequence is SESKV *(15)*. Evidence has shown that the interaction of PDZ sequences in the β-ARs with PDZ-binding proteins can profoundly affect the cellular trafficking of these receptors.

One example of a PDZ-binding protein that interacts with the β-ARs is the ezrin-radixin-moesin (ERM)-binding phosphoprotein-50 (EBP50), which is also known as NHERF (Na$^+$/H$^+$ exchange regulatory factor). Cao and associates *(16)* demonstrated that the rapid recycling of β_2-AR from early endosomes back to the cell surface is dependent on the receptor interaction with EBP50. By mutating a serine in the PDZ-binding motif of the β_2-AR, the authors were able to disrupt interaction of the receptor with EBP50. The mutated receptor was rapidly internalized. However, unlike the wild-type receptor, the alanine-containing mutant was transported to lysosomes and degraded. In addition, these investigators demonstrated that the mutated serine residue (S411) could be phosphorylated by GRK5, and that this phosphorylation promoted the rapid lysosomal degradation of the β_2-AR. Because phosphorylation of this serine is not necessary for the β-arrestin binding, the authors concluded that this regulatory effect of GRK5 is independent of the arrestin-based internalization pathway. Overall, these results support the conclusion that EBP50 plays a vital role in the rapid recycling of the β_2-AR to the cell surface via a PDZ domain-dependant interaction, and that this interaction might be modified by receptor phosphorylation *(16,17)*.

In addition to EBP50, in vitro data demonstrated interactions between the β-ARs and other PDZ-binding proteins. For example, Hu et al. *(15,18)* demonstrated an interaction between the C-terminal-binding domain of the β_1-AR and PSD-95, resulting in a decrease in receptor internalization. PSD-95 contains multiple PDZ domains and has been shown to complex with the N-methyl-D-aspartate receptor *(19)* and the Kv 1.4 potassium channel *(20)*. Phosphorylation of serine in the terminal SESKV sequence by GRK5 blocks the association of the β_1-AR with PSD-95, resulting in increased receptor internalization. In addition, Xu and coworkers *(21)* showed that MAGI-2 (membrane-associated guanylate kinase inverted-2; also known as S-SCAM for synaptic scaffolding molecule) binds to the PDZ domain of the β_1-AR and enhances the internalization of the β_1-AR. Thus, PSD-95 and MAGI-2 have reciprocal effects on β_1-AR internalization.

The interaction between the β-AR and PDZ proteins can significantly affect the physiological response of the receptor to agonist activation. For example, Xiang et al. *(22)* used cardiomyocytes cultured from the hearts of a β_1-/β_2-AR double-knockout line of mice to show that the effect of agonist activation on contractile rate depended on the subtype of β-AR transfected into the cardiomyocytes. Transfection of β_2-AR resulted in a brief increase in contractile rate followed by a more sustained period of negative chronotropy. The period of negative chronotropy depended on G_i activation and receptor internalization *(22)*. In contrast, transfection with the β_1-AR only increased the contractile rate. However, transfection with a β_1-AR receptor containing a mutated PDZ interaction sequence incapable of interacting with PSD-95 resulted in a biphasic effect to agonist that was similar to that seen following transfection of the wild-type β_2-AR. The β_2-AR does not interact with the PSD-95; therefore, this type of regulatory activity does not occur for this receptor.

Although the PDZ domain of the β_2-AR does not couple to the PSD-95, there is evidence for a physiological role of other PDZ-binding proteins in regulating β_2-AR function. In particular, Xiang et al. *(23)* and Kobilka *(9)* showed that the specific interaction between the β_2-AR and EBP50 affects the signaling of this subtype. Agonist treatment of cardiomyocytes isolated from the β_1/β_2-AR double-knockout mice transfected with the wild-type β_2-AR resulted in the expected biphasic effect on contractile rate (*see* above). In contrast, expression of a β_2-AR in which the last three C-terminal amino acids were mutated to alanines significantly increased the initial positive chronotrophic effect but did not enhance the subsequent negative effects on contractile rate. The authors concluded that disrupting the interaction between the β_2-AR and EBP50 inhibited receptor recy-

cling after agonist-induced internalization, thus preventing its ability to couple
to G_i and produce negative chronotrophic effect. The authors could not rule out
the possibility that other proteins bind to the C-terminus of the receptor, such as
the membrane fusion regulatory protein N-ethylmaleimide-sensitive factor (NSF)
(17), and have a similar effect on the rapid recycling of the receptor to the cell
surface.

Although not completely understood, the role of the interaction between the
β-ARs and these novel binding partners could be to regulate the recycling and
degrading of the β-AR independent of the arrestin/clathrin pathways. As depicted
in Fig. 3, the interaction with proteins like EBP50, NSF, PSD-95, and MAGI-2
could circumvent the clathrin-coated pit pathway and target the receptor for
continued residence near the cell surface (PSD-95), rapid internalization and
recycling (EBP50, NSF), or rapid receptor degradation (MAGI-2). Furthermore,
the differential ability of these proteins to interact with the $β_1$- and $β_2$-AR suggests
a further level of complexity in the regulatory activity of the β-AR.

2.3.2. β-AR–Caveolae Interactions

Caveolae are membrane structures that serve multiple regulatory functions
(24,25). However, there is still a great deal unknown regarding the regulatory
activity of these membrane domains (24,25). Several groups have shown that the
$β_1$-AR is predominantly localized to caveolae, whereas only a small fraction of
the $β_2$-AR is localized in caveolae (24,25). Agonist activation disrupts the caveolar localization of the $β_2$-AR. This divergence in caveolar localization behavior is thought to contribute to the noted differences in the regulatory activities
between these receptors. For example, neonatal myocytes cultured from $β_1$-AR
and $β_2$-AR double-knockout mice were transfected with either receptor, and the
effect on contractile rate was studied (26). Disruption of the caveolar localization
of the $β_2$-AR with filipin converted the biphasic effect (see above), with an
increase in rate followed by a decrease in contractile rate to a prolonged monophasic (26). In contrast, filipin had no effect on the $β_1$-AR response. These authors
concluded that the caveolar localization of the $β_2$-AR is essential for its typical
signaling properties.

Rapacciuolo et al. (27) demonstrated that, following agonist activation, the
$β_1$-AR can undergo both caveolar-mediated as well as clathrin-mediated internalization. Indeed, these authors showed that both internalization pathways make
an approximately equal contribution to $β_1$-AR internalization. These authors
further showed that the nature of the protein kinase that phosphorylated the
receptor determined its internalization fate. For example, PKA-mediated phosphorylation of the $β_1$-AR resulted in internalization via the caveolae pathway. In
contrast, GRK phosphorylation led to the expected arrestin/clathrin internalization pathway.

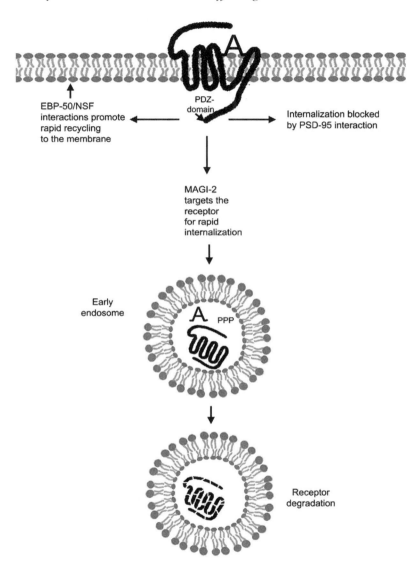

Fig. 3. Effect of novel binding proteins on the intracellular localization and trafficking properties of the β-ARs.

2.4. Summary

Figure 1 presents a model in which receptor activation is envisioned as linear and highly dependent on random collisions between receptor and G protein. It is apparent that signaling is not that of an elementary or capricious event. Indeed, the internalization scheme presented in Fig. 2 is also too simplistic to account for recent observations. It seems clear that receptor activation of signaling does not take place only on the cell surface and that receptor internalization is not only involved in signal inactivation. Rather, the signaling and internalization pathways converge. This is illustrated in part in Fig. 2, which shows how clathrin-mediated internalization can trigger non-GPCR signaling. However, newly discovered receptor–protein complexes argue for a far more complicated relationship between internalization and signaling. For example, PDZ-type interactions could "short circuit" the clathrin internalization pathway and "fast track" receptor resensitization and reinsertion into the cell membrane.

3. The α_1-Adrenergic Receptors

Three α_1-ARs (α_{1A}, α_{1B}, and α_{1D}) have been isolated, cloned, and characterized *(1,2)*. Similar to the observations made with the β-ARs, the cellular localization and trafficking properties of the three α_1-ARs do not conform to the dogmatic thinking regarding GPCRs.

3.1. The Cellular Localization of the α_1-ARs

Using a peptide antibody that specifically recognizes a sequence in the C-terminus of the α_{1B}-AR, Fonseca et al. *(28)* showed that the α_{1B}-AR stably transfected in HEK-293 cells is localized predominantly on the cell membrane. Similarly, an α_{1B}-AR/green fluorescent protein (GFP) fusion protein transiently transfected into COS-7 cells was primarily localized to the cell membrane *(29)*. In contrast, an α_{1A}-AR/GFP construct was localized in intracellular compartments. Intracellular α_{1A}-AR expression was confirmed using antibodies directed against a FLAG-tagged epitope inserted into the α_{1A}-AR *(29)*. Commercially available peptide antibodies that recognize the C-terminus of the α_1-AR subtypes (Santa Cruz Biotech. Santa Cruz, CA) were used to localize these receptors in stably transfected Rat1 fibroblasts *(30,31)*. Using this approach, the α_{1B}-AR was detected mainly on the cell surface, consistent with previous observations. These authors also noted that although a portion of the α_{1A}-ARs was expressed intracellularly, a significant cell surface population could be observed *(29)*. Surprisingly, the α_{1D}-AR was predominantly localized intracellularly in a perinuclear endosomal compartment *(30,31)*. Overexpression of wild-type β-arrestin or the dominant negative form of arrestin had no effect on the intracellular expression of the α_{1D}-AR *(32)*. Similar localization patterns were obtained using α_1-AR/GFP fusion proteins transfected into HEK-293 cells *(32,33)*. Together, data obtained using heterologous expression systems indicate a high degree of subtype-specific regulation of cellular localization.

It is highly relevant to show that the differential cellular localization of the three α_1-ARs occurs in cells that natively express these receptors. The difficulty

**A Alpha1B-AR/GFP
adenovirus**   **B Alpha1D-AR/GFP
adenovirus**

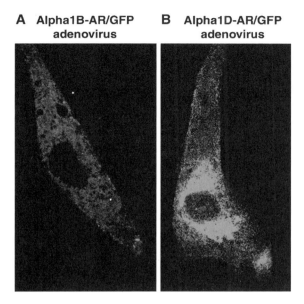

Fig. 4. Confocal imaging of human aortic smooth muscle cells transfected with an adenovirus containing either (**A**) the α_{1B}-AR or (**B**) α_{1D}-AR. To facilitate imaging, each receptor was expressed as a fusion protein with GFP. *See* Color Plate 1 following p. 148.

with studying natively expressing cells such as vascular smooth muscle cells or cardiomyocytes is that these cells are difficult to transfect with conventional methods and the available antibodies have only limited potency, making detection of endogenous receptor difficult. The intracellular expression of the α_1-ARs in vascular smooth muscle was observed in a unique series of studies using BODIPY-FL-labeled prazosin to image α_1-AR subtypes in cultured prostate smooth muscle cells *(34)*. These authors noted intracellular expression for each of the three subtypes and estimated that, in smooth muscle cells, 40% of the total α_1-AR population is expressed intracellularly.

We developed adenoviral constructs of the human α_{1B}-AR and the α_{1D}-AR coupled with GFP. These constructs infected human aortic smooth muscle cells (Cascade Biologics, Portland, OR) with approx 70% efficiency *(35)*. Confocal images of infected cells (Fig. 4; *see* Color Plate 1 following p. 148.) show that the α_{1B}-AR/GFP is primarily expressed on the cell surface of vascular smooth muscle cells, although some cytoplasmic expression is also observed. This localization pattern agrees with the work of MacKenzie et al. *(34)*.

The basal intracellular localization of the α_{1D}-AR was also examined using adenoviral-mediated transfer into human aortic smooth muscle cells (*see* Fig. 4 and Color Plate 1 following p. 148). In agreement with studies from heterologous expression systems, we observed that a significant portion of the α_{1D}-ARs were located in intracellular compartments. In addition to the expected intracellular localization, we noted cell surface expression of this receptor. Why the α_{1D}-AR is expressed predominantly intracellularly is not understood. Numerous reports indicated that this receptor is consititutively active (31,36,37). This constitutive activity could account for the intracellular localization by promoting continuous endocytosis from the cell membrane to the intracellular space. Studies using receptor constructs indicated that amino acids 1–79 of the extracellular N-terminus of the α_{1D}-AR contain a sequence(s) that regulates cell surface localization (38,39). Deleting this sequence greatly increased the cell surface expression of the α_{1D}-AR, whereas replacing analogous regions of either the α_{1A}- or the α_{1B}-AR with the 1–79 sequence of the α_{1D}-AR significantly decreased expression of these receptors.

Although these experiments with adenoviral transfer of the human α_{1B}- and α_{1D}-ARs receptors into human cells are preliminary, they do suggest that there may be differences in α_1-AR expression in human cells when compared to heterologous systems. The α_{1D}-AR may be expressed on the cell surface to a greater degree in human cells, and the α_{1B}-AR is expressed in intracellular compartments.

3.2. Agonist-Mediated Phosphorylation, Internalization, and Desensitization of the α_1-ARs

Our understanding of the phosphorylation, internalization, and desensitization of the α_1-ARs is not nearly as well developed as for the β-ARs. Critical aspects related to these phenomena have been reviewed (40–42). For example, Diviani et al. (43) observed that serines 404, 408, and 410 in the α_{1B}-AR were phosphorylated by GRK following stimulation with epinephrine. These same serines along with serines 394 and 400 were also phosphorylated following treatment with phorbol ester, indicating that they are also protein kinase C (PKC) sites in the α_{1B}-AR (44).

Agonist-mediated internalization of the α_{1B}-AR was initially described in the 1980s (45,46). More recently, Fonseca et al. (28) used immunocytochemistry to show that the α_{1B}-AR is internalized in an agonist-dependent manner to compartments also containing the transferrin receptor. Additional studies by Wang et al. (47) identified subdomains of the C-terminus of the α_{1B}-AR that were essential for receptor internalization and downregulation. Truncation of the receptor after amino acid 366 yielded an α_{1B}-AR that could neither be internalized nor downregulated. Deletion studies have shown that internalization and downregulation of the α_{1B}-AR are regulated by different sequences in the C-terminus (47).

In addition to requiring GRK-mediated phosphorylation, Diviani et al. (48) noted that the α_{1B}-AR internalized in an arrestin-dependent manner. This conclusion was supported by the work of Chalothorn and associates *(33)*, demonstrating that overexpression of a dominant negative form of arrestin completely blocked α_{1B}-AR internalization. Consistent with other internalization studies, an intact C-terminus was necessary for interaction of α_{1B}-AR with arrestin *(49)*.

In contrast to the α_{1B}-AR, much less is known about the phosphorylation, internalization, and desensitization properties of the other α_1-ARs. The α_{1A}-AR is phosphorylated following agonist activation, although not to the same extent as the α_{1B}-AR *(50)*. As predicted from the relative extent of phosphorylation, the α_{1B}-AR was desensitized to a greater degree than was the α_{1A}-AR. Chalothorn et al. *(33)* compared agonist-mediated receptor internalization of the α_{1B}- and α_{1A}-AR/GFPs in living transiently transfected HEK-293 cells. The α_{1B}-AR is rapidly internalized with a significant intracellular signal observed within 5 min. On the other hand, the α_{1A}-AR was internalized at a much slower rate, with 30 min to 1 h required to observe significant receptor internalization *(33)*. Like the α_{1B}-AR, internalization of the α_{1A}-AR receptor was blocked by cotransfection with a dominant negative form of arrestin *(33)*. Together, these data suggest that α_{1A}-AR and α_{1B}-AR are differentially phosphorylated and desensitized following agonist treatment.

Inserting the C-terminus of the α_{1B}-AR into the α_{1A}-AR resulted in a receptor chimera that was more extensively phosphorylated and desensitized than the wild-type α_{1A}-AR *(50)*. These results indicate that C-terminal sequences control the phosphorylation and desensitization of the α_1-ARs. Price et al. *(51)* demonstrated that the α_{1A}-AR was internalized and desensitized in an apparent GRK2-dependent manner. In contrast to the results with α_{1B}-AR or those obtained by Vazquez-Prado et al. *(50)*, Price et al. *(51)* showed that neither agonist-mediated internalization nor desensitization of the α_{1A}-AR was dependent on sequences in the C-terminal tail.

Probably the least well studied of the α_1-ARs in terms of phosphorylation, desensitization, or internalization is the α_{1D}-AR. No internalization of those α_{1D}-ARs expressed on the cell surface has been observed *(31,32)*. Yang and coworkers *(52)* used stably transfected fibroblasts to show that the increase in inositol phosphates mediated by the α_{1A}- and α_{1B}-ARs could be desensitized; the increase mediated by the α_{1D}-AR was refractory to agonist-mediated desensitization. In contrast to these results, Garcia-Sainz et al. *(53)* used stably transfected fibroblasts to show that the α_{1D}-AR could be phosphorylated and desensitized following exposure to norepinephrine. Thus, desensitization of the α_{1D}-AR is very different from that of the other α_1-ARs.

3.3. Summary

Our understanding of the cellular trafficking properties of the α_1-AR subtypes is not nearly as refined as for the β-ARs. We also do not know if these receptors internalize using analogous protein pathways and binding partners as do the β-ARs or if novel α_1-AR/protein interactions contribute to non-G protein-based signaling. We do know that these receptors are phosphorylated and internalized in an arrestin-dependent manner. It has also been demonstrated that following internalization, both the α_{1A}- and α_{1B}-ARs can be found co-localized with β-arrestin *(32)*. In addition, Diviani et al. *(54)* noted a direct interaction between the μ_2 of the AP2 complex and the α_{1B}-AR. Interestingly, the AP2 complex usually interacts with GPCRs via arrestins. Therefore, in addition to the regulated interaction with the AP2 complex via arrestins, the α_{1B}-AR could internalize via direct interaction with AP2. Also not clear is whether the association of α_1-AR with arrestins and their subsequent internalization can trigger non-G protein signaling as it does for the β-ARs. Such a possibility was suggested by Alcantara-Hernandez et al. *(55)*, who noted that a novel association between PKC and the α_{1B}-AR forms following agonist activation may participate in receptor desensitization. Another interaction that is poorly described relates to the caveolar localization of α_1-ARs. Fujita et al. *(56)* found that α_1-ARs were localized in caveolae. Subsequently, it was noted that the α_{1B}-AR subtype could be localized to a caveolar subdomain *(57)*.

It is tempting to speculate that the cellular trafficking properties of the α_1-ARs will be similar to those observed for the β-AR system. Although the overall trafficking and regulatory patterns are similar, each of the adrenergic receptor subtypes has shown a tendency to develop distinctly unique avenues of regulatory activities. Therefore, it would not be much of a surprise if we find that the trafficking patterns of the α_1-ARs are different in significant ways from those observed for the β-AR.

4. The α_2-Adrenergic Receptors

4.1. Cellular Localization of the α_2-AR

Similar to the α_1-ARs, our knowledge of the cellular trafficking properties of the α_2-AR family is not as nearly refined as that for the β-ARs. Three α_2-ARs (α_{2A}, α_{2B}, and α_{2C}) have been isolated, cloned, and characterized. An overview of the nature of the α_2-AR subtypes, their localization, and their cellular trafficking properties has been published *(58)*. Reminiscent of the α_1-ARs, subtypes of the α_2-ARs are differentially localized within the cell. Indeed, results from studies conducted with polarized Madin-Darby canine kidney cells showed that the α_2-ARs are selectively expressed on the basolateral surface (exposed to the blood) as opposed to the apical aspect (exposed to urine) of these renal cells *(59,60)*. In investigating the mechanism for this differential localization, Wozniak and Limbird *(60)* noted that α_{2A}-AR is inserted directly and selectively into the basolateral membrane. The targeting of this receptor to the basolateral aspect is determined by a sequence as yet poorly defined near the lipid–α_{2A}-AR interface;

the retention at the basolateral surface is dependent on sequences in the third intracellular loop *(61)*. In contrast to the adenosine A_1-receptor, which requires microtubules for selective basolateral expression, the basolateral expression of both α_{2B}- and α_{2C}-ARs is achieved by differences in receptor half-lives. Initially, both α_{2B}- and α_{2C}-ARs are expressed equally on the basolateral and apical membranes. However, as a result of specific sequences in the third intracellular loop, both α_{2B}- and α_{2C}-ARs have much longer half-lives for retention on the basolateral surface when compared to the apical aspect of the membrane *(60,62)*. Because of the more rapid loss from the apical membrane, a selective basolateral localization for the α_{2B}- and α_{2C}-ARs is achieved.

Evidence has suggested that interactions between the third intracellular loop of the α_2-ARs and spinophilin, a multidomain protein thought to be involved in the assembly of protein complexes, may contribute to the selective basolateral localization of these receptors *(63,64)*. Brady et al. *(64)* also demonstrated that, in embryo fibroblasts from spinophilin null mice, the α_{2B}-AR internalized at a much faster rate than that observed in fibroblasts from wild-type mice. These results suggest that, like PSD-95 or NSF interactions with the β-AR, novel protein interactions with the α_2-AR family can affect receptor distribution and agonist-mediated internalization. In addition to the cell surface expression, the α_{2C}-AR is localized in intracellular compartments such as the endoplasmic reticulum and the Golgi *(60,65)*.

4.2. Agonist-Mediated Internalization, Phosphorylation, and Desensitization of the α_2-ARs

Internalization of the α_{2B}-AR subtypes has been extensively studied in heterologous systems. These data have consistently shown that this receptor is rapidly internalized following agonist activation *(65–69)*. DeGraff et al. *(70)* demonstrated that the internalization of the α_{2B}-AR in transiently transfected COS-1 cells could be enhanced by overexpressing either β-arrestin-1 or -2. Conversely, the internalization could be blocked by cotransfection with a dominant negative form of dynamin *(70)*. Olli-Lahdesmaki et al. *(71)* demonstrated that α_{2B}-AR endocytosis could be blocked by treatment with hyperosmotic sucrose, indicating that this receptor internalized in a clathrin-dependent manner. Together, these data suggest that a pathway involving arrestin coupling of the receptor and clathrin internalizes the α_{2B}-AR.

Data with the α_{2A}-AR are more controversial. In stably transfected CHO cells, Eason and Liggett *(66,67)* noted that the α_{2A}-AR could be internalized following agonist activation. In contrast, in transfected HEK-293 cells, α_{2A}-AR internalization was not observed *(65,71)*. Despite the demonstration that the α_{2A}-AR binds arrestin, internalization of the α_{2A}-AR could only be marginally enhanced by arrestin overexpression *(70,72,73)*. Furthermore, in contrast to the α_{2B}-AR, α_{2A}-

AR endocytocsis was only partially blocked by inhibiting clathrin-coated pit endocytosis with hyperosmotic sucrose. A complete blockade of internalization was accomplished by treatment with filipin, an agent that inhibits caveolae-mediated internalization. These data suggest that the α_{2A}-AR is internalized via both clathrin- and caveolae-mediated pathways and could account for the observations of DeGraff et al. *(70)* that noted only a modest effect of arrestin overexpression on α_{2A}-AR endocytosis.

Both the α_{2A}- and α_{2B}-ARs have been shown to undergo agonist-mediated phosphorylation and desensitization *(66,67)*. Jewell-Motz and Liggett *(74)* showed that an acidic environment within the C-terminus (amino acids 294–309) was necessary for the GRK-dependent phosphorylation and agonist-mediated desensitization of the α_{2B}-AR. Similarly, an EESSSS motif in the C-terminus of the α_{2A}-AR was found to be critical for the GRK-dependent phosphorylation and agonist-mediated desensitization of this receptor. Liang et al. *(75)* demonstrated that PKC could also phosphorylate the α_{2A}-AR. Mutation of serine 360 resulted in a significant decrease in PKC phosphorylation and agonist-dependent desensitization. Therefore, pathways independent of GRK can desensitize the α_{2A}-AR. Another novel desensitization pathway involving the α_{2A}-AR was found by Bawa et al. *(76)*. These workers noted that treatment of BE (2)-C human neuroblastoma cells with epinephrine resulted in α_{2A}-AR desensitization that was mediated by GRK3, and α_{2A}-AR downregulation was produced as a consequence of activating β_2-AR. Eason and associates *(77)* showed that a palmitoylated cysteine in the C-terminus was necessary for agonist-mediated desensitization of the human α_{2A}-AR. This residue is missing in the human α_{2C}-AR.

Results of studies with the human α_{2C}-AR indicate that this receptor neither phosphorylated nor desensitized following agonist activation *(66,67)*. In contrast, work from Bylund's laboratory showed that the opossum α_{2C}-AR is phosphorylated by GRK and undergoes agonist-dependent desensitization *(69,78)*. Deupree and coworkers *(78)* then demonstrated that the opossum receptor contains the sequence EESTSE. This sequence is also contained within the α_{2A}-AR and is phosphorylated by GRK. The human α_{2C}-AR contains DESSAAAAE, suggesting that hydroxyl amino acids in an acidic environment were necessary for the receptor to undergo GRK-mediated phosphorylation.

4.3. Perspective

Like the α_1-ARs, the α_2-AR family has unique localization and cellular trafficking properties. Both receptor families have a subtype that is localized to intracellular compartments. Whether this intracellular localization has functional consequences or is an artifact of the methods used to localize these receptors is not known. Unknown also is whether the α_2-AR participates in the activation of non-G protein-dependent signaling pathways. However, we do know that activation of ERK1/2 by the α_2-AR does not depend on receptor internalization *(68,70)*. Whether the α_2-AR can be regulated by interactions with novel binding partners such as PSD-95, NSF, or MAGI-2 is unknown.

References

1. Piascik MT, Perez DM. α_1-Adrenergic receptors: new insights and directions. J Pharmacol Exp Ther 2001;298:403–410.
2. Zhong H, Minneman KP. α_1-Adrenoceptor subtypes. Eur J Pharmacol 1999;375: 261–276.
3. Kaumann AJ, Engelhardt S, Hein L, Molenaar P, Lohse M. Abolition of (–)-CGP 12177-evoked cardiostimulation in double β_1/β_2-adrenoceptor knockout mice. Obligatory role of β_1-adrenoceptors for putative β_4-adrenoceptor pharmacology. Naunyn Schmiedebergs Arch Pharmacol 2001;363:87–93.
4. Claing A, Laporte SA, Caron MG, Lefkowitz R. Endocytosis of G protein-coupled receptors: roles of G protein-coupled receptor kinases and β-arrestin proteins. Prog Neurobiol 2002;66:61–79.
5. Krupnick JG, Benovic JL. The role of receptor kinases and arrestins in G protein-coupled receptor regulation. Annu Rev Pharmacol Toxicol 1998;38:289–319.
6. Pierce KL, Premont RT, Lefkowitz RJ. Seven-transmembrane receptors. Nat Rev Mol Cell Biol 2002;3:639–650.
7. Luttrell LM. G protein-coupled receptor signalling in neuroendocrine systems. J Mol Endocrinol 2003;30:117–126.
8. Sorkin A, Zastrow M. Signal transduction and endocytosis: close encounters of many kinds. Nature 2002;3:600–613.
9. Kobilka BK. Agonist-induced conformational changes in the β_2 adrenergic receptor. J Pept Res 2002;60:317–321.
10. Naga Prasad SV, Laporte SA, Chamberlain D, Caron MG, Barak L, Rockman HA. Phosphoinositide 3-kinase regulates β_2-adrenergic receptor endocytosis by AP-2 recruitment to the receptor/β-arrestin complex. J Cell Biol 2002;158:563–575.
11. Daaka Y, Luttrell LM, Lefkowitz RJ. Switching of the coupling of the β_2-adrenergic receptor to different G proteins by protein kinase A. Nature 1997;390:88–91.
12. Luttrell LM, Ferguson SS, Daaka Y, et al. β-Arrestin-dependent formation of β_2 adrenergic receptor-Src protein kinase complexes. Science 1999;283:655–661.
13. Fan G, Shumay E, Malbon CC, Wang H. c-Src tyrosine kinase binds the β_2-adrenergic receptor via phospho-Tyr-350, phosphorylates G-protein-linked receptor kinase 2, and mediates agonist-induced receptor desensitization. J Biol Chem 2001;276:13,240–13,247.
14. Hung A, Sheng M. PDZ domains: structural modules for protein complex assembly. J Biol Chem 2002;277:5699–5702.
15. Hu LA, Chen W, Premont RT, Cong M, Lefkowitz RJ. G protein-coupled receptor kinase 5 regulates β_1-adrenergic receptor association with PSD-95. J Biol Chem 2002;277:1607–1613.
16. Cao TT, Deacon HW, Reczek D, Bretscher A, von Zastrow M. A kinase-regulated PDZ-domain interaction controls endocytic sorting of the β_2-adrenergic receptor. Nature 1999;401:286–290.

17. Cong M, Perry SJ, Hu LA, Hanson PI, Claing A, Lefkowitz RJ. Binding of the β_2 receptor to n-ethylmaleimide-sensitive factor regulates receptor recycling. J Biol Chem 2001;276:45,145–45,152.

18. Hu LA, Tang Y, Miller WE, et al. β_1-Adrenergic receptor association with PSD-95. Inhibition of receptor internalization and facilitation of β_1-adrenergic receptor interaction with N-methyl-D-aspartate receptors. J Biol Chem 2000;275:38,659–38,666.

19. Christopherson KS, Hillier BJ, Lim WA, Bredt DS. PSD-95 assembles a ternary complex with the N-methyl-D-aspartic acid receptor and a bivalent neuronal NO synthase PDZ domain. J Biol Chem 1999;274:27,467–27,473.

20. Imamura F, Maeda S, Doi T, Fujiyoshi Y. Ligand binding of the second PDZ domain regulates clustering of PSD-95 with the Kv1.4 potassium channel. J Biol Chem 2002;277:3640–3646.

21. Xu J, Paquet M, Lau AG, Wood JD, Ross CA, Hall RA. β_1-Adrenergic receptor association with the synaptic scaffolding protein membrane-associated guanylate kinase inverted-2 (MAGI-2). J Biol Chem 2001;276:41,310–41,317.

22. Xiang Y, Devic E, Kobilka B. The PDZ binding motif of the β_1 adrenergic receptor modulates receptor trafficking and signaling in cardiac myocytes. J Biol Chem 2002;277:33,783–33,790.

23. Xiang Y, Kobilka B. The PDZ-binding motif of the β_2-adrenoceptor is essential for physiologic signaling and trafficking in cardiac myocytes. Proc Natl Acad Sci USA 2003;100:10,776–10,781.

24. Razani B, Woodman SE, Lisanti MP. Caveolae: from cell biology to animal physiology. Pharmacol Rev 2002;54:431–467.

25. Hnasko R, Lisanti MP. The biology of caveolae: lessons from caveolin knockout mice and implications for human disease. Mol Interventions 2003;3:445–456.

26. Xiang Y, Rybin VO, Steinberg SF, Kobilka B. Caveolar localization dictates physiologic signaling of β_2-adrenoceptors in neonatal cardiac myocytes. J Biol Chem 2002;277:34,280–34,286.

27. Rapacciuolo A, Suvarna S, Barki-Harrington L, et al. Protein kinase A and G protein-coupled receptor kinase phosphorylation mediates β_1 adrenergic receptor endocytosis through different pathways. J Biol Chem 2003;278:35,403–35,411.

28. Fonseca MI, Button DC, Brown RD. Agonist regulation of α_{1B}-adrenergic receptor subcellular distribution and function. J Biol Chem 1995;270:8902–8909.

29. Hirasawa A, Sugawara T, Awaji T, Tsumaya K, Ito H, Tsujimoto G. Subtype-specific differences in subcellular localization of α_1-adrenoceptors: chlorethylclonidine preferentially alkylates the accessible cell surface α_1-adrenoceptors irrespective of the subtype. Mol Pharmacol 1997;52:764–770.

30. Hrometz SL, Edelmann SE, McCune DF, et al. Expression of multiple α_1-adrenoceptors on vascular smooth muscle: correlation with the regulation of contraction. J Pharmacol Exp Ther 1999;290:452–463.

31. McCune DF, Edelmann SE, Olges JR, et al. Regulation of the cellular localization and signaling properties of the α_{1B}- and α_{1D}-adrenoceptors by agonists and inverse agonists. Mol Pharmacol 2000;57:659–666.

32. Chalothorn D, McCune DF, Edelmann SE, Garcia-Cazarin ML, Tsujimoto G, Piascik MT. Differences in the cellular localization and agonist-mediated internal-

izization properties of the α_1-adrenoceptor subtypes. Mol Pharmacol 2002;61:1008–1016.

33. Chalothorn D, McCune DF, Edelmann SE, et al. Differential cardiovascular regulatory activities of the α_{1B}- and α_{1D}-adrenoceptor subtypes. J Pharmacol Exp Ther 2003;305:1045–1053.

34. Mackenzie JF, Daly CJ, Pediani JD, McGrath JC. Quantitative imaging in live human cells reveals intracellular α_1-adrenoceptor ligand-binding sites. J Pharmacol Exp Ther 2000;294:434–443.

35. Garcia-Cazarin ML, Edelmann SE, Smith J, Kraner SD, Piascik MT. Construction of adenoviral vectors expressing the α_1-adrenoceptors for the efficient transfection of vascular smooth muscle cells. FASEB J 2004;18:5401.

36. Garcia-Sainz JA, Torres-Padilla ME. Modulation of basal intracellular calcium by inverse agonists and phorbol myristate acetate in rat-1 fibroblasts stably expressing α_{1d}-adrenoceptors. FEBS Lett 1999;443:277–281.

37. Gisbert R, Noguera MA, Ivorra MD, D'Ocon P. Functional evidence of a constitutively active population of α_{1D}-adrenoceptors in rat aorta. J Pharmacol Exp Ther 2000;295:810–817.

38. Pupo AS, Uberti MA, Minneman KP. N-terminal truncation of human α_{1D}-adrenoceptors increases expression of binding sites but not protein. Eur J Pharmacol 2003;462:1–8.

39. Hague C, Chen Z, Pupo AS, Schulte N, Toews ML, Minneman K. The N-terminus of the human α_{1D}-adrenergic receptor prevents cell surface expression. J Pharmacol Exp Ther 2004;309:388–397.

40. Garcia-Sainz JA, Vazquez-Prado J, del Carmen Medina L. α_1-Adrenoceptors: function and phosphorylation. Eur J Pharmacol 2000;389:1–12.

41. Cotecchia S, Bjorklof K, Rossier O, Stanasila L, Greasley P, Fanelli F. The α_{1b}-adrenergic receptor subtype: molecular properties and physiological implications. J Recept Signal Transduct Res 2002;22:1–16.

42. Toews ML, Prinster SC, Schulte NA. Regulation of α_{1B} adrenergic receptor localization, trafficking, function, and stability. Life Sci 2003;74:379–389.

43. Diviani D, Lattion AL, Cotecchia S. Characterization of the phosphorylation sites involved in G protein-coupled receptor kinase- and protein kinase C-mediated desensitization of the α_{1B}-adrenergic receptor. J Biol Chem 1997;272:28,712–28,719.

44. Iacovelli L, Franchetti R, Grisolia D, De Blasi A. Selective regulation of G protein-coupled receptor-mediated signaling by G protein-coupled receptor kinase 2 in FRTL-5 cells: analysis of thyrotropin, α_{1B}-adrenergic, and A1 adenosine receptor-mediated responses. Mol Pharmacol 1999;56:316–324.

45. Leeb-Lundberg LM, Cotecchia S, DeBlasi A, Caron MG, Lefkowitz RJ. Regulation of adrenergic receptor function by phosphorylation. I. Agonist-promoted desensitization and phosphorylation of α_1-adrenergic receptors coupled to inositol phospholipid metabolism in DDT1 MF-2 smooth muscle cells. J Biol Chem 1987; 262:3098–3105.

46. Cowlen MS, Toews ML. Evidence for α_1-adrenergic receptor internalization in DDT1 MF-2 cells following exposure to agonists plus protein kinase C activators. Mol Pharmacol 1988;34:340–346.

47. Wang J, Wang L, Zheng J, Anderson JL, Toews ML. Identification of distinct carboxyl-terminal domains mediating internalization and down-regulation of the hamster α_{1B}-adrenergic receptor. Mol Pharmacol 2000;57:687–694.
48. Diviani D, Lattion AL, Larbi N, et al. Effect of different G protein-coupled receptor kinases on phosphorylation and desensitization of the α_{1B}-adrenergic receptor. J Biol Chem 1996;271:5049–5058.
49. Mhaouty-Kodja S, Barak LS, Scheer A, et al. Constitutively active α_{1b} adrenergic receptor mutants display different phosphorylation and internalization features. Mol Pharmacol 1999;55:339–347.
50. Vazquez-Prado J, Medina LC, Romero-Avila MT, Gonzalez-Espinosa C, Garcia-Sainz JA. Norepinephrine- and phorbol ester-induced phosphorylation of α_{1a}-adrenergic receptors. Functional aspects. J Biol Chem 2000;275:6553–6559.
51. Price RR, Morris DP, Biswas G, Smith MP, Schwinn DA. Acute agonist-mediated desensitization of the human α_{1a}-adrenergic receptor is primarily independent of carboxyl terminus regulation. Implications for regulation of α_{1a} AR splice variants. J Biol Chem 2002;277:9570–9579.
52. Yang M, Ruan J, Voller M, Schalken J, Michel MC. Differential regulation of human α_1-adrenoceptor subtypes. Naunyn Schmiedebergs Arch Pharmacol 1999;359:439–446.
53. Garcia-Sainz JA, Vazquez-Cuevas F, Romero-Avila M. Phosphorylation and desensitization of α_{1d}-adrenergic receptors. Biochem J 2001;353:603–610.
54. Diviani D, Lattion AL, Abuin L, Staub O, Cotecchia S. The adaptor complex 2 directly interacts with the α_{1b}-adrenergic receptor and plays a role in receptor endocytosis. J Biol Chem 2003;278:19,331–19,340.
55. Alcantara-Hernandez R, Leyva-Illades D, Garcia-Sainz JA. Protein kinase C-α_{1b}-adrenoceptor coimmunoprecipitation: effect of hormones and phorbol myristate acetate. Eur J Pharmacol 2001;419:9–13.
56. Fujita T, Toya Y, Iwatsubo K, et al. Accumulation of molecules involved in α_1-adrenergic signal within caveolae: caveolin expression and the development of cardiac hypertrophy. Cardiovasc Res 2001;51:709–716.
57. Toews ML, Prinster SC, Schulte NA. Regulation of α_{1B} adrenergic receptor localization, trafficking, function, and stability. Life Sci 2003;74:379–389.
58. Saunders C, Limbird LE. Localization and trafficking of α_2-adrenergic receptor subtypes in cells and tissues. Pharmacol Ther 1999;84:193–205.
59. Keefer JR, Limbird LE. The α_{2A}-adrenergic receptor is targeted directly to the basolateral membrane domain of Madin-Darby canine kidney cells independent of coupling to pertussis toxin-sensitive GTP-binding proteins. J Biol Chem 1993;268:11,340–11,347.
60. Wozniak M, Limbird LE. The three α_2-adrenergic receptor subtypes achieve basolateral localization in Madin-Darby canine kidney II cells via different targeting mechanisms. J Biol Chem 1996;271:5017–5024.
61. Keefer JR, Kennedy ME, Limbird LE. Unique structural features important for stabilization vs polarization of the α_{2A}-adrenergic receptor on the basolateral membrane of Madin-Darby canine kidney cells. J Biol Chem 1994;269:16,425–16,432.

62. Saunders C, Limbird LE. Microtubule-dependent regulation of α_{2B} adrenergic receptors in polarized MDCKII cells requires the third intracellular loop but not G protein coupling. Mol Pharmacol 2000;57:44–52.

63. Richman JG, Brady AE, Wang Q, Hensel JL, Colbran RJ, Limbird LE. Agonist-regulated interaction between α_2-adrenergic receptors and spinophilin. J Biol Chem 2001;276:15,003–15,008.

64. Brady AE, Wang Q, Colbran RJ, Allen PB, Greengard P, Limbird LE. Spinophilin stabilizes cell surface expression of α_{2B}-adrenergic receptors. J Biol Chem 2003; 278:32,405–32,412.

65. Daunt DA, Hurt C, Hein L, Kallio J, Feng F, Kobilka BK. Subtype-specific intracellular trafficking of α_2-adrenergic receptors. Mol Pharmacol 1997;51:711–720.

66. Eason MG, Liggett SB. Subtype-selective desensitization of α_2-adrenergic receptors. Different mechanisms control short and long term agonist-promoted desensitization of α_2C10, α_2C4, and α_2C2. J Biol Chem 1992;267:25,473–25,479.

67. Eason MG, Liggett SB. Functional α_2-adrenergic receptor-Gs coupling undergoes agonist-promoted desensitization in a subtype-selective manner. Biochem Biophys Res Commun 1993;193:318–323.

68. Schramm NL, Limbird LE. Stimulation of mitogen-activated protein kinase by G protein-coupled α_2-adrenergic receptors does not require agonist-elicited endocytosis. J Biol Chem 1999;274:24,935–24,940.

69. Jones SB, Leone SL, Bylund DB. Desensitization of the α_2 adrenergic receptor in HT29 and opossum kidney cell lines. J Pharmacol Exp Ther 1990;254:294–300.

70. DeGraff JL, Gagnon AW, Benovic JL, Orsini MJ. Role of arrestins in endocytosis and signaling of α_2-adrenergic receptor subtypes. J Biol Chem 1999;274:11,253–11,259.

71. Olli-Lahdesmaki T, Scheinin M, Pohjanoksa K, Kallio J. Agonist-dependent trafficking of α_2-adrenoceptor subtypes: dependence on receptor subtype and employed agonist. Eur J Cell Biol 2003;82:231–239.

72. von Zastrow M, Link R, Daunt D, Barsh G, Kobilka B. Subtype-specific differences in the intracellular sorting of G protein-coupled receptors. J Biol Chem 1993;268:763–766.

73. Wu G, Krupnick JG, Benovic JL, Lanier SM. Interaction of arrestins with intracellular domains of muscarinic and α_2-adrenergic receptors. J Biol Chem 1997; 272:17,836–17,842.

74. Jewell-Motz EA, Liggett SB. An acidic motif within the third intracellular loop of the α_2C2 adrenergic receptor is required for agonist-promoted phosphorylation and desensitization. Biochemistry 1995;34:11,946–11,953.

75. Liang M, Eason MG, Theiss CT, Liggett SB. Phosphorylation of ser360 in the third intracellular loop of the α_{2A}-adrenorecptor during protein kinase C-mediated desensitization. Eur J Pharmacol 2002;437:41–46.

76. Bawa T, Altememi GF, Eikenburg DC, Standifer KM. Desensitization of α_{2A}-adrenoceptor signalling by modest levels of adrenaline is facilitated by β_2-adrenoceptor-dependent GRK3 up-regulation. Br J Pharmacol 2003;138:921–931.

77. Eason MG, Jacinto MT, Theiss CT, Liggett SB. The palmitoylated cysteine of the cytoplasmic tail of α_{2A}-adrenergic receptors confers subtype-specific agonist-promoted downregulation. Proc Natl Acad Sci USA 1994;91:11,178–11,182.

78. Deupree JD, Borgeson CD, Bylund DB. Down-regulation of the α_{2C} adrenergic receptor: involvement of a serine/threonine motif in the third cytoplasmic loop. BMC Pharmacol 2002;2:9.

5

Adrenergic Receptors in Clinical Medicine

Martin C. Michel and Paul A. Insel

Summary

The sympathetic nervous system is a main regulator of homeostasis and mediates most of its effects via the nine subtypes of α_1-, α_2-, and β-adrenergic receptors. Although recent years have witnessed major progress in the identification of adrenergic receptor subtypes with specific cell and tissue functions in experimental animals, similar progress for human tissues remains limited. At present, most data are available for β-adrenergic receptor subtypes in the human heart, but substantial information is available regarding urogenital tissues, particularly the prostate and the bladder. The discovery of a specific role of α_{1A}-adrenergic receptors in the human prostate has led to the development of selective antagonists that effectively treat prostate symptoms without major effects on blood pressure. Hence, α_1-adrenergic antagonists have largely replaced surgery as the primary treatment of the highly prevalent condition of benign prostatic hyperplasia. It is hoped that better phenotyping of other human tissues will contribute to similar progress in other disease states.

Key Words: Adrenergic receptor; artery; bladder; clinical; heart; lung; prostate.

1. Introduction

Adrenergic receptors play an important role in several aspects of clinical medicine. This is perhaps not surprising given the importance of the autonomic, particularly the sympathetic, nervous system in the regulation of virtually every organ system in the body. Physiological regulation of these organ systems occurs in response to norepinephrine as the sympathetic postganglionic synaptic neu-

From: *The Receptors: The Adrenergic Receptors: In the 21st Century*
Edited by: D. Perez © Humana Press Inc., Totowa, NJ

rotransmitter and epinephrine as a hormone released into the circulation by chromaffin cells, primarily located in the adrenal medulla. Such regulation is determined by two key factors: the concentration of neuronally released and circulating catecholamines and expression and functional activity of the various adrenergic receptors (and receptor subtypes) that bind and respond to those amines. Thus, normal function of the cardiovascular, pulmonary, endocrine-metabolic, genitourinary, and other systems is influenced by "sympathoadrenal (adrenergic) tone."

Clinical disorders in those and other organ systems can be associated with altered sympathetic nervous system activity (and, in turn, tissue and circulating levels of catecholamines) or with altered expression and activity of adrenergic receptors. Such diseases include settings with prominently enhanced levels of catecholamines, such as chromaffin cell tumors (pheochromocytoma) and disorders with more modest (and thus sometimes more difficult to document) changes in circulating or tissue catecholamines. Examples of the latter include essential hypertension and congestive heart failure, two widely prevalent cardiovascular disorders. The ability of catecholamines to desensitize and downregulate adrenergic receptors creates a conundrum in trying to assess and define primary vs secondary roles for altered receptor expression and function in clinical settings.

Because of their widespread expression in human tissues and ability to have an impact on numerous physiological systems, adrenergic receptors have proved to be highly useful pharmacological targets. Knowledge regarding the presence and function of human adrenergic receptors, especially of various receptor subtypes (Table 1) is incomplete, particularly when compared to results from animal studies, including murine knockouts of most of the receptor subtypes. Nevertheless, completion of the human genome project has shown definitively that humans express genes for only nine adrenergic receptor subtypes ($\alpha_{1A,B,D}$, $\alpha_{2A,B,C}$, $\beta_{1,2,3}$) *(1)*. The principal reason for the lack of information regarding tissue expression of the various receptor subtypes is the lack of appropriate pharmacological agents that can specifically identify functional protein for each of the subtypes. Considerable data exist regarding detection of messenger ribonucleic acid (mRNA) of the receptor subtypes, but it is questionable whether there will be precise correspondence between mRNA and protein expression. Moreover, data from studies with experimental animals does not necessarily predict expression and function of adrenergic receptors in humans *(2–5)*.

Agonists and antagonists for each of the types and certain subtypes of adrenergic receptors have been used to treat many clinical disorders (Table 2). Detailed discussion of the physiological roles of adrenergic receptors and the identity and uses of all the agonists and antagonists directed to these receptors is beyond the scope of this chapter. Such information is available in textbooks of physiology and

Table 1

Presence and Function of Adrenergic Receptor Subtypes

Tissue	Response	Subtype	Confirmed in Humans
• Postjunctional (sympathetic) neurons	α_2 inhibition of transmitter release	Mostly α_{2A}	Yes
	β enhancement of transmitter release	Mostly β_2	Yes
• Heart	β inotropy, chronotropy, dromotropy, bathmotropy	$\beta_1 = \beta_2 >> \beta_3$	Yes
	α_1 weak inotropy	?	Yes
	α_2 prejunctional inhibition	mostly α_{2A}	Yes
• Blood vessels	α_1 smooth muscle contraction	Variable	Limited
	α_2 direct smooth muscle contraction, indirect relaxation via endothelium	Variable	Limited
	β smooth muscle relaxation	$\beta_2 \geq \beta_1$; β_3 unclear	Yes
• Lung	β smooth muscle relaxation	Only β_2	Yes
• Liver	Stimulation of gluconeogenesis	Mostly α_{1A}	Yes
	Stimulation of glycogenolysis	Mostly β_2	Yes
• Gut	α_2 inhibition of smooth muscle contraction	mostly α_{2A}	No
• Pancreatic islet cells	β stimulation of insulin and glucagon secretion	β_2	Yes
	α_2 inhibition of insulin secretion	Mostly α_{2A}	Limited
• Adipocytes	α_2 inhibition of lipolysis	Mostly α_{2A}	Yes
	β stimulation of lipolysis and thermogenesis	$\beta_1 > \beta_2 > \beta_3$	Yes
• Leukocytes	β inhibition of immune and inflammatory function	Only β_2	Yes

(Continued on next page)

Table 1 (Continued)
Presence and Function of Adrenergic Receptor Subtypes

Tissue	Response	Subtype	Confirmed in Humans
• Platelets	α_2 enhancement of aggregation	Only α_{2A}	Yes
• Skeletal muscle	β stimulation of tremor	β_2	Yes
	β stimulation of glucose K$^+$ uptake, lipolysis	Mostly β_2	Yes
• Kidney	α_2 inhibition of renin release and modulation of tubular function	Mostly α_{2A}	Limited
	β stimulation of renin release	β_1	Yes
• Uterus	β smooth muscle relaxation	Mostly β_2	Yes
• Prostate	α_1 smooth muscle contraction	Mostly α_{1A}	Yes
	α_2 present but unknown function	Mostly α_{2A}	Yes
	β smooth muscle relaxation	Mostly β_2	Yes
• Bladder	α_1 (mainly in diseased tissue)	Variable	Yes
	α_2 present but unknown function	Mostly α_{2A}	Yes
	β smooth muscle relaxation	Mostly β_3	Yes
• Penis	α_1 smooth muscle contraction	$\alpha_{1A} > \alpha_{1B} > \alpha_{1D}$	Yes
	α_2 present but unknown function	Mostly α_{2A}	Yes
	β smooth muscle relaxation	β_2/β_3	Yes
• Pineal gland	α_1 stimulation of melatonin secretion/release	? α_{1B}	Limited
	β stimulation of melatonin secretion/release	$\beta_1 > \beta_2$	Yes
	α_2 inhibition of melatonin secretion/release	?	Limited

Note: The table describes human data; where insufficient information from humans is available, animal data was given as an indication.

132

Table 2
Use of Adrenergic Agonists and Antagonists in Human Disease

Disease	Type	Purpose	Examples
Cardiovascular diseases			
• Arrhythmias	β-Antagonists	Reduce sinoatrial rate and atrioventricular conductance	Propranolol, Sotalol
• Arterial hypertension	β-Antagonists	Reduce cardiac output and renin release	Atenolol, Bisprolol, Metoprolol
	$α_1$-Antagonists	Reduce peripheral resistance	Doxazosin, Terazosin
	$α_2$-Agonists	Central (and peripheral prejunctional) reduction of sympathetic activity	Clonidine
• Coronary heart disease (also secondary prevention of myocardial infarction)	β-Antagonists	Reduce heart rate and hence increase oxygen supply and reduce oxygen demand	Atenolol, Bisprolol Metoprolol
• Congestive heart failure	β-Agonists	Acute inotropic support	Dobutamine, Orciprenaline
	β-Antagonists	Prevention of sudden death	Bisoprolol, Carvedilol, Metoprolol
• Shock	β-Agonists	Enhance cardiac output, redistribute blood volume, bronchodilation	Epinephrine
Respiratory diseases			
• Asthma, Chronic obstructive pulmonary disease	$β_2$-Agonists	Reduce bronchial smooth muscle tone	Formeterol, Salbutamol, Salmeterol, Terbutaline
• Rhinitis	α-agonists	Acutely reduce secretion	Oxymetazoline, Xylometazoline

(Continued on next page)

Table 2 (Continued)
Use of Adrenergic Agonists and Antagonists in Human Disease

Disease	Type	Purpose	Examples
Endocrine diseases			
• Hyperkalemia	β_2-Agonists	Promote cellular potassium uptake	Salbutamol, Terbutaline
• Hyperthyroidism	β-Antagonists	Reduce peripheral sympathetic hyperresponsiveness	Propranolol
• Pheochromocytoma	α-Antagonists	Reduce norepinephrine-induced vasoconstriction	Phenoxybenzamine
Urogenital diseases			
• Benign prostatic hyperplasia	α_1-Antagonists	Reduce bladder outlet resistance (relaxation of prostate smooth muscle)	Alfuzosin, Doxazosin Tamsulosin, Terazosin
• Erectile dysfunction	α_2-Antagonists	Relax penile smooth muscle (central effect?)	Yohimbine
• Neurogenic voiding dysfunction	α-Antagonists	Unknown mechanism of action	Phenoxybenzamine
• Premature labor	β_2-Agonists	Reduce uterine smooth muscle tone	Fenoterol, Ritodrine, Terbutaline
Neuropsychiatric diseases and conditions			
• Alcohol and morphine withdrawal	α_2-Agonists	Central (and peripheral prejunctional) reduction of sympathetic activity	Clonidine
• Anesthesia	α_2-Agonists	Pain reduction, cardiovascular stabilization	Clonidine
• Depression	α_2-Antagonists	Enhance noradrenaline release	Mianserin
• Migraine	β-Antagonists	Reduce number of attacks	Metoprolol, Propranolol
• Stagefright	β-Antagonists	Reduce tachycardia and tremor	Propranolol
Other uses			
• Glaucoma	β-Antagonists	Reduce intraocular pressure	Timolol

Note: Not all of the listed examples are first-line treatment within the indicated disease pharmacology or in other sources *(6–8)*. In addition, numerous recent reviews describe information regarding clinical development and indications for the use of adrenergic receptor agonists and antagonists *(9–17)*. Therefore, in this chapter we briefly summarize the role of adrenergic receptors in cardiovascular and pulmonary medicine and then focus on urogenital disease, a field in which the last decade has witnessed substantial progress and growing clinical utility for drugs that target adrenergic receptors.

2. Adrenergic Receptors in Cardiovascular Medicine

The most extensively studied human tissue regarding adrenergic receptors is the heart, in which β-adrenergic receptors mediate positive chronotropic, inotropic, dromotropic, and bathmotropic effects (i.e., increased rate, force, excitability, and conductivity) *(18)*. Although β_1-adrenergic receptors appear to dominate in the human heart for most of these functions, β_2-adrenergic receptors can contribute to a relevant degree, particularly in the atria. It has also been suggested that β_3-adrenergic receptors mediate negative inotropic response (albeit probably not in response to endogenous catecholamines) in the human heart *(19)*, but others have not confirmed these findings. In addition, a propranolol-resistant state of the β_1-adrenergic receptor exists; this was previously sometimes referred to as a β_4-adrenergic receptor *(20)*.

β-Adrenergic agonists have been used for acute inotropic support, but their long-term use in patients with chronic heart failure appears detrimental *(21)*. On the other hand, β-adrenergic antagonists, particularly those selective for β_1-adrenergic receptors, have been very useful for the treatment of coronary heart disease, including the secondary prevention of myocardial infarction, as well as for hypertension and certain arrhythmias. β-Adrenergic receptor antagonists are useful drugs for the chronic treatment of congestive heart failure *(22–24)*.

In contrast, α_1-adrenergic receptors exert only a minor, if any, role in the human heart, and the subtype involved has not been studied in detail. α_2-Adrenergic receptors inhibit transmitter release from sympathetic and parasympathetic nerve fibers, and although no postsynaptic role has been identified for them in the human heart, data have indicated a role for an α_{2B}-adrenergic receptor genetic variant in acute coronary events and sudden death, suggesting that this variant may be a risk factor for cardiovascular disease *(25–27)*. Such an effect might result from enhanced tendency for coronary artery thrombosis; of note, though, the receptor subtype that promotes activation and aggregation of platelets by catecholamines is the α_{2A}-subtype *(28)*.

The presence of α_1-adrenergic receptor subtypes has been mapped in the human vasculature at the mRNA level *(29)*, but few vessels have been studied functionally. In resistance vessels, α_{1A}-adrenergic receptors appear to dominate the response to exogenously applied agonists *(30,31)*, but other subtypes may contribute, particularly in larger vessels *(29,32)*. An understanding of the role of α_2-adrenergic receptors in human blood vessels has been hampered by the fact that receptors on vascular smooth muscle cells can mediate contraction, whereas those on the endothelium mediate vasodilation. Little information is available regarding the α_2-adrenergic receptor subtypes involved. Although it is generally assumed that vasodilation occurs via β_2-adrenergic receptors, β_1-receptors may contribute in certain blood vessels *(33,34)*. Limited information is known regarding the role of β_3-adrenergic receptors in human blood vessels, but extrapolating from animal studies, it is likely that this subtype contributes to vasodilation in humans *(35,36)*.

Some time ago, we proposed that an altered expression of α_1-or α_2-adrenergic receptors might play a role in the pathogenesis of essential hypertension *(37)*. This proposal was based on evidence for increased α-adrenergic receptor expression in spontaneously hypertensive rats (mainly in the kidney), which preceded the blood pressure elevation and absence of this increase in animal models of acquired hypertension. Similarly, an increase in expression of α_{2A}-adrenergic receptors on platelets of hypertensive patients had been noted, and this increase was present in normotensive offspring of hypertensive patients. However, later genetic studies in both rats and humans failed to confirm a pathogenetic role for α_2-adrenergic receptors in essential hypertension *(38,39)*. The expression of β-adrenergic receptors had also been found to be altered in hypertension, including in animal models of acquired hypertension *(40)*; similar changes in humans were reversed on blood pressure normalization *(41)*. Taken together, available studies do not support a major role of adrenergic receptors in the pathogenesis of essential hypertension. However, a number of studies have explored the possibility that genetic variants of adrenergic receptors might contribute to the development, prognosis, or therapeutic response of hypertensive patients, an intriguing hypothesis for which no firm consensus has yet been reached *(42,43)*.

The α- and β-adrenergic antagonists have been used for many years to lower blood pressure in patients with arterial hypertension, but more recent data have questioned this use, particularly for α_1-adrenergic receptor antagonists. The arm of the ALLHAT (Antihypertensive and Lipid-Lowering Treatment to Prevent Heart Attack Trial) study that involved administration of those agents was stopped prematurely because the α-adrenergic antagonist used (doxazosin) did not provide benefits relative to a thiazide diuretic and may have been associated with a greater incidence of hypertension-associated complications *(44)*. Therefore, α_1-adrenergic receptor antagonists are no longer recommended as first-line monotherapy for hypertensive patients. More recently, based on new results and a reevaluation of those from older studies, it has been proposed that β-adrenergic receptor antagonists may also provide less benefit than other classes of antihypertensive drugs *(45)*. Nevertheless, β-adrenergic receptor antagonists remain a widely accepted choice for the first-line treatment of hypertension.

In addition to their possible role in contributing to hypertension, disease-related changes in adrenergic receptors have been hypothesized to accompany or underlie other cardiovascular disorders. Of particular interest is the possibility that antibodies directed against β-adrenergic receptors might play a role in cardiomyopathy. Certain clinical observations and studies with experimental animals have supported this possibility, but evidence for such a role is not yet definitive *(46,47)*. In addition, in limb ischemia, hyperresponsiveness of skeletal muscle resistance arteries to noradrenaline is accompanied by enhanced α_1-adrenergic receptor reserve without a change in the profile of receptor subtypes *(48)*.

3. Adrenergic Receptors in Pulmonary Medicine

All three subtypes of α_1-adrenergic receptors (particularly the α_{1A}-subtype) and all three subtypes of α_2-adrenergic receptors are expressed in human lung at the mRNA level, but no major role in the regulation of human airway function has been described *(49–53)*. Among the β-adrenergic receptors, β_1- and β_2-adrenergic receptors coexist in the human lung; the β_3-subtype appears to be absent *(53)*. β_2-Adrenergic receptors are more abundant than β_1-adrenergic receptors in all pulmonary cell types (except in pulmonary blood vessels) and are apparently the only subtype on airway smooth muscle cells *(53)*. Accordingly, relaxation of airway smooth muscle is a prototypical function of β_2-adrenergic receptors, and β_2-selective agonists have been used for many years as bronchodilator drugs in asthma, chronic obstructive pulmonary disease, and other pulmonary conditions. Short-acting β-adrenergic agonists, such as salbutamol or terbutaline, are well established as acute bronchodilators, whereas long-acting β-adrenergic agonists, such as salmeterol or formoterol, are preferentially used alone or together with inhaled corticosteroids in prophylaxis and as suppressors of chronic bronchoconstriction *(54,55)*. The expression and responsiveness of airway β_2-adrenergic receptors can be regulated by a variety of factors that include genetics, age, disease states, and, possibly most important in therapeutics, drug treatment *(43,56,57)*. The last includes desensitization on treatment with β-adrenergic agonists and sensitization (or prevention of desensitization) in patients treated with inhaled or systemically administered glucocorticoids. β_2-Adrenergic receptors on inflammatory cells, which have products that influence bronchial airway cell function and which are responsive to glucocorticoids, appear to show greater propensity for desensitization than do the receptors on airway smooth muscle *(58,59)*.

4. Adrenergic Receptors in the Urogenital Tract

The expression pattern of adrenergic receptors and their subtypes within the urogenital tract varies greatly among the individual tissues. The human kidney expresses few α_1-adrenergic receptors (and these are primarily on renal arteries and of the α_{1A} subtype; *29*), but a large number of α_2-adrenergic receptors, particularly the α_{2A}-subtype, are involved in the regulation of vascular resistance, inhibition of renin release, and modulation of tubular function *(60)*. Hence, blood pressure lowering by α_2-adrenergic agonists is accompanied by smaller alterations of renal perfusion than that by other classes of blood pressure-lowering drugs.

Healthy human bladder expresses few α_1-adrenergic receptors; these are predominantly of the α_{1D}-subtype, but their physiological role remains to be determined *(61)*. Some data obtained with experimental animals raise the possibility that bladder dysfunction is accompanied by enhanced action of these receptors, and that such regulation may involve a subtype switch *(62)*. Human bladder also expresses a large number of α_2-adrenergic receptors, largely belonging to the α_{2A}-subtype, for which no physiological postjunctional function has as yet been identified *(63)*. β-Adrenergic receptors are considered the main physiological mediator for relaxation of bladder smooth muscle, hence allowing accommodation of increasing volumes of urine at acceptable pressure during the filling phase of the micturition cycle *(64)*. In humans, this appears to occur predominantly, if not exclusively, through a β_3-subtype *(65)*. The finding that few other human tissues are so enriched in β_3-adrenergic receptors makes these receptors attractive as a target for drugs that treat bladder dysfunction *(66)*. Accordingly, several β_3-selective agonists are currently in clinical development for the treatment of the overactive bladder syndrome and urinary urge incontinence.

The bladder outflow tract, particularly the urethra, also expresses several types of adrenergic receptors. α_{1A}-Adrenergic receptor-mediated urethral contraction may contribute to bladder outlet resistance and the maintenance of continence. α-Adrenergic agonists have been used "off label" to treat stress urinary incontinence *(67)*, but the best-studied drug, phenylpropanolamine, was withdrawn from the market by the Food and Drug Administration because of concerns of increased risk for stroke during treatment. An α_{1A}-selective partial agonist, Ro 115-1240, demonstrated efficacy without cardiovascular effects in a placebo-controlled study of women with stress incontinence *(68)*, but its clinical development has been stopped.

Hyperplastic growth of the prostate, an important part of the male bladder outflow tract, occurs with increasing age; the resultant enlargement, benign prostatic hyperplasia (BPH), is frequently associated with bothersome symptoms *(69)*. This hyperplasia represents growth of stromal and, to a lesser extent, glandular-epithelial elements and is accompanied by a dynamic component:

increased smooth muscle tone within the prostatic capsule and bladder outlet, largely as a consequence of adrenergic innervation *(70)*. The human prostate contains a large number of α_2-adrenergic receptors, mostly of the α_{2A}-subtype, and all three β-adrenergic receptors, but their function remains unclear *(63,71)*. The human prostate also expresses α_1-adrenergic receptors, predominantly of the α_{1A}-subtype, as detected both at the mRNA and protein levels and primarily located on smooth muscle cells; thus, α_{1A}-adrenergic receptors are the main, if not exclusive, subtype that mediates prostatic contraction *(70,72)*. As a consequence, α_1-adrenergic antagonists have become a mainstay of medical treatment of BPH.

BPH, a histological diagnosis, affects the majority of elderly men by causing lower urinary tract symptoms (LUTS) that affect both the voiding and storage phase of the micturition cycle. In the past, BPH was treated surgically, but with the advent and success of α_1-adrenergic antagonists, the majority of patients now primarily receive this form of medical treatment. The use of α_1-adrenergic receptor antagonists to treat LUTS suggestive of BPH was originally based on the concept that α_1-adrenergic receptors, particularly of the α_{1A}-subtype, mediate contraction of the prostate, bladder neck, and urethra and hence contribute to the dynamic (phasic) component of increased bladder outlet resistance *(70)*. However, α_1-adrenergic antagonists have only moderate effects in the treatment of BPH-associated obstruction but are considerably more effective in alleviating irritative LUTS, implying that symptoms of BPH that occur during the storage phase of the micturition cycle are unlikely to result directly from obstruction. Therefore, it is currently thought that an additional component contributes to symptom relief in BPH patients, possibly blockade of α_{1D}-adrenergic receptors located in the bladder or the spinal cord *(72)*.

Inhibitors of the enzyme 5α-reductase (e.g., finasteride and dutasteride) are the other current main option for medical treatment of BPH. Four comparative studies with a duration of 6 mo to longer than 4 yr demonstrated that α_1-adrenergic receptor antagonists are more effective than 5α-reductase inhibitors in relieving BPH symptoms *(73–76)*. Although 5α-reductase inhibitors are inferior in relieving symptoms, they prevent prostatic growth and can reduce BPH complications, such as acute urinary retention, over periods of 4 yr and longer *(76,77)*. Because of their different mechanisms of action, it is not surprising that the combined administration of an α_1-adrenergic receptor antagonist and a 5α-reductase inhibitor has significantly greater long-term effects on BPH progression than either drug alone *(76)*.

Prior to their use in BPH patients, α_1-adrenergic receptor antagonists were used in the treatment of arterial hypertension. Therefore, α_1-antagonists originally developed for the treatment of hypertension, such as doxazosin and terazosin, lower blood pressure when used to treat BPH patients; as a result, such patients can have blood pressure-related side effects, such as orthostasis, dizziness, and asthenia. Interestingly, alfuzosin, which is chemically similar to doxazosin and terazosin, largely lacks these side effects and has a tolerability similar to placebo despite exhibiting some blood pressure lowering *(78)*. Tamsulosin is a chemically different α_1-antagonist with selectivity for α_{1A}- and α_{1D}- relative to α_{1B}-adrenergic receptors *(79)*. In therapeutically equivalent doses, tamsulosin causes much less vasodilation than do other α_1-adrenergic receptor antagonists *(80)* and even when given in combination with anti-hypertensive drugs causes little blood pressure lowering *(81)*. Accordingly, its tolerability is close to placebo, including in patients with comorbidities or who are taking multiple medications *(81,82)*. Whether this tolerability and relative lack of vascular effects of tamsulosin are explained by its subtype selectivity or its pharmacokinetic properties remains unclear, but slow-release formulations of other α_1-antagonists also show improved tolerability *(83,84)*. Taken together, these data show that α_1-adrenergic receptor antagonists are an effective form of medical treatment for LUTS resulting from BPH, and that subtype selectivity or pharmacokinetic factors can provide selectivity for the urogenital relative to the cardiovascular system.

The human penis expresses various subtypes of α-adrenergic receptors that are involved in smooth muscle contraction *(85,86)*. Nevertheless, the α_2-antagonist yohimbine has only moderate efficacy in treating erectile dysfunction *(87)*, and α_1-adrenergic receptor antagonists have failed to demonstrate efficacy relative to placebo in clinical trials for this indication *(9)*. β_2 and β_3-Adrenergic receptors have been shown to relax corpus cavernosum smooth muscle and thus are suggested as possible targets for treatment of erectile dysfunction *(88)*.

The human uterus expresses α_1-adrenergic receptors that mediate contraction, but specific roles of individual subtypes and the overall contribution to myometrial tone are not well established *(89)*. All three α_2-adrenergic receptor subtypes are also expressed; their expression is highly regulated during pregnancy, with protein expression of the α_{2A}-subtype predominating at term *(90)*. The relaxant action of β-adrenergic receptors opposes the contractile responses of myometrial α-adrenergic receptors. Among the β-adrenergic receptors, expression of the β_2-subtype dominates in the human myometrium, but the other two subtypes can also be detected *(91)*. There is considerable intersubject variability in expression of β_2-adrenergic receptors, with a decrease in expression at term that likely contributes to an enhancement in uterine tone at that time *(92,93)*. β-Adrenergic agonists have been used for many years to treat preterm labor, but myometrial β_2-adrenergic receptors undergo rapid desensitization and downregulation on agonist treatment *(94)*. Accordingly, β_2-adrenergic agonists have only moderate efficacy, particularly when used for more than a few days *(10)*. It has been suggested that β_3-adrenergic agonists might provide an alternative approach for such tocolytic therapy, but no clinical assessment of such agents has been undertaken *(95)*.

5. Conclusions and Future Perspective

Many physiological functions have been linked to specific subtypes of α_1-, α_2-, and β-adrenergic receptors in various animal species. Because of the obvious reason of limited access, particularly regarding healthy tissue, similar progress for human adrenergic receptors has been slower and in many cases limited to the characterization of expression of RNA for the receptor subtypes. A more extensive characterization of protein and function for all the human adrenergic receptor subtypes is needed to identify specific targets for possible therapeutic intervention.

The interindividual variability in responsiveness to adrenergic agonists and antagonists presents not only a major challenge, but also an important opportunity for the future use of such drugs. Part of this variability has a genetic basis (i.e., polymorphisms and other variants in the genes encoding the adrenergic receptor subtypes) *(42,43,96–98)*. Although variation in the genes for the adrenergic receptors (or their signaling machinery) have the potential to influence tissue responsiveness to adrenergic drugs, variants in the genes that encode drug-metabolizing enzymes also may influence adrenergic drug responses. Another type of interindividual variability derives from differences in the regulation of adrenergic receptor expression and responsiveness that result from physiological factors such as age, pregnancy, and pathophysiological conditions such as heart failure or asthma and from drug treatment *(6)*. This has been best documented for the heart *(18)* and airways *(56)*. These intrinsic (genetic) and extrinsic (disease, drug treatment) factors are likely to interact, but only limited data are available regarding such interaction *(43,99)*. It thus remains unclear whether information gleaned from assessment of interindividual differences will allow "personalized medicine" (i.e., beyond individual trial and error) in terms of the clinical administration of adrenergic agonists and antagonists. Of particular importance for the future, especially since the completion of the human genome, will be to determine whether intrinsic differences (i.e., genetic variants) or extrinsic factors are more important for interindividual variability. The ability to predict phenotype based on a given genotype, especially in terms of combinations of variants defined by genetic haplotypes, is an area that is just beginning to be explored.

Acknowledgment

Work in Dr. Insel's and Dr. Michel's laboratories is supported by grants from the National Institutes of Health and the Deutsche Forschungsgemeinschaft, respectively.

References

1. Vassilatis DK, Hohmann JG, Zeng H, et al. The G protein-coupled receptor repertoires of human and mouse. Proc Natl Acad Sci USA 2003;100:4903–4908.
2. Price DT, Lefkowitz RJ, Caron MG, Berkowitz D, Schwinn DA. Localization of mRNA for three distinct α_1-adrenergic receptor subtypes in human tissues: implications for human α-adrenergic physiology. Mol Pharmacol 1994;45:171–175.
3. Berkowitz DE, Price DT, Bello EA, Page SO, Schwinn DA. Localization of messenger RNA for three distinct α_2-adrenergic receptor subtypes in human tissues. Evidence for species heterogeneity and implications for human pharmacology. Anesthesiology 1994;81:1235–1244.
4. Thomas RF, Liggett SB. Lack of β_3-adrenergic receptor mRNA expression in adipose and other metabolic tissues in the adult human. Mol Pharmacol 1993;43:343–348.
5. Eason MG, Liggett SB. Human α_2-adrenergic receptor subtype distribution: widespread and subtype-selective expression of α_2C10, α_2C4, and α_2C2 mRNA in multiple tissues. Mol Pharmacol 1993;44:70–75.
6. Insel PA. Adrenergic Receptors in Man. New York: Dekker, 1987.
7. Hoffman BB. Catecholamines, sympathomimetic drugs, and adrenergic receptor antagonists. In: Hardman JG, Limbird LE, eds.,Goodman and Gilman's Pharmacological Basis of Therapeutics. 10th ed. New York: McGraw-Hill, 2001:215–268.
8. Insel PA, Feldman RD. Norepinephrine Receptors in Encyclopedia of Endocrine Diseases. Vol. 3.San Diego, CA: Elsevier, 2004, pp. 375–382.
9. Kendall MJ. Clinical trial data on the cardioprotective effects of β-blockade. Basic Res Cardiol 2000;95 Suppl 1:I25–I30.
10. Berkman ND, Thorp JMJ, Lohr KN, et al. Tocolytic treatment for the management of preterm labor: a review of the evidence. Am J Obstet Gynecol 2003;188:1648–1659.
11. Nishina K, Mikawa K, Uesugi T, et al. Efficacy of clonidine for prevention of perioperative myocardial ischemia. A critical appraisal and meta-analysis of the literature. Anesthesiology 2002;96:323–329.
12. Limmroth V, Michel MC. The prevention of migraine: a critical review with special emphasis on β-blockers. Br J Clin Pharmacol 2001;52:237–243.
13. Andersson K-E, Stief CG. Oral α adrenoceptor blockade as a treatment of erectile dysfunction. World J Urol 2001;19:9–13.
14. Ahmed I, Takeshita J. Clonidine. A critical review of its role in the treatment of psychiatric disorders. CNS Drugs 1996;6:53–70.
15. Bravo EL. Pheochromocytoma: an approach to antihypertensive management. Ann N Y Acad Sci 2002;970:1–10.
16. Gowing L, Farrell M, Ali R, White J. α_2-Adrenergic Agonists for the Management of Opioid Withdrawal. Chichester, UK: Wiley, 2004.
17. Boyd RE. α_2-Adrenergic receptor agonists as analgesics. Curr Top Med Chem 2001;1:193–197.
18. Brodde O-E, Michel MC. Adrenergic and muscarinic receptors in the human heart. Pharmacol Rev 1999;51:651–689.

19. Gauthier C, Tavernier G, Trochu JN, et al. Interspecies differences in the cardiac negative inotropic effects of β_3-adrenoceptor agonists. J Pharmacol Exp Ther 1999;290:687–693.

20. Joseph SS, Lynham JA, Molenaar P, Grace AA, Colledge WH, Kaumann AJ. Intrinsic sympathomimetic activity of (–)-pindolol mediated through a (–)-propranolol-resistant site of the β_1-adrenoceptor in human atrium and recombinant receptors. Naunyn-Schmiedeberg's Arch Pharmacol 2003;368:496–503.

21. Amidon TM, Parmley WW. Is there a role for positive inotropic agents in congestive heart failure: focus on mortality. Clin Cardiol 1994;17:641–647.

22. Squire IB, Barnett DB. The rational use of β-adrenoceptor blockers in the treatment of heart failure. The changing face of an old therapy. Br J Clin Pharmacol 2000;49:1–9.

23. Bristow, M. Antiadrenergic therapy of chronic heart failure. Surprises and new opportunities. Circulation 2003;107:1100–1102.

24. Packer M. Do β-blockers prolong survival in heart failure only by inhibiting the β_1-receptor? A perspective on the results of the COMET trial. J Cardiac Fail 2003;9:429–443.

25. Snapir A, Heinonen P, Tuomainen TP, et al. An insertion/deletion polymorphism in the α_{2B}-adrenergic receptor gene is a novel genetic risk factor for acute coronary events. J Am Coll Cardiol 2001;37:1516–1522.

26. Snapir A, Mikkelsson J, Perola M, Penttila A, Scheinin M, Karhunen PJ. Variation in the α_{2B}-adrenoceptor gene as a risk factor for prehospital fatal myocardial infarction and sudden cardiac death. J Am Coll Cardiol 2003;41:190–194.

27. Etzel JP, Rana BK, Wen G, et al. Genetic analysis of the human α_{2B}-adrenergic receptor: identification of a particular genotype as a possible cardiovascular risk factor. Unpublished manuscript.

28. O'Rourke MF, Iversen LJ, Lomasney JW, Bylund DB. Species orthologs of the α_{2A} adrenergic receptor: the pharmacological properties of the bovine and rat receptors differ from the human and porcine receptors. J Pharmacol Exp Ther 1994;271:735–740.

29. Rudner XL, Berkowitz BA, Booth JV, et al. Subtype specific regulation of human vascular α_1-adrenergic receptors by vessel bed and age. Circulation 1999;100:2336–2343.

30. Jarajapu YPR, Johnston F, Berry C, et al. Functional characterization of α_1-adrenoceptor subtypes in human subcutaneous resistance arteries. J Pharmacol Exp Ther 2001;299:729–734.

31. Jarajapu YPR, Coats P, McGrath JC, Hillier C, MacDonald A. Functional characterization of α_1-adrenoceptor subtypes in human skeletal muscle resistance arteries. Br J Pharmacol 2001;133:679–686.

32. Giessler C, Wangemann T, Silber R-E, Dhein S, Brodde O-E. Noradrenaline-induced contraction of human saphenous vein and human internal mammary artery: involvement of different α-adrenoceptor subtypes. Naunyn-Schmiedeberg's Arch Pharmacol 2002;166:104–109.

33. Ferro A, Kaumann AJ, Brown MJ. β_1- and β_2-adrenoceptor-mediated relaxation in human internal mammary artery and saphenous vein: unchanged β- and α-adrenoceptor-responsiveness after chronic β_1-adrenoceptor blockade. Br J Pharmacol 1993;109:1053–1058.

34. Abdelmawla AH, Langley RW, Szabadi E, Bradshaw CM. Comparison of the effects of nadolol and bisoprolol on the isoprenaline-evoked dilatation of the dorsal hand vein in man. Br J Clin Pharmacol 2001;51:583–589.
35. Authier C, Langin D, Balligand J-L. β_3-Adrenoceptors in the cardiovascular system. Trends Pharmacol Sci 2000;21:426–431.
36. Guimaraes S, Moura D. Vascular adrenoceptors: an update. Pharmacol Rev 2001; 53:319–356.
37. Michel MC, Insel PA, Brodde O-E. Renal α-adrenergic receptor alterations: a cause of essential hypertension? FASEB J 1989;3:139–144.
38. Michel MC, Jäger S, Casto R, et al. On the role of renal α-adrenergic receptors in spontaneously hypertensive rats. Hypertension 1992;19:365–370.
39. Michel MC, Plogmann C, Philipp T, Brodde O-E. Functional correlates of α_{2A}-adrenoceptor gene polymorphism in the HANE study. Nephrol Dial Transplant 1999;14:2657–2663.
40. Brodde O-E, Michel MC. Adrenergic receptors and their signal transduction mechanisms in hypertension. J Hypertension 1992;10 Suppl 7:S133–S145.
41. Feldman RD, Lawton WJ, McArdle WL. Low sodium diet corrects the defect in lymphocyte β-adrenergic responsiveness in hypertensive subjects. J Clin Invest 1987;79:290–294.
42. Koopmans RP, Insel PA, Michel MC. Pharmacogenetics of hypertension treatment: a structured review. Pharmacogenetics 2003;12:705–713.
43. Kirstein SL, Insel PA. Autonomic nervous system pharmacogenomics: a progress report. Pharmacol Rev 2004;56:31–52.
44. ALLHAT Officers. Major cardiovascular events in hypertensive patients randomized to doxazosin vs chlorthalidone. The Antihypertensive and Lipid-Lowering Treatment to Prevent Heart Attack Trial (ALLHAT). JAMA 2000;283:1967–1975.
45. Messerli FH, Beevers DG, Franklin SS, Pickering TG. β-Blockers in hypertension-the emperor has no clothes: an open letter to present and prospective drafters of new guidelines for the treatment of hypertension. Am J Hypertens 2003;16:870–873.
46. Christ T, Wettwer E, Dobrev D, et al. Autoantibodies against the β_1 adrenoceptor from patients with dilated cardiomyopathy prolong action potential duration and enhance contractility in isolated cardiomyocytes. J Mol Cell Cardiol 2001;33: 1515–1525.
47. Jahns R, Boivin V, Hein L, et al. Direct evidence for a β_1-adrenergic receptor-directed autoimmune attack as a cause of idiopathic dilated cardiomyopathy. J Clin Invest 2004;113:1419–1429.
48. Jarajapu YP, McGrath JC, Hillier C, MacDonald A. The α_1-adrenoceptor profile in human skeletal muscle resistance arteries in critical limb ischaemia. Cardiovasc Res 2003;57:554–562.
49. Eason MG, Liggett SB. Human α_2-adrenergic receptor subtype distribution: widespread and subtype-selective expression of α_2C10, α_2C4, and α_2C2 mRNA in multiple tissues. Mol Pharmacol 1993;44:70–75.
50. Weinberg DH, Trivedi P, Tan CP, et al. Cloning, expression and characterization of human α adrenergic receptors α_{1A}, α_{1B} and α_{1C}. Biochem Biophys Res Commun 1994;201:1296–1304.

51. Berkowitz DE, Price DT, Bello EA, Page SO, Schwinn DA. Localization of messenger RNA for three distinct α_2-adrenergic receptor subtypes in human tissues. Evidence for species heterogeneity and implications for human pharmacology. Anesthesiology 1994;81:1235–1244.

52. Spina D, Rigby PJ, Paterson JW, Goldie RG. α_1-Adrenoceptor function and autoradiographic distribution in human asthmatic lung. Br J Pharmacol 1989;97:701–708.

53. Mak JCW, Nishikawa M, Haddad E-B, et al. Localisation and expression of β-adrenoceptor subtype mRNAs in human lung. Eur J Pharmacol 1996;302:215–221.

54. Ram FSF, Sestini P. Regular inhaled short acting β_2 agonists for the management of stable chronic obstructive pulmonary disease: Cochrane systematic review and meta-analysis. Thorax 2003;58:580–584.

55. Jackson CM, Lipworth B. Benefit-risk assessment of long-acting β_2 agonists in asthma. Drug Safety 2004;27:243–270.

56. Shore SA, Moore PE. Regulation of β-adrenergic responses in airway smooth muscle. Resp Physiol Neurobiol 2003;137:179–195.

57. Litonjua AA, Silverman EK, Tantisira KG, Sparrow D, Sylvia JS, Weiss ST. β_2-Adrenergic receptor polymorphisms and haplotypes are associated with airways hyperresponsiveness among nonsmoking men. Chest 2004;126:66–74.

58. Barnes PJ. Effect of β-agonists on inflammatory cells. J Allergy Clin Immunol 1999;104:S10–S17.

59. Adcock IM, Maneechotesuwan K, Usmani O. Molecular interactions between glucocorticoids and long-acting β_2-agonists. J Allergy Clin Immunol 2002;110:S261–S268.

60. Michel MC, Rump LC. α-Adrenergic regulation of human renal function. Fundam Clin Pharmacol 1996;10:493–503.

61. Malloy BJ, Price DT, Price RR, et al. α_1-Adrenergic receptor subtypes in human detrusor. J Urol 1998;160:937–943.

62. Hampel C, Dolber PC, Smith MP, et al. Modulation of bladder α_1-adrenergic receptor subtype expression by bladder outlet obstruction. J Urol 2002;167:1513–1521.

63. Goepel M, Wittmann A, Rübben H, Michel MC. Comparison of adrenoceptor subtype expression in porcine and human bladder and prostate. Urol Res 1997;25:199–206.

64. Andersson K-E, Arner A. Urinary bladder contraction and relaxation: physiology and pathophysiology. Physiol Rev 2004;84:935–986.

65. Yamaguchi O. β_3-Adrenoceptors in human detrusor muscle. Urology 2002;59 Suppl 5A:25–29.

66. Andersson K-E. Treatment of overactive bladder: other drug mechanisms. Urology 2000;55 Suppl 5A:51–57.

67. Alhasso A, Glazener CMA, Pickard R, N'Dow J. Adrenergic drugs for urinary incontinence in adults. The Cochrane Library 1. Chichester, UK: Wiley, 2004.

68. Musselman DM, Ford APDW, Gennevois DJ, et al. A randomized crossover study to evaluate Ro 115-1240, a selective $\alpha_{1A/L}$-adrenoceptor partial agonist in women with stress urinary incontinence. BJU Int 2004;93:78–83.

69. Emberton M, Andriole GL, de la Rosette JJMCH, et al. Benign prostatic hyperplasia: a progressive disease of aging men. Urology 2003;61:267–273.
70. Berkowitz DE, Nardone NA, Smiley RM, et al. Distribution of β_3-adrenoceptor mRNA in human tissues. Eur J Pharmacol 1995;289:223–228.
71. Michel MC. Potential role of α_1-adrenoceptor subtypes in the aetiology of LUTS. Eur Urol Suppl 2002;1:5–13.
72. Roehrborn CG, Schwinn DA. α_1-Adrenergic receptors and their inhibitors in lower urinary tract symptoms and benign prostatic hyperplasia. J Urol 2004;171:1029–1035.
73. Lepor H, Williford WO, Barry MJ, et al. The efficacy of terazosin, finasteride, or both in benign prostatic hyperplasia. N Engl J Med 1996;335:533–539.
74. Kirby R, Roehrborn CG, Boyle P, et al. Efficacy and tolerability of doxazosin and finasteride, alone or in combination, in treatment of symptomatic benign prostatic hyperplasia: the Prospective European Doxazosin and Combination Therapy (PREDICT) trial. Urology 2003;61:119–126.
75. Debruyne FM, Jardin A, Colloi D, et al. Sustained-release alfuzosin, finasteride and the combination of both in the treatment of benign prostatic hyperplasia. Eur Urol 1998;34:169–175.
76. McConnell JD, Roehrborn CG, Bautista O, et al. The long-term effect of doxazosin, finasteride, and combination therapy on the clinical progression of benign prostatic hyperplasia. N Engl J Med 2003;349:2387–2398.
77. McConnell JD, Bruskewitz R, Walsh P, et al. The effect of finasteride on the risk of acute urinary retention and the need for surgical treatment among men with benign prostatic hyperplasia. N Engl J Med 1998;338:557–563.
78. Michel MC, Flannery MT, Narayan P. Worldwide experience with alfuzosin and tamsulosin. Urology 2001;58:508–516.
79. Michel MC, de la Rosette JJMCH. Efficacy and safety of tamsulosin in the treatment of urological diseases. Exp Opin Pharmacother 2004;5:151–160.
80. Schäfers RF, Fokuhl B, Wasmuth A, et al. Differential vascular α_1-adrenoceptor antagonism by tamsulosin and terazosin. Br J Clin Pharmacol 1999;47:67–74.
81. Michel MC, Mehlburger L, Bressel H-U, Schumacher H, Schäfers RF, Goepel M. Tamsulosin treatment of 19,365 patients with lower urinary tract symptoms: does comorbidity alter tolerability? J Urol 1998;160:784–791.
82. Michel MC, Bressel H-U, Goepel M, Rübben H. A 6-month large-scale study into the safety of tamsulosin. Br J Clin Pharmacol 2001;51:609–614.
83. Kirby RS, Andersen M, Gratzke P, Dahlstrand C, Hoye K. A combined analysis of double-blind trials of the efficacy and tolerability of doxazosin-gastrointestinal therapeutic system, doxazosin standard and placebo in patients with benign prostatic hyperplasia. BJU Int 2001;87:192–200.
84. van Kerrebroeck P, Jardin A, Laval K-U, van Cangh P, ALFORTI Study Group. Efficacy and safety of a new prolonged release formulation of alfuzosin 10 mg once daily vs alfuzosin 2.5 mg thrice daily and placebo in patients with symptomatic benign prostatic hyperplasia. Eur Urol 2000;37:306–313.
85. Goepel M, Krege S, Price DT, Michelotti GA, Schwinn DA, Michel MC. Characterization of α-adrenoceptor subtypes in the corpus cavernosum of patients undergoing sex change surgery. J Urol 1999;162:1793–1799.

86. Costa P, Soulie-Vassal ML, Sarrazin B, Rebillard X, Navratil H, Bali JP. Adrenergic receptors on smooth muscle cells isolated from human penile corpus cavernosum. J Urol 1993;150:859–863.
87. Ernst E, Pittler MH. Yohimbine for erectile dysfunction: a systematic review and meta-analysis of randomized clinical trials. J Urol 1998;159:433–436.
88. Cirino G, Sorrentino R, d'Emmanuele di Villa Bianca R, et al. Involvement of β_3-adrenergic receptor activation via cyclic GMP- but not NO-dependent mechanisms in human corpus cavernosum function. Proc Natl Acad Sci USA 2003;100: 5531–5536.
89. Breuiller-Fouche M, Doualla-Bell F, Maka K, Geny B, Ferre F. α_1 Adrenergic receptor: binding and phosphoinositide breakdown in human myometrium. J Pharmacol Exp Ther 1991;258:82–87.
90. Adolfsson PI, Dahle LO, Berg G, Svensson SP. Characterization of α_2-adrenoceptor subtypes in pregnant human myometrium. Gynecol Obstet Invest 1998;45:145–150.
91. Bardou M, Loustalot C, Cortijo J, et al. Functional, biochemical and molecular biological evidence for a possible β_3-adrenoceptor in human near-term myometrium. Br J Pharmacol 2000;130:1960–1966.
92. Sakakibara T, Inoue Y, Uzue S, et al. Diversity of inhibitory responses to β_2-stimulants shown by term-pregnant human myometria in vitro is partly due to differences in receptor density. Am J Obstet Gynecol 2002;186:997–1004.
93. Chanrachakul B, Matharoo-Ball B, Turner A, et al. Reduced expression of immunoreactive β_2-adrenergic receptor protein in human myometrium with labor. J Clin Endocrinol Metab 2003;88:4997–5001.
94. Engelhardt S, Zieger W, Kassubek J, Michel MC, Lohse MJ, Brodde O-E. Tocolytic therapy with fenoterol induces selective down-regulation of β-adrenergic receptors in human myometrium. J Clin Endocrinol Metab 1997;82:1235–1242.
95. Dennedy MC, Houlihan DD, McMillan H, Morrison JJ. β_2- and β_3-adrenoreceptor agonists: human myometrial selectivity and effects on umbilical artery tone. Am J Obstet Gynecol 2002;187:641–647.
96. Michel MC, Insel PA. Receptor gene polymorphisms: lessons on functional relevance from the β_1-adrenoceptor. Br J Pharmacol 2003;138:279–282.
97. Leineweber K, Büscher R, Bruck H, Brodde O-E. β-Adrenoceptor polymorphisms. Naunyn-Schmiedeberg's Arch Pharmacol 2004;369:1–22.
98. Small KM, McGraw DW, Liggett SB. Pharmacology and physiology of human adrenergic receptor polymorphisms. Annu Rev Pharmacol Toxicol 2003;43: 381–411.
99. Bruck H, Leineweber K, Beilfuß A, et al. Genotype-dependent time course of lymphocyte β_2-adrenergic receptor down-regulation. Clin Pharmacol Ther 2003; 74:255–263.

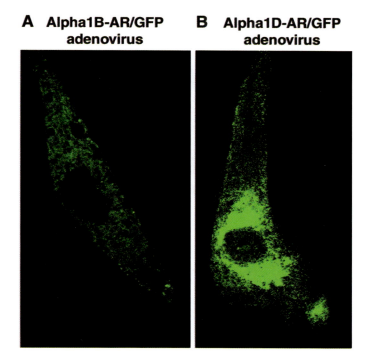

Color Plate 1, Fig. 4, Chapter 4. Confocal imaging of human aortic smooth muscle cells transfected with an adenovirus. To facilitate imaging, each receptor was expressed as a fusion protein with GFP. (*See* pp. 117–118.)

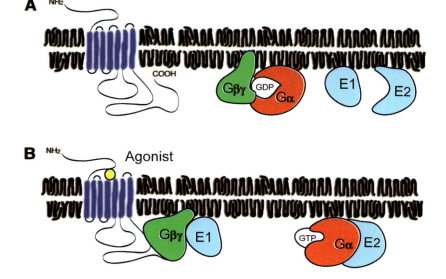

Color Plate 2, Fig. 1, Chapter 11. Classical AR signaling. (*See* full caption and discussion on p. 294.)

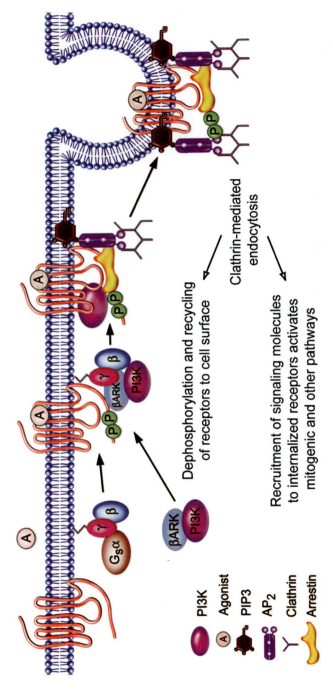

Color Plate 3, Fig. 2, Chapter 11. Major mechanisms involved in β-AR desensitization and internalization. (*See* full caption on p. 296 and discussion on p. 295.)

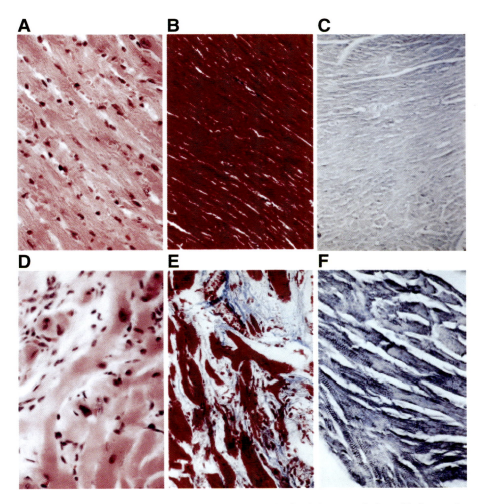

Color Plate 4, Fig. 5, Chapter 11. Histopathological characteristics of left ventricular specimens taken from mice overexpressing the human β_1-AR. The upper panels show (**A**) HE stain, (**B**) Masson's Trichrome stain, and (**C**) signal for epitope-tagged human β_1-AR protein in control hearts. The lower panels (**D–F**) show representative sections from transgenic mice overexpressing the human β_1-AR. (*See* pp. 306–308; from ref. *95*, © 2000, with permission from Elsevier.)

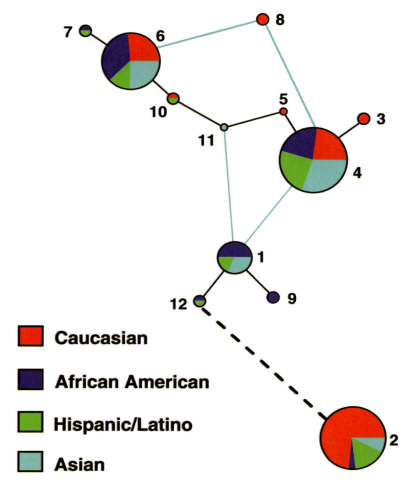

Color Plate 5, Fig. 2, Chapter 13. Phylogenetics of β_2-AR haplotypes. Each circle represents a haplotype with an area that correlates with its frequency in the test population. Sections within each circle show the distribution by race. Connecting lines: solid black, single-site differences; solid blue, two-site differences; dashed, more than two-site differences. Analysis was by the minimum spanning network algorithm. (*See* pp. 340–341; reprinted with permission.)

PART III

IMAGING ADRENERGIC
RECEPTORS AND THEIR FUNCTION

6

Use of Fluorescent Ligands and Receptors to Visualize Adrenergic Receptors

John C. McGrath and Craig J. Daly

Summary

This chapter reviews and compares the strengths, limitations, and potential for development of the two major methodologies employed to visualize the locations and properties of adrenergic receptors: fusion proteins of receptors with fluorescent protein tags and fluorescent ligands. In each case, the three subfamilies of adrenergic receptors (β, α_1, and α_2) are considered. Emphasis is placed on time sequence imaging in live cells, providing insights to receptor mobilization and regulation. The use of recombinant fusion proteins such as green fluorescent protein has been mainly confined to cell culture; fluorescent ligands can also be utilized in native tissues. It is shown how the two approaches can validate each other and provide complementary information. The importance of appropriate image acquisition and quantitative image analysis is stressed if meaningful data are to be acquired. These approaches have resulted in the recent discovery of more diverse adrenergic receptor locations in both unexpected tissue types and subcellular locations. Finally, the ability to exploit the changing fluorescent properties of interacting fluorophores to elucidate interactions between receptor molecules, such as dimerization or chaperoning, are considered. It is concluded that we have entered a new phase in which visualization of adrenergic receptors in multidimensional analysis is providing new insights to receptor biology, and that visualization in live heterogeneous organs and tissues is bringing this to the physiological level.

Key Words: β-, α_1-, and α_2-Adrenergic receptors; confocal microscopy; fluorescent ligands; green fluorescent protein; image analysis.

From: *The Receptors: The Adrenergic Receptors: In the 21st Century*
Edited by: D. Perez © Humana Press Inc., Totowa, NJ

1. Introduction

Knowledge of the organ, tissue, and subcellular location of adrenergic receptors (ARs) has recently been given some interesting new directions through the use of fluorescent labels. Essentially, this has won new information on receptor distribution at the tissue level plus dynamic data on receptor mobility/trafficking at the cellular level. Essentially, ARs have now been found in cells not previously considered, and the cell surface membrane is no longer considered their dominant location.

The discovery of the three families of ARs depended entirely on classical agonist–antagonist–response pharmacology, as did the first division of the β-AR family into two subtypes. This was enabled by the convenient availability of bioassay tissues for each receptor type that responded with unique characteristics to selective agonists, antagonists, or both. It was implicit in this that the different receptors resided on different cell types and mediated different types of responses. In the immediate precloning era, the proliferation of further subtypes was accomplished using radioligand binding to build on the established functional pharmacology of antagonists. This relied on aberrations from the expected affinity series to predict receptor subtypes, so it no longer required isolation of a specific cellular response and could be achieved in tissues with cellular heterogeneity. When cloning methodology became available, the antagonist series was paramount in distinguishing the characteristics of reexpressed receptors. Reverse pharmacology was then employed to seek native receptors with the binding characteristics of the clones. This turned out to be nontrivial because the selectivity of the available antagonists was more difficult to establish in functional terms in native tissues than in binding.

It would have helped at that point if antibodies to the receptors could have been employed to map the location of the receptor subtypes by immunohistochemistry. In retrospect, two factors stand out as confounding this and diverting the visualization of ARs along the alternative routes of epitope labeling and fluorescent ligand binding. These factors are apparent nonselectivity and actual heterogeneity, which may be different sides of the same coin.

Regarding apparent nonselectivity, although a number of laboratories made the attempt, it proved difficult to find "satisfactory" antibodies to selectively label each subtype with certainty. They often proved satisfactory in purified membranes or cell clones only to fail in native tissues, labeling many cell types when they were expected to target only a subpopulation. In some cases, this may have involved a lack of antibody selectivity because of high conservation of sequence among G protein-coupled receptors (GPCRs).

For actual heterogeneity, in retrospect, difficulties with antibodies may also have been partly caused by the receptors actually present, unexpectedly, on diverse cell types where no function for them had been established or where a particular receptor was masked, in functional experiments, by the presence of another member of the same subfamily.

As it turned out, the use of fluorescent ligands and fluorescent epitopes coupled with simultaneous improvements in microscope technology meant that the visualization of ARs could be accomplished in live cells and tissue. This gave immediate access not only to subcellular localization, but also to receptor trafficking and to the ability to tie localization of receptors to the pharmacological properties of the drugs that activate or block them. This chapter sets out how our current knowledge of ARs was informed by these approaches.

2. General Use of Green Fluorescent Protein and G Protein-Coupled Receptor Fusion Proteins

The ARs, particularly β_2 were among the first examples of GPCR for which green fluorescent proteins (GFP) fusion proteins were employed to visualize receptor location *(1)*. Recent reviews of the general use of GFP–GPCR fusion proteins cover the general issues *(2)*. These are essentially the validation of the fusion protein vs the wild-type receptor with respect to ligand binding and localization in the cell to exclude, respectively, interference with the binding pocket and mislocation from, for example, aggregation of the receptor in an inappropriate location because of the properties of the GFP. Validation of localization, of course, can be tricky if the point under investigation is that localization is not known. In general, this is most satisfactory if both a fluorescent ligand and receptor antibody are available, and in recombinant systems, an antibody to an additional epitope is generally the most satisfactory solution. Some early work may still require revalidation.

In nonactivated cells, once validated, GFP–GPCRs inform on localization of receptors. Indeed, this can be used as an efficient means of identifying effectively transfected cells to clone them. However, there is a danger of prejudice concerning the desirable characteristics of cells to be cloned. GFP–GPCRs transfected into native tissues or used transgenically may hold out a more fruitful use in establishing the cellular localization of receptors.

The most widespread use of GFP–GPCR fusion proteins is in the study of the mechanisms underlying agonist-induced internalization and recycling of receptors. This is confined to situations in which the net distribution of receptors throughout cells is altered in a clearly visualizable manner. It cannot inform on the subtler situation for which accelerated recycling occurs without a net change of receptor distribution (i.e., outward equals inward movement, although at an accelerated rate).

Because data from modern microscopes usually starts as digital data, images are pictorial representations of this to aid analysis, but the data are there for other forms of quantitative analysis. With GFP–GPCR fusion proteins, the obvious applications of quantitative analysis are quantification of the receptors in a particular location, such as a comparison of the receptor density in different parts of the cell or a global comparison of, say, surface and intracellular receptors and their net redistribution following agonist-activated internalization. Moreover, this can be done in three dimensions (3D) to capture an entire cell's complement of receptors, whereas with two dimensions (2D) they may not redistribute in the same plane. This can then be extended to the time dimension in either 2D or 3D, which can assess the rate of the process under analysis.

2.1. Application of GFP to β-ARs

The β_2-AR was the first of the family of ARs to be cloned. Consequently, this subtype has been most widely studied and manipulated by genetic techniques. Despite the relatively large size (238 aa) of the GFP, Barak et al. *(1)* created a human β_2–GFP fusion protein that retained full function when transiently expressed in HEK-293 cells. In addition, agonist and antagonist binding to the β_2–GFP fusion protein was almost identical to that of the native receptor. The β_2–GFP construct distributed mainly on the cell surface under stable conditions and relocated to endosomal compartments on agonist stimulation *(1)*. Similar characteristics were observed when the construct was expressed in HeLa cells, in which agonist stimulation caused receptor relocation to endosomes and lysosomes *(3)*. The human β_1–GFP fusion has also been shown to retain its native pharmacology and cellular distribution *(4)*. Following agonist stimulation, the phosphorylated receptor can bind β-arrestin, leading to internalization. However, the β_1–AR has been shown to exhibit a low affinity for β-arrestin, therefore making this subtype relatively resistant to internalization. Work by Shiina et al. *(5)* demonstrated this difference in β_1-AR and β_2-AR internalization through the use of GFP–arrestin expression in HEK-293 cells.

β-ARs are expressed on a wide range of native cell types; therefore, caution is advised when extrapolating the mechanisms of receptor turnover in model cells (i.e., HEK-293, HeLa, etc.) to that of native tissue. Nevertheless, GFP fusions expressed in cells are still an excellent model for the study of GPCR internalization and degradation (for review, *see* ref. *6*).

The hypothesis that β_1-ARs downregulate in response to antidepressant treatment has been studied using a β_1-AR–GFP fusion expressed in C6 glioblastoma cells *(7)*. These authors reported almost identical dissociation constants for [^{3}H]CGP-12177 binding at the native and GFP fusion with β_1-AR. Furthermore, approx 22% of β_1–GFP ARs internalized within 3 min of agonist (isoprenaline) treatment. From a methodological viewpoint, this study is interesting in that it used image restoration and 3D segmentation of confocal volumes to estimate the degree of receptor internalization.

2.2. Application of GFP to α_1-ARs

Fully functional GFP fusion proteins have been made for all three α_1-AR subtypes *(8)*. Differences in the cellular distribution between α_1-AR subtypes have been a notable issue *(see* Chapter 4). One of the earliest reports of α_1-AR–GFP subtype distribution in cells suggested that the α_{1B}-AR was predominantly located on the surface, and the α_{1A}-AR was mainly intracellular *(9)*. The membrane-located hamster α_{1B}–GFP was next shown to have identical binding properties to the WT receptor (expressed in mouse αT3 cells) and to undergo agonist-induced internalization *(10)*. This is consistent with the α_{1B}-AR belonging to the same class of receptor as the β_2-AR (as classified in *11*) in displaying higher affinity for β-arrestin-2. Interestingly, Oakley et al. *(11)* also show differential distribution of the arrestin–GFP isoforms within the cell cytoplasm and nucleus.

Chalothorn et al. *(8)* conducted a comprehensive study of the cellular distribution of GFP-linked α_B-AR subtypes in HEK-293 cells. This study demonstrated a preferential surface membrane location of α_{1B}-ARs, an intracellular predominance of α_{1D}-ARs, and a heterogeneous distribution of α_{1A}-ARs, although this was not quantified, relying solely on interpretation of pictures. Agonist-induced internalization was more readily observed for α_{1B}-ARs, with little or no internalization of α_{1D}-AR, so this was attributed to the initial location of the receptors, with α_{1D}-AR having little scope for internalization. This is in line with an earlier study (nonimaging) of differential agonist-induced downregulation of the human α_1-AR subtypes in which the α_{1D}-AR was relatively resistant and the α_{1B}-AR had greatest sensitivity *(12)*. The difference in initial localization of subtypes has been associated with the different degree of constitutive activity of the subtypes, with α_{1D}-AR having the greatest activity and thus a greater degree of self-internalization *(13)*.

Two subsequent studies concentrated on the potential role of oligomerization on the spontaneous or activated internalization of α_1-AR subtypes *(see* Chapter 3). Both used confocal imaging and GFP and CFP constructs to enable co-localization of different subtypes. Stanasila et al. *(14)*, using fluorescence resonance energy transfer (FRET), demonstrated that oligomerization of the α_1-AR subtypes correlated with their ability to cointernalize on exposure to the agonist. The α_{1A}-selective agonist oxymetazoline induced the cointernalization of the α_{1A}- and α_{1B}-AR, whereas the α_{1B}-AR could not cointernalize with the NK1 tachykinin or CCR5 chemokine receptors. They proposed that oligomerization might therefore represent an additional mechanism regulating the physiological responses mediated by the α_{1A}- and α_{1B}-AR subtypes. Hague et al. *(15)*, studying all three subtypes using probe co-localization, indicated differential interactions and possible dimerization between α_1-subtypes, such that $\alpha_{1B/D}$ heterodimerization promotes surface expression of α_{1D}-AR whereas $\alpha_{1A/D}$ does not.

Overall, studies with GFP-linked α_1-ARs expressed in model cell lines appear to provide almost unanimous support for a predominantly intracellular location of the α_{1A}- and α_{1D}-subtypes and a mainly cell surface location for α_{1B}. It is interesting that, in the one native system in which attempts have been made to study the function of all three α_1-AR subtypes (i.e., contraction of vascular smooth muscle), α_{1A} and α_{1D} have the dominant role, and that of α_{1B} is minor *(16)*. This suggests either that a balance in favor of intracellular rather than surface receptors is a physiologically normal situation or that recombinant cell systems do not reflect accurately the true physiological situation. This may be further informed by visualization of receptors in native systems as discussed in Section 3.

2.3. Application of GFP to α_2-ARs

At this time, there are no data on GFP–α_2-AR fusion proteins. Information on the differential distribution of α_2-AR subtypes was obtained in cell cultures using antibodies to epitope tags *(17)*. There is a lack of published imaging data on the subcellular distribution of α_2-AR.

2.4. Transfection of Native Tissues

The ability to transfect cell cultures efficiently with fully functional GFP-linked AR subtypes prompted us to attempt an in vitro transfection of the cells in a blood vessel. We chose the α_{1B}-AR–GFP that cell culture work suggested might have a cell surface location. The vessel employed was the mouse mesenteric artery, which has a functional response that is mainly through α_{1A}-AR but for which there is evidence for the presence of α_{1B} because its receptor pharmacology changes in the α_{1B}-KO *(16)*. We also had evidence from other blood vessels that the vascular adventitial cell population was altered in α_{1B}-AR-KO mice *(18,19)*, suggesting a trophic influence of this receptor. In vitro transfection using the lipofection method incorporating the use of Tfx™-50 (promega) showed a diffuse pattern of fluorescence from the α_{1B}-AR–GFP on mesenteric arterial smooth muscle cells (Fig. 1C). Thus, when artificially transfected, the receptors distributed themselves on the smooth muscle cell surface as previously demonstrated in cell culture. This was done on vessels from the α_{1B}-AR-KO mouse in an attempt to minimize competition from native receptors.

This still leaves the question of whether the native receptors adopt this distribution. We took two separate approaches to this. First, we carried out the transfection with the α_{1B}-AR–GFP fusion protein under its own promoter *(20)*. This proved negative in vascular smooth muscle, presumably because the native expression level is low, but positive expression was found in adventitial cells. This not only showed that the transfection/promoter system was effective when the native expression level was high, but also suggested that α_{1B}-AR expression

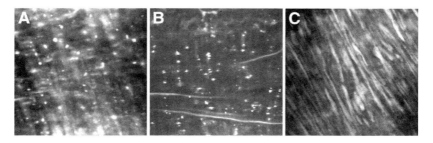

Fig. 1. α_1-AR distribution in mouse mesenteric artery: (**A**) WT showing 30-nm QAPB (BODIPY FL-prazosin) binding; (**B**) α_{1B}-AR-KO showing 30-nm QAPB binding; (**C**) α_{1B}-KO following in vitro transfection with α_{1B}-AR–GFP.

level is low in vascular smooth muscle and thus that the expression level was artificially high with the first transfection method.

We then took a separate approach to visualizing the native α_1-AR population using a fluorescent ligand for α_1-ARs related to the α_1-AR antagonist prazosin (BODIPY FL-prazosin, also known as QAPB) (*see* Section 3). This showed that α_1-AR subtypes existed in both clustered and diffuse arrangements in smooth muscle cells of WT mouse mesenteric artery (Fig. 1A). In the α_{1B}-KO mouse, receptors remaining (presumably α_{1A}) existed almost entirely as intracellular clusters (Fig. 1B) similar to those observed in transfected cells *(8)*. This suggested that the native α_{1B}-AR exists in a more diffuse (i.e., less-clustered) arrangement, as shown by the transfected α_{1B}-AR–GFP receptors. A caveat here, of course, is that the change caused by knocking out the α_{1B}-AR does not necessarily represent the straightforward loss of the image of α_{1B}-AR because the oligomerization studies showed that one subtype may alter the disposition of others.

In vitro transfection for 5 d of the GFP–α_{1B}-AR under its mouse promoter showed a readily detectable fluorescence signal in adventitial cells, including cells with long processes, previously identified as "sensory nerves." Cells that were readily identified as fibroblasts, from their morphology, showed a distribution of GFP-based fluorescence very similar to cultured fibroblasts transfected with ARs, with a high-intensity punctuate intracellular fluorescence. The sensory nerves showed perinuclear fluorescence together with fluorescence extending for a limited distance along their elongated processes, consistent with a time-dependent distribution of newly synthesized receptors. Both cell phenotypes bound fluorescent α-AR ligands at similar sites, and the sensory nerves showed binding along the full length of their processes. The transfection process was shown to be effective in all cells of the cultured vessel, as indicated by transfection with GFP alone. Thus, the limitation of the GFP– α_{1B}-promoter construct to a high-intensity signal in the adventitial cells can be attributed to this as the main source of native α_{1B} expression in these vessels. This is consistent with the classical functional pharmacology, which shows that the main contractile response in the vascular smooth muscle is caused by α_{1A}-AR *(16)*. The localization of the α_{1B}-AR to the adventitial cells focuses attention toward functions that have been tentatively ascribed to these cells, including a role in vascular remodeling *(21)*.

This section indicates that is possible to transfect cells with GFP fusion proteins of the AR families. The co-localization of these proteins with fluorescent ligands provides a link that allows comparison with native cell systems that do not possess such useful tags but that bind the fluorescent ligands. However, an additional utility is provided by the ability to label receptors in native systems with GFP, which provides the opportunity for receptor translocation studies in native cells. This has been accomplished on two levels. First, by in vitro transfection of native tissues or cells (*see* Fig. 1C) and second by creating transgenic mice harboring the GFP–AR constructs (*see* Chapter 7).

3. Fluorescent Ligands for Adrenergic Receptors

Fluorescent ligands offer significant advantages over traditional methods of ligand binding and immunohistochemistry *(22)*. Historically, fluorescent ligands were used as stains in a more histological approach rather than used as high-affinity markers for receptors on live cells. The number of studies employing the use of fluorescent ligands has increased markedly over the last few years and now involves the use of both fluo-antagonist and fluo-agonists *(18)*. Multiple fluo-ligands are now used in combination in ever-more-elaborate studies. An excellent example is the study by Pick et al. *(23)*, who used different colored ligands to track the time-course of expression of the 5-HT3 receptor in isolated cells. Similar approaches, using fluo-ligand combinations, have revealed the clustering and mobility of nicotinic acetylcholine and opioid receptors *(24,25)*.

The pH sensitivity of some fluorophores may be of use in determining their fate during transport though endosomal compartments of varying pH. In the vast majority of studies using fluo-ligands, internalized receptor appears in a perinuclear region. Using a combination of red and green BODIPY-deltorphin analogs it has been shown that μ- and δ-receptors take different routes to the perinuclear region *(26)*. The accumulation of receptor subtypes in one cellular compartment, not necessarily associated with degradation, raises interesting questions about possible functional interactions at this site. It would be interesting to perform detailed co-localization studies in the early endosomes and recycling regions. Green and red forms of somatostatin have already been used to demonstrate receptor oligomerization by FRET *(27)*, presenting an alternative to GFP labeling of the receptors and therefore possible use in native tissues.

Fluorescent derivatives of drugs that bind to the ligand recognition site of GPCRs are employed, in principle, in exactly the same way as radioligands and are subject to the same considerations. In addition, their affinity for the receptor is more likely to be changed by the bulkier fluorescent tag than by the trivial changes inherent in a radioactive isotope, so this must be assessed. Another factor, itself an advantage, is that, in native systems, the pharmacology of the compound can be established so that when it is visualized there is a high probability of a direct connection between the label and the pharmacological action in question.

If live cells are employed, another useful issue, sometimes employed in radioligand binding is that, because the ligand approaches and binds to the receptor on its extracellular face, the ligand would be expected to be visualized at the cell surface unless the receptor moves inside with the ligand attached. This issue is exploited in studies of receptor internalization. One of the most widespread uses of fluorescent ligands has been the internalization of fluorescent agonists, which activate the receptor and are subsequently carried inside when this activation leads to internalization. A condition for such an experiment is that the ligand should not be able to enter the cell unless attached to the receptor. This leads to another feature of the test molecule that must be validated, its permeability into the cell, independent of receptors. For most purposes, impermeability is desirable. This is a general property expected of GPCR ligands, which are generally charged molecules that penetrate cells, if at all, via carrier-mediated processes. However, fluorescent moieties are often highly lipophilic. Being covalently bound to otherwise hydrophilic molecules may alter their cellular distribution (e.g., concentrate them in liposomes).

Quantitative analysis of fluorescent ligand data can cover the same ground as for GFP–GPCRs and enables two further gains. First, when receptors are redistributed, GFP–GPCRs show only the net redistribution, but a ligand attached to the internalizing receptor shows which receptors internalize even if the net distribution remains unaltered because of recycling balancing the overall picture. Second, the binding of the fluorescent ligand to the receptor is subject to competition. Thus, the prevention or reversal of binding by competitor nonfluorescent ligands can provide quantitative information on the binding site's properties, for example, (1) indicating some modification of binding under a particular set of circumstances or (2) allowing the subtype of a receptor to be determined when the fluorescent ligand has a degree of promiscuity but highly subtype-specific competitor ligands are available.

An advantage for fluorescent ligands over ^{3}H ligands is the ability to visualize binding to whole tissues without the need for tissue fixation, freezing, or membrane disruption. This enables ligand binding to be viewed *in situ* among varying cell types and at varying tissue depths if confocal microscopy is used (Fig. 2A,B).

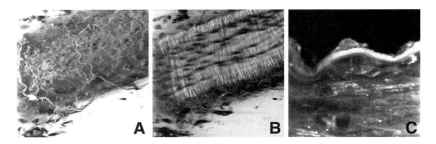

Fig. 2. QAPB (α_1-AR–ligand) and CGP12177 (β-AR–ligand) binding to segments of mouse and rat mesenteric artery: **(A)** 30-nm QAPB binding to the adventitia of mouse mesenteric artery; **(B)** 30-nM QAPB binding to mesenteric artery viewed from the luminal surface, showing smooth muscle cell binding (vertical light stripes) and the presence of nuclear "syto" stain in endothelial cells (horizontal dark ovals); **(C)** CGP12177 (1 µM) binding to cut ring segments of fixed rat mesenteric artery. Endothelial cells are separated from the (lower) smooth muscle cells by the highly fluorescent internal elastic lamina; both cell types show ligand-induced fluorescence.

We have identified a surprisingly high degree of "adrenoceptor" binding in the adventitia of mouse arteries (particularly mesentery; *see* Fig. 2A). The presence of binding to cells with long processes (Fig. 2A) is of interest as their function (possibly sensory nerves) is not entirely clear at this time.

Figure 2 shows the binding of a fluorescent prazosin analog (α_1-antagonist) to a segment of unfixed "live" mesenteric artery. Ligand binding is viewed from either the adventitial surface (Fig. 2A) or luminal surface (Fig. 2B) in combination with a fluorescent nuclear stain.

3.1. Application of Fluorescent Ligands for β-AR Studies

The earliest studies of β-ARs using a fluorescent form of propranolol (9-AAP and DAPN) indicated that the receptors existed in a clustered conformation *(28,29)*. Later studies with NBD-alprenolol (fluorescent form) demonstrated that β-ARs were both mobile and clustered *(30)*. However, the fluorescent antagonists NBD-alprenolol and NBD-pindolol were subsequently shown to be both nonselective and noncompetitive *(31)*.

A further significant development was the synthesis of a fluorescent form of the hydrophilic β-AR ligand CGP12177 *(32)*. These authors synthesized both a BODIPY and FITC version of CGP12177 and found that the BODIPY form exhibited similar binding characteristics when compared with the native form. Our own work with both these compounds also observed significant photobleaching of the FITC form; the BODIPY form was far more stable under fluorescence excitation.

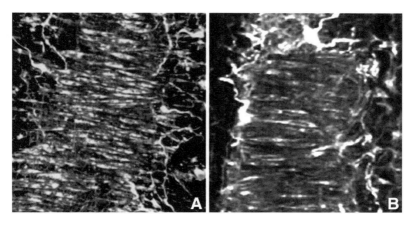

Fig. 3. BODIPY TMR-CGP12177 (1 μ*M*) binding to segments of rat mesenteric artery: **(A)** more intracellular clustered binding in medial smooth muscle; **(B)** more membrane-bound locations of CGP binding. Note also β-AR on adventitial cells with long processes (possibly sensory nerves).

Red and green BODIPY CGP12177 were until recently commercially available and were used by Baker et al. *(33)*, on recombinant human β$_2$-AR. In their studies on CHO-K1 cells, the compound was confined to the location of the plasmalemmal membrane, suggesting that it did not penetrate the cell, as expected of a lipophilic antagonist ligand that binds to a receptor that does not internalize unless activated.

BODIPY TMR CGP12177 was employed by us and colleagues on pressure-fixed, small mesenteric resistance rat arteries and segments of rat aorta. The fluorescent ligand was shown to be an antagonist of the β$_1$-AR that mediates vasodilation in mesenteric artery. The fluorescent ligand was localized to the medial smooth muscle cells and adventitial cells. It was concluded that the receptors on the mesenteric artery smooth muscle cells were responsible for the vaso-dilation to β-AR agonists such as isoprenaline. Although this may seem unsur-prising, it is in fact the first demonstration of visualization of β-AR on vascular smooth muscle cells at high resolution. The receptors were distributed both on the cell surface and at perinuclear intracellular sites (Fig. 3), a distribution that is very similar to that for α$_1$-AR on similar cells (*22*; *see* Section 3.2).

The compound was also used to visualize β-AR in cardiac myocytes. In this case, it was difficult to obtain high-resolution images of receptors on the cell surface, but after incubation for 60 min, they could be visualized at distinct intracellular sites, which thus represent the highest density of β-ARs in cardiac

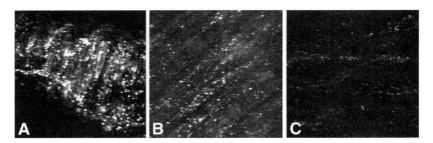

Fig. 4. QAPB (100 n*M*) binding to rat mesenteric artery and anococcygeus muscle (**A**) mesenteric artery medial smooth muscle cells; (**B**) anococcygeus smooth muscle; (**C**) anococcygeus in the presence of 10-μ*M* YM12617, a high-affinity α_1-AR antagonist.

myocytes. This is not altogether surprising because these cells are mostly occupied by contractile proteins, leaving little space for other essential organelles, such as mitochondria and endoplasmic reticulum, which are thus confined to limited regions throughout the cell but particularly perinuclear.

3.2. Application of Fluorescent Ligands for α_1-AR Studies

Over 10 yr ago, the first fluorescent form of the α_1-AR antagonist prazosin was synthesized and supplied by Molecular Probes Incorporated. The fluorophore of choice was BODIPY FL because of its relative pH insensitivity and stability under excitation (i.e., photobleached more slowly than FITC). Our first observations confirmed that BODIPY FL-prazosin bound to the medial smooth muscle cells of small resistance arteries and strips on anococcygeus in a manner consistent with the orientation of the cells (Fig. 4). In addition to the expected cell surface, we also observed significant amounts of intracellular clustered binding that could be inhibited by preincubation with nonfluorescent antagonists (Fig. 4; *34*). One interesting observation (and powerful advantage) was that the BODIPY FL-prazosin appeared to fluoresce more (or only) when bound. This characteristic made it possible to visualize antagonist binding without washing and thus at true equilibrium. Therefore, it was possible to construct binding-induced fluorescence intensity (concentration) curves and compare these with ligand binding of [³H]prazosin on membranes of identical cells. We found that image analysis-based methods of antagonist binding gave very similar results to those of traditional ligand binding (*35*).

The α_1-AR subtypes have been implicated in the pathogenesis of benign prostatic hyperplasia, so prostatic smooth muscle cells were a natural target for investigation with this technique. Two drugs, which were favored therapeutically, were doxazosin (nonselective) and YM12617 (α_{1A}-selective tamsulosin).

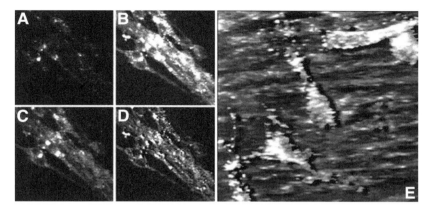

Fig. 5. QAPB (BODIPY FL-prazosin) binding to neuronal cells: **(A)** autofluorescence from neurons cultured from mouse cortex functionally characterized as containing α_{2D}-adrenoceptors; **(B)** binding of QAPB (5 nM) to cultured neurons; **(C)** QAPB in the presence of rauwolscine (10 μM); **(D)** subtraction of image C from B showing the area of displacement (i.e., specific binding to α_2-adrenoceptors). Panel **(E)** shows a simulated fluorescence projection of a section of anococcygeus muscle incubated with 30 nM QAPB. The nerve cells on the surface of the muscle exhibit strong fluorescence, which is reversed by rauwolscine (*see* Fig. 6).

Doxazosin is a quinazoline and structurally related to prazosin (and therefore BODIPY FL-prazosin). In addition, YM12617 inhibits BODIPY FL-prazosin binding to rat anococcygeus smooth muscle (our unpublished observations, (1995; Fig 4). Therefore, it was of interest to examine the receptor distribution in isolated human prostate smooth muscle cells. We observed and quantified significant amounts of intracellular binding in these cells, and this was eliminated by the selective α_{1A}-AR antagonist RS100329 *(36,37)*, which is consistent with the belief held by some workers that α_{1A}-ARs are located in mainly intracellular locations *(9)*.

In most blood vessels, the presence of more than one AR subtype can be detected. However, α_{1A}-ARs are widely believed to be the main subtype involved in activation of resistance artery smooth muscle (for review, *see* ref. *38*). The small arteries of rat skeletal muscle exhibit mainly an α_{1A}-AR profile *(39)* and express large quantities of intracellular receptor, as identified by the binding of BODIPY FL-prazosin *(40;* Fig. 5*)*.

3.3. Application of Fluorescent Ligands for α_2-AR Studies

Immunohistochemical or immunofluorescence techniques have demonstrated a differential distribution and agonist-mediated internalization of the α_2-AR subtypes *(41,42)*. Because antibodies generally require tissue fixation for access and GFP fusions are not forthcoming, it would be useful to have fluorescent ligands. However, presently we are not aware of any commercially available fluorescent ligands for α_2-ARs. Our own preliminary work with BODIPY FL-prazosin has indicated that this compound has a relatively low affinity for the rabbit prejunctional α_{2A}- (pKd 6.08) and mouse α_{2D}-AR (pKd 6.06). These values correlate well with those of prazosin at the same sites (5.83 and 6.53, respectively). In binding experiments, BODIPY FL-prazosin showed slightly higher affinity than prazosin at all three subtypes (pKi): α_{2A}, 7.83; α_{2B}, 7.34; α_{2D}, 7.78. The affinity of prazosin for the same sites was 6.13, 7.61, and 6.27, respectively. Thus, BODIPY FL-prazosin can recognize α_2-ARs with moderate to low affinity but is not subtype selective. It can therefore be used to visualize α_2-AR provided that precautions are taken to eliminate or take into account binding to α_1-AR.

Although our binding and functional studies indicated that BODIPY FL-prazosin was a weak α_2-AR ligand, fluorescence studies showed that 5-nm binding to cultured neurons was reversed by rauwolscine (Fig. 5). Using image subtraction, we found that specific binding sites were localized at the perinuclear region (presumably intracellular) and in clusters (Fig. 5D). In addition, binding to anococcygeus was observed within the smooth muscle and surface-located neuronal cells (Fig. 5E). The binding-induced fluorescence to these anococcygeus neuronal cells could be reversed by addition of rauwolscine (Fig. 6).

We have observed, in endothelial cells of mouse carotid artery, BODIPY FL-prazosin binding that is inhibited by the α_2-antagonist rauwolscine. The presence of α_2-ARs on vascular endothelium is not new *(43–45)*, but its visualization is. In addition, a report has suggested the presence of α_{1D}-ARs on the endothelium *(46)*, so as methodology improves, we can anticipate visualization of α_1-ARs on endothelium.

4. Visualization Techniques and Quantitative Image Analysis

The generation of images in scientific research is now commonplace. We can image virtually the whole spectrum of biomolecular activity, from a whole body magnetic resonance imaging scan to a visual map of gene activity on a microarray. Clinical diagnoses are derived from magnetic resonance imaging, positron emission tomography, computerized tomography, ultrasound, and X-ray images. Molecular processes are viewed using blots, gels, microarrays, and digital images. Therefore, we can image everything from drug binding through cell signaling to tissue metabolism. The importance of imaging in the pharmaceutical industry was highlighted in two articles in *Drug Discovery World (47)* and *PharmaGenomics (48)*. Both articles reflected the way in which basic imaging techniques play a huge role in drug discovery, with almost 70% of

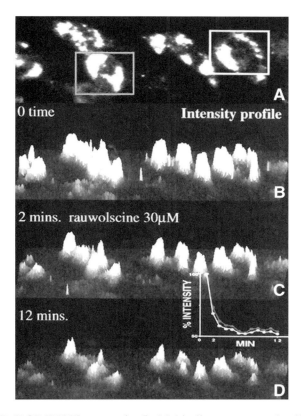

Fig. 6. QAPB (BODIPY FL-prazosin, 5 n*M*) binding to neuronal cells on the surface of a section of rat anococcygeus: (**A**) *xy* view of fluorescence at time-point zero, before addition of rauwolscine; (**B**) intensity profile plot of image a showing varying fluorescence intensity as peaks; (**C**) 2 min after addition of rauwolscine (30 μ*M*), the height of the peaks is reduced; (**D**) after 12 min, the maximum reduction in fluorescence (peak height) is achieved. The two rectangular areas shown in A have their respective fluorescence intensity measured and plotted over time (*see* inset) to show the development of fluorescence intensity reduction.

experiments resulting in image formation. However, there are two key factors: (1) image quality must be high and accurately reflect the biological process, and (2) some form of quantitative or qualitative analysis must be possible.

With the drug–receptor complex, we have a moving target. Both entities are recycled within cells, and both are candidates for degradation. Therefore, imaging this process is a multidimensional problem (four dimensions [4D] over time and multiple dimensions if more than one probe is visualized). The first (and most important) issue is removal of optical artifacts and calibration of the data.

At the most basic level, the data can be visualized (rendered) as an image volume viewed at varying angles and manually compressed or stretched to fit. Alternatively, a more mathematical approach can be taken if the optical aberrations can be measured. In 3D fluorescence microscopy, this measurement is known as the point spread function (psf), and a process of deconvolution can be used to correct any aberrations with a known psf. Once corrected, the data can be rendered for viewing and measurement with confidence.

With respect to studying ARs (or any GPCRs), there are a few key processes we wish to visualize and measure. These can be achieved only with high-quality imaging and can be broadly viewed as follows:

Receptor density:

It is necessary first to establish how the signal relates to the proportion of receptor. For instance, is the concentration of the probe proportional to the concentration of the receptor? Do all of the probes occupy all/only the receptors. How is nonspecific binding assessed? How is the detection device controlled for making comparative studies?

Receptor location:

If sufficiently high resolution (without aberration) can be achieved, then establishing the subcellular location is not difficult. Some questions then arise. Does the receptor co-localize with markers for specific cell organelles? If this involves co-localization (or FRET), do the optical parameters of the various probes overlap? Is there a need to correct for this? As receptors move around in vesicles, can they be tracked?

Optical illusion:

A common issue arises if, say, most receptors are widely distributed at a low density, but a minority are highly concentrated. Oversimplistic interpretation of an image may detect only the latter. This can be a particular factor when interpreting images of receptors that are "expected" to be on the cell surface. Consider a cell as a water-filled sphere. If a quantity of paint is spread over the surface, it will be more visible than if is diluted in the cell water. Setting an inappropriately low threshold will show only surface receptors.

Receptor function:

There are many probes that report on cell activation via the concentration of other cellular molecules (e.g., calcium). We have simultaneously visualized fluo-antagonist binding and agonist-induced Ca^{2+} activation in single cells. Ideally, we would combine receptor density, location, and functional experiments to determine exactly which receptors, at what location, drive a particular form of activation. The individual components of this process can be digitally captured. However, visualization of such a complex multidimensional process has not yet been achieved.

4.1. Imaging ARs

As outlined in this chapter, ARs can be visualized using fluorescent antibodies *(9,17,42)*, protein conjugates *(1,3,4,8)*, or ligands *(33,35)*. Each technique has its own set of advantages and disadvantages. However, all present similar issues for effective visualization and quantification.

Once a 2D image or 3D volume is captured, it can be processed, visualized, and measured. A simple 2D image can be very informative as it can show, at a given tissue or cell depth, the pattern of diffuse or clustered receptor distribution (*see* Figs. 1 and 4). In a whole tissue, a single 2D image, if carefully selected from the midregion, can show the receptor distribution in individual cells and even the distribution of receptors at the outer edge of the tissue (*see* Fig. 3). Our interpretation of our own image data, collected over many different cell and tissue types, is that the overall distribution of receptors in model cell systems and native tissues is similar. In particular, we have seen a large amount of intracellular ARs in every tissue we have examined. In contrast to some model cells expressing GFP-fused ARs, we have never seen native cells that express receptor at the cell surface exclusively. Although the location of native and recombinant receptors appears similar, it is uncertain if the mechanisms of sequestration and internalization are the same. Ideally, this process would be studied in cells *in situ* and would necessitate the use of 3D and 4D imaging.

There are several software packages and modules available to enable volume rendering, co-localization of multiple probes, particle tracking, and isosurface modeling to visualize and measure structures of interest (i.e., receptor-containing vesicles). A limited number of studies have examined AR distribution using 3D imaging *(7,36,37)*. We are unaware of any 4D studies that have used advanced imaging and particle tracking to study receptor turnover in living tissues. This is one of our goals for the future.

The resolution of confocal microscopy is not high enough to resolve actual protein structure. Therefore, ligand–receptor or receptor–G protein complexes are resolved as "hot spots" of intense light at high ligand concentrations and as diffuse scatterings of bright points at low concentrations. Isosurfaces are an ideal way to display these different conditions (*see* Fig. 7). Once a surface is generated, the software can report the surface area and volume of a selected object. In addition, the distance an object travels over time can be plotted and measured. Although such software is available, it has not yet been properly exploited in applications of receptor sequestration and recycling.

An additional complexity is the possibility of protein–protein interactions during the cascade of receptor-recycling events. We now know that receptor subtypes can form oligomers, and this has become an area of great interest. The visualization of protein–protein interactions can be achieved using simple co-localization studies *(15)* or FRET *(14)*. Co-localisation is a process whereby

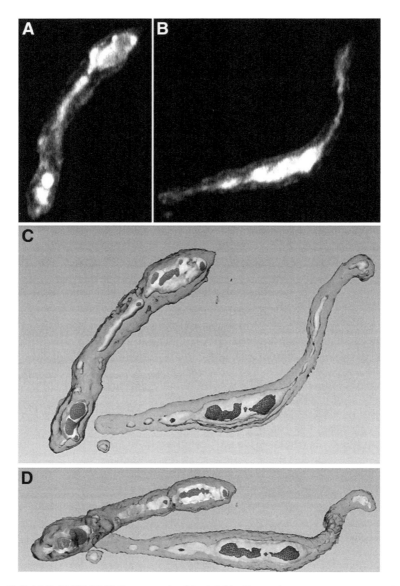

Fig. 7. QAPB (BODIPY FL-prazosin, 30 nM) binding to isolated smooth muscle cells. **(A,B)** Single orthoslice views of two individual cells B)show binding to the surface membrane and prominent binding to intracellular sites. The optical slices are the midpoint images of a full serial section collected by confocal microscopy. **(C,D)** The surface-rendered models of both cells are shown from different viewing angles. Three threshold levels have been rendered in each cell to show the low-intensity binding-induced fluorescence (generally cell surface), midrange intensity (light color intracellular surface), or high intensity (dark surface). (Images generated from data collected by Y. P. R. Jarajapu.)

the relative amounts of two overlapping fluorescent signals are measured. However, overlapping fluorescent signals can also be problematic if the requirement is to see separate signals. To address this a technique of spectral unmixing has been developed which holds the promise of having the ability, for instance, to separate a GFP signal from a broad "green" autofluorescence signal. In addition, it may be necessary to conduct co-localization studies of multiple 4D volumes if the fate of two or more subtypes is to be tracked following agonist stimulation. This provides an interesting technical challenge for both image capture and analysis.

In summary, there is huge potential to be gained in working with images. However, analysis of images is fraught with danger if sufficient care has not been taken during the acquisition and postprocessing/correction stages.

5. Conclusion

Fluorescence techniques have been used in various formats for the study of receptors for over 30 yr. In the past, the experimental result was a 2D micrograph. Today, the result can be in the form of a 4D movie. This creates many exciting possibilities for future research. Receptors can be engineered to be endogenously fluorescent, constitutively active, nonfunctional, or a host of other mutant forms. Advances in microscopy, live cell imaging, and image analysis make it possible to visualize the life cycle of the receptor. If the images acquired are accurate, then we can begin to understand more fully the relationships that exist between the various AR subtypes. For a given tissue, we would want to know how the individual receptor subtypes are distributed in different cell types: Do they undergo internalization? Do they dimerize? Are intracellular receptors functionally coupled? What happens when one or more are knocked out? How do these features relate to disease? Through the use of fluorescent ligands, antibodies, and proteins used in combination with high-performance computing and microscopy, we can now begin to answer these questions and more.

Acknowledgments

We are grateful to colleagues and postgraduate and postdoctoral researchers for their important input into our various research projects over the years. In particular, we acknowledge Silvia Arribas, Anna Briones, Christine Brown, Jose Maria Gonzales, Y. P. R. Jarajapu, Janet Mackenzie, Raquel Miguel, Majid Shafaroudi, Ulrika Trendelenburg, Elisabet Vila, and Alison Woollhead for their contributions to the data alluded to or presented in this chapter. We also acknowledge the support of Tenovus Scotland, the British Heart Foundation, Wellcome Trust, the Medical Research Council, the Biotechnology and Biological Sciences Research Council, and the European Commission.

References

1. Barak LS, Ferguson SSG, Zhang J, Martenson C, Meyer T, Caron MG. Internal trafficking and surface mobility of a functionally intact β_2-adrenergic receptor-green fluorescent protein conjugate. Mol Pharmacol 1997;51:177–184.
2. Milligan G. The use of receptor G-protein fusion proteins for the study of ligand activity. Receptors Channels 2002;8:309–317.
3. Kallal L, Gagnon AW, Penn RB, Benovic JL. Visualization of agonist-induced sequestration and down-regulation of a green fluorescent protein-tagged β_2-adrenergic receptor. J Biol Chem 1998;273: 322–328.
4. McLean A, Milligan G. Ligand regulation of green fluorescent protein-tagged forms of the human β_1- and β_2-adrenoceptors;comparisons with the unmodified receptors. Br J Pharmacol 2000;130:1825–1832.
5. Shiina T, Kawasaki A, Nagao T, Kuros H. Interaction with β-arrestin determines the difference in internalization behavior between β_1- and β_2-adrenergic receptors. J Biol Chem 2000;275:29,082–29,090.
6. Kallal L, Benovic JL. Using green fluorescent proteins to study G-protein-coupled receptor localisation and trafficking. Trends Pharmacol Sci 2000;21: 175–180.
7. Burgi S, Baltensperger K, Honegger UE. Antidepressant-induced switch of β_1-adrenoceptor trafficking as a mechanism for drug action. J Biol Chem 2003;278: 1044–1052.
8. Chalothorn D, McCune DF, Edelmann SE, Garcia-Cazarin ML, Tsujimoto G, Piascik MT. Differences in the cellular localization and agonist-mediated internalization properties of the α_1-adrenoceptor subtypes. Mol Pharmacol 2002;61: 1008–1016.
9. Hirasawa A, Awaji T, Xu Z, Shinoura H, Tsujimoto G. Subtype-specific differences in subcellular localization and chlorethylclonidine inactivation of α_1-adrenoceptors. Mol Pharmacol 1997;52:764–770.
10. Awaji T, Hirasawa A, Kataoka M, et al. Real-time optical monitoring of ligand-mediated internalization of α_{1b}-adrenoceptor with green fluorescent protein. Mol Endocrinol 1998;12:1099–1111.
11. Oakley RH, Laporte SA, Holt JA., Caron M, Barak L. Differential affinities of visual arrestin, βarrestin1, and arrestin2 for G protein-coupled receptors delineate two major classes of receptors. J Biol Chem 2000;275:17,201–17,210.
12. Yang M, Ruan J, Voller M, Schalke J, Michel MC. Differential regulation of human α_1-adrenoceptor subtypes. Naunyn Schmiedebergs Arch Pharmacol 1999; 359:439–446.
13. Chalothorn D, McCune DF, Edelmann SE, et al. Differential cardiovascular regulatory activities of the α_{1B}- and α_{1D}-adrenoceptor subtypes. J Pharmacol Exp Ther 2003;305:1045–1053.
14. Stanasila L, Perez JB, Vogel H, Cotecchia S. Oligomerization of the α_{1a}- and α_{1b}-adrenergic receptor subtypes. Potential implications in receptor internalization. J Biol Chem. 2003;278:40,239–40,251.
15. Hague C, Uberti MA, Chen Z, Hall RA, Minneman KP. Cell surface expression of α_{1d}-adrenergic receptors is controlled by heterodimerization with α_{1b}-adrenergic receptors. J Biol Chem 2004;279:15,541–15,549.

16. Daly CJ, Deighan C, McGee A, et al. A knockout approach indicates a minor vasoconstrictor role for vascular α_{1B}-adrenoceptors in mouse. Physiol Genomics 2002;9:85–91.
17. Uhlen S, Axelrod D, Keefer JR, Limbird L, Neubig RR. Membrane organisation and mobility of α_2-adrenoceptors in MDCK cells. Pharmacol Commun 1995;6: 155–167.
18. Daly CJ, McGrath JC. Fluorescent ligands, antibodies and proteins for the study of receptors. Pharmacol Ther 2003;100:101–118.
19. McGrath JC, Pediani JD, Macmillan J, et al. Adventitial cells are identified as the major location of vascular α_{1B}-adrenoceptors and may drive vascular remodelling. Br J Pharmacol 2002;137:21P.
20. Zuscik MJ, Piascik MT, Perez DM. Cloning, cell-type specificity, and regulatory function of the mouse α_{1b}-adrenergic receptor promoter. Mol Pharmacol 1999;56: 1288–1297.
21. Mu HM, Zhu ZM, Wang HY, Wang LJ. Effect of removal of the adventitia on vascular remodeling and vasoconstriction in rabbits. Acta Physiol Sin 2003;55: 290–295.
22. McGrath JC, Arribas SM, Daly CJ. Fluorescent ligands for the study of receptors. Trends Pharmacol Sci 1996;17:393–399.
23. Pick H, Preuss A, Mayer M, Wohland T, Hovius R, Vogel H. Monitoring expression and clustering of the ionotropic 5HT3 receptor in plasma membranes of live biological cells. Biochemistry 2003;42:877–884.
24. Akaaboune M, Grady RM, Turney S, Sanes JR, Lichtman JW. Neurotransmitter receptor dynamics studied in vivo by reversible photo-unbinding of fluorescent ligands. Neuron 2002;34:865–876
25. Arttamangkul S, Alvarez-maubecin, Thomas G, Williams JT, Grandy DK. Binding and internalization of fluorescent opioid peptide conjugates in living cells. Mol Pharmacol 2000;58:1570–1580.
26. Beaudet A, Nouel D, Stroh T, Vandenbulcke F, Dal-Farra C, Vincent JP. Fluorescent ligands for studying neuropeptide receptors by confocal microscopy. Braz J Med Biol Res 1998;31:1479–1489.
27. Patel RC, Kumar U, Lamb DC, et al. Ligand binding to stomatostatin receptors induces receptor-specific oligomer formation in live cells. Proc Natl Acad Sci USA 2002;99:3294–3299.
28. Atlas D, Melamed E, Lahav M. Direct localisation of β adrenoceptor sites in rat cerebellum by a new fluorescent analogue of propranolol. Nature 1976;261:420–421.
29. Atlas D, Melamed, E. Direct mapping of β-adrenergic receptors in the rat central nervous system by a novel fluorescent β-blocker. Brain Res 1978;150:377–385.
30. Henis YI, Hekman M, Elson EL, Helmreich EJ. Lateral motion of β receptors in membranes of cultured liver cells. Proc Nat Acad Sci USA 1982;79:2907–2911.
31. Rademaker B, Kramer K, Bast A, Timmerman H. Irreversible binding of the fluorescent β-adrenoceptor probes alprenolol-NBD and pindolol-NBD to specific and non-specific binding sites. Res Commun Chem Pathol Pharmacol 1988;60: 147–159.
32. Heithier H, Hallmann, D, Boege F, et al. Synthesis and properties of fluorescent β-adrenoceptor ligands. Biochemistry 1994;33:9126–9134.

33. Baker JG, Hall I, Hill SJ. Pharmacology and direct visualisation of BODIPY TMR-CGP: a long acting fluorescent β_2-adrenoceptor agonist. Br J Pharmacol 2003;139: 232–242.

34. McGrath JC, Daly CJ. Viewing adrenoceptors;past, present, and future; commentary and a new technique. Pharmacol Commun 1995;6:269–279.

35. Daly CJ, Milligan CM, Milligan G, Mackenzie JF, McGrath JC. Cellular localisation and pharmacological characterisation of functioning α_1-adrenoceptors by fluorescent ligand binding and image analysis reveals identical binding properties of clustered and diffuse populations of receptors. J Pharmacol Exp Ther 1998;286:984–990.

36. McGrath JC, Mackenzie JF, Daly CJ. Pharmacological implications of cellular localisation of α_1-adrenoceptors in native smooth muscle cells. J Autonom Pharmacol 1999;19:303–310.

37. Mackenzie JF, Daly CJ, Pediani JD, McGrath JC. Quantitative imaging in live human cells reveals intracellular α_1-adrenoceptor ligand-binding sites. J Pharmacol Exp Ther 2000;294:434–443.

38. Guimaraes S, Moura D. Vascular adrenoceptors: an update. Pharmacol Rev 2001; 53:319–356.

39. Jarajapu YPR, Coats P, McGrath JC, Hillier C, MacDonald A. Functional characterization of α_1-adrenoceptor subtypes in human skeletal muscle resistance arteries. Br J Pharmacol 2001;133:679–686.

40. Jarajapu YPR, Macdonald A, Hillier C, McGrath JC, Mackenzie JF, Daly CJ. Quantitative imaging of QAPB-associated fluorescence in smooth muscle cells from human skeletal muscle resistance arteries. Br J Pharmacol 2002;135:303P.

41. Daunt DA, Hurt C, Hein L, Kallio J, Feng F, Kobilka BK. Subtype-specific intracellular trafficking of α_2-adrenergic receptors. Mol Pharmacol 1997;51:711–720.

42. Olli-Lahdesmaki T, Kallio J, Scheinin M. Receptor subtype-induced targeting and subtype-specific internalization of human α_2-adrenoceptors in PC12 cells. J Neurosci 1999;19:9281–9288.

43. Cocks TM, Angus JA. Endothelium-dependent relaxation of coronary arteries by noradrenaline and serotonin. Nature 1983;305:627–630.

44. Vanhoutte PM, Miller VM. α_2-Adrenoceptors and endothelium-derived relaxant factor. Am J Med 1989;87:1S–5S.

45. Vanhoutte PM. Endothelial adrenoceptors. J Cardiovasc Pharmacol 2001;38: 796–808.

46. Filippi S, Parenti A, Donnini S, Granger HJ, Fazzini A, Ledda F. α_{1D}-Adrenoceptors cause endothelium-dependent vasodilatation in the rat mesenteric vascular bed. J Pharmacol Exp Ther 2001;296:869–875.

47. Dunkle R. Role of image informatics in accelerating drug discovery. Drug Discov World Winter 2004:75–82.

48. Sinskey AJ, Finkelstein SN, Cooper SM. Medical imaging in drug discovery. PharmaGenomics 2004;4:20–26.

7

Localization of Adrenergic Receptor Subtypes and Transgenic Expression of Fluorescent-Tagged Receptors

Dianne M. Perez

Summary

Although the adrenergic receptors have been cloned since the late 1980s and early 1990s, analysis of the expression of the subtypes in specific tissues and cell types has been hampered because of the lack of high-affinity and high-avidity antibodies. Most of the antibodies currently available have limited use in transfected systems in which receptor density is high but give poor results when used to determine endogenous expression. This limitation in antibody avidity is common in membrane proteins and in G protein-coupled receptors (GPCRs) because of poor protein purification and membrane epitope recognition. Although analysis of ligand binding to tissue homogenates yields an estimate of the tissue content of the various adrenergic receptor subtypes, it does not have sufficient resolution to determine cell type distribution. Currently, methods useful for determining receptor localization are *in situ* hybridization histochemistry and receptor autoradiography. This chapter reviews the localization of the various adrenergic receptors using these methods. I also introduce the concept and utility of using transgenic mice expressing fluorescent-tagged adrenergic receptor subtypes to determine the cell type-specific localization of these receptors using the α_1-adrenergic receptor as a model system.

Key Words: Adrenergic receptor; autoradiography; brain; fluorescent; green fluorescent protein; hybridization; *in situ* hybridization; RNA; localization; transgenics.

From: *The Receptors: The Adrenergic Receptors: In the 21st Century*
Edited by: D. Perez © Humana Press Inc., Totowa, NJ

1. Introduction

Although many studies have used radioligand binding on cell lines or tissues to determine the localization of the adrenergic receptor (AR) subtypes, I only review the distribution based on either *in situ* hybridization histochemistry or receptor autoradiography because these are the only methods that can determine cellular localization. The use of *in situ* hybridization histochemistry in particular can discern subtype specificity. I also limit discussion of AR localization based on polymerase chain reaction (PCR) data because of the vast potential for contamination at both the ribonucleic acid (RNA) and tissue levels. Also, PCR cannot determine exactly where in the tissue the receptor is located. The limitation of *in situ* hybridization is that the distribution of messenger RNA (mRNA) may not define protein localization because the mRNA can be transported from cell bodies. The use of radioligands for autoradiography is also limited by the lack of discrimination of the subtypes and high background binding. In general, most tissues contain multiple AR subtypes and multiple members within each subfamily. In the brain, all of the ARs are prominent in the gray areas, with very little expression in the white matter. Dominant expression of a particular subtype cannot yet be ascertained until the receptor protein for all subtypes can be quantitated. Unless specified, all localizations discussed below are in the rat.

2. Localization Based on *In Situ* Hybridization or Receptor Autoradiography: α_1-Adrenergic Receptors

2.1. Brain

The distribution of α_1-AR subtypes in the brain has been determined by either receptor autoradiography or *in situ* hybridization to mRNAs *(1–3)*. Most studies have used rat brain, but analyses in the mouse and other species indicate that they are similar to the rat *(4)*. One of the most important differences noted between species, however, was the high density of total α_1-ARs in human and monkey hippocampi; in all other species, such as the rat and mouse, the total α_1-AR density was low. The distribution of the α_1-AR subtypes in this study was not performed. Although there are numerous discrepancies between published studies, the general pattern of α_1-AR expression is consistent.

Autoradiography is performed using a nonselective antagonist (either [^{3}H]prazosin or [^{125}I]-2-[-(3-iodo-4-hydroxyphenyl)-ethylaminomethyl tetralone ([^{125}I]HEAT). Therefore, the particular α_1-AR subtype involved cannot be determined. Although some studies used somewhat selective antagonists such as WB4101 or 5-methylurapidil to discriminate α_{1a}-ARs (10- to 100-fold α_{1a}-selective), these compounds cannot distinguish between the α_{1b}- and α_{1d}-ARs. Therefore, we know the general patterns of α_1-AR subtype expression but cannot be conclusive because of the use of nonselective compounds or the transport of the mRNA. AR distribution for all subtypes determined via these methods is summarized in Tables 1 and 2.

In cats, the highest levels of total α_1-AR density, labeled with [^{3}H]prazosin, were found in laminae II, IX, and X of the cerebral cortex *(5)*. The highest levels of α_{1A}-AR mRNA expression were seen in the olfactory bulb, tenia tectae, horizontal diagonal band/magnocellular preoptic area, zona incerta, ventromedial hypothalamus, lateral mammillary nuclei, ventral dentate gyrus, piriform cortex, medial and cortical amygdala, magnocellular red nuclei, pontine nuclei, superior and lateral vestibular nuclei, brain stem reticular nuclei, and several cranial nerve motor nuclei. Using *in situ* hybridization and combining a probe for choline acetyltransferase mRNA with a probe specific for the α_{1A}-AR, the α_{1A}-AR mRNA was determined to be expressed in cholinergic motor neurons. Prominent α_{1A}-AR signals were also seen in the neocortex, claustrum, lateral amygdala, ventral cochlear nucleus, raphe magnus, and the ventral horn of thoracic spinal cord *(6)*. Consistently, the α_{1A}-AR was primarily localized in the olfactory bulb, intermediate layers of the cortex, but inconsistently in the hippocampus and the reticular nucleus of the thalamus according to the 1993 studies of McCune et al. *(2)*.

The α_{1B}-AR is expressed in intermediate and deep layers of the cortex, thalamus, hippocampus, dorsal raphe, and cerebellum *(2)*. The distribution of α_{1B}-AR immunoreactivity has been determined in female rat brain regions involved in stress and neuroendocrine function. The pattern of immunolabeling seen resembles that obtained in previous *in situ* hybridization studies. Several hypothalamic areas that control pituitary function show intense immunolabeling, including the paraventricular nucleus (PVN) of the hypothalamus, the supraoptic nucleus, and the median eminence. α_{1B}-AR immunoreactivity is also observed in large pyramidal neurons of layer V of the cerebral cortex and the frontal cortex. Virtually all of the thalamic regions are labeled, especially the lateral and ventral areas. In addition, labeled cells are present in hippocampus, the medial septum, the horizontal and vertical limbs of the diagonal band of Broca, and the caudate putamen. Finally, some midbrain and hindbrain regions important for motor function are immunoreactive *(7)*. However, most investigators in the field believe that these antibodies are not sensitive and specific enough to detect endogenous protein, but they are mentioned here because this is the only report of their use in the brain, and the pattern of expression is consistent with the RNA studies.

The PVN of the hypothalamus contains a number of neuroendocrine cell groups involved in the hormonal stress response. Ascending noradrenergic afferents to the PVN, acting through α_1-ARs, are thought to play a role in stress-induced activation of the hypothalamic-pituitary-adrenal axis. The α_{1D}-AR subtype is the most prominently expressed mRNA in the PVN. In sections through the PVN, nearly all oxytocin neurons expressed the α_{1D}-AR mRNA, suggesting a direct role for α_1-ARs in the regulation of oxytocin secretion *(8)*.

Table 1
Distribution of Adrenergic Receptor Subtypes in the Brain Via *In Situ* or Autoradiography

Tissue	α_{1A}	α_{1B}	α_{1D}	α_{2A}	α_{2B}	α_{2C}	β_1	β_2	β_3
Cerebral cortex	++r	+++r	++r	++m,r	+h	++m,r	++r	++r	ND
Hippocampus									
• Dentate gyrus	++r	+h	++r	+h	+m,h	++r,h	+r	+r	ND
• CA1	+r	—	++r	+m,r,h	+m,h	+m,r,h	+r	++r,gp	ND
• CA3	+h	—	++r	+m,r	+m	+m	—	+r	ND
Basal ganglia									
• Caudate/putamen	—	+r	—	—	+m	++m,r	++r	+r	ND
• Globus pallidus	+r	ND	ND	—	—	+r	+r	+r	ND
• Islands of Calleja	ND	ND	ND	—	+m	++m,r	ND	ND	ND
• Claustrum	++r	ND	++m,r	+m	+m,r	ND	ND	+r	ND
Cerebellum									
• Granule cell layer	—	ND	ND	++m,r	—	—	ND	ND	ND
• Molecular layer	—	ND	ND	—	—	—	ND	ND	ND
• Purkinje layer	—	ND	ND	—	++m	—	ND	ND	ND
• Cerebellar nuclei	+r	+r	+r	++m,r	—	+m,r	+r	+r	ND
Olfactory									
• Anterior olfactory nuclei	+r	ND	ND	++m,r	—	++m,r	++r	ND	ND
• Piriform cortex	++r	—	—	+m,r	+m	++m,r	+r	++r	ND
• Olfactory tubercle	ND	ND	ND	ND	—	ND	—	++r	ND
• Bulb	++r	+r	+++r	+m	—	++m,r	+r	++r	ND
Amygdaloid	++r	ND	ND	++m,r	—	+m,r	++r	+r	ND
Thalamus									
• Dorsal lateral geniculate nuclei	—	+++r	+r	+m	++m,r	+m	+r	+r	ND
• Reticular thalmic nuclei	—	—	++r	++r	+m	—	+r	—	ND
• Intralaminar nuclei	—	++r	ND	—	++m,r	—	+r	ND	ND
• Paraventricular thalmic nuclei	—	++r	ND	+r	+m,r	—	+r	+r	ND

Tissue	α_{1A}	α_{1B}	α_{1D}	α_{2A}	α_{2B}	α_{2C}	β_1	β_2	β_3
Hypothalamus									
• Periventricular hypothalmic nuclei	++r	+r	—	+m,r	—	+m	—	ND	ND
• Dorsomedial hypothalamic nuclei	—	+r	—	++m,r	—	+m	—	—	ND
• Posterior	ND	ND	ND	++m,r	—	+m	ND	ND	ND
• Mammillary nuclei	++r	ND	ND	++m,r	—	+m	ND	ND	ND
• Lateral	++r	ND	ND	++m,r	—	+m	ND	ND	ND
• Preoptic	++r	+r	ND	+m,r	—	+m,r	ND	ND	ND
• Paraventricular hypothalamic nuclei	ND	+r	+++r	++m	—	+m,r	ND	ND	ND
Midbrain									
• Superior colliculus	+r	ND	ND	+m,r	—	+r	+r	+r	ND
• Inferior colliculus	—	ND	ND	+m,r	—	+m,r	ND	ND	ND
• Dorsal raphe nuclei	+r	+++r	—	+m,r	—	+r	—	—	ND
• Substantia nigra	—	ND	ND	+m	—	+r	+r	+r	ND
• Central gray	+r	ND	ND	++r	—	—	ND	ND	ND
Brain stem and pons									
• Locus coeruleus	ND	—	—	+++m,r	—	+r	—	—	ND
• Dorsal motor	ND	+r	ND	+m,r	—	+r	ND	ND	ND
• Lateral reticular nuclei	++r	ND	ND	++m,r	—	++r	ND	ND	ND
• Motor trigeminal nuclei	+++r	ND	ND	+m,r	—	+r	ND	ND	ND
• Reticulotegmental nuclei pons	++r	ND	ND	++m,r	—	++r	ND	ND	ND
• Inferior olive	ND	—	+++r	++m	—	—	—	—	ND
Pineal gland	+++r	+r	—	—	+r	+++r	+r	ND	ND
Spinal cord	++r	++r	++r	++r	—	+r	+r	+r	ND
Pituitary	ND	ND	ND	ND	ND	ND	+r,h,rb	+++r,h,rb	ND

gp, guinea pig; h, human; m, mouse; ND, not determined; r, rat; rb, rabbit; —, not detected; +, low expression; ++ medium expression; +++, high expression.

Table 2

Distribution of Adrenergic Receptor Subtypes in Peripheral Tissues Via *In Situ* or Autoradiography

Tissue	α_{1A}	α_{1B}	α_{1D}	α_{2A}	α_{2B}	α_{2C}	β_1	β_2	β_3
Bladder	+r,h	—	—	ND	ND	ND	+h	+h	+++h
Kidney									
• Cortex	+r,h	+r,h	+r,h	ND	—	ND	+r,gp	+r,gp	ND
• Glomeruli	+h	+h	+h	ND	—	ND	++r,gp	ND	ND
• Proximal tubule	+r	+r	+r	ND	+r	ND	—	++gp	ND
• Distal tubule	ND	ND	ND	ND	—	ND	+r,gp	ND	ND
Urethra									
• Proximal	++h	++h	++h	ND	ND	ND	ND	ND	ND
• Distal	++h	+h	+h	ND	ND	ND	ND	ND	ND
Prostate									
• Stromal	+++h	+h	+h	ND	ND	ND	—	—	ND
• Glandular	+h	+++h	+h	ND	ND	ND	+r	+r	ND
Lung									
• Pulmonary blood vessels	ND	ND	ND	ND	ND	ND	+h	++r,h	—
• Airway epithelium	ND	ND	ND	ND	ND	ND	—	++r.h	—
• Smooth muscle									
Small airways	ND	ND	ND	ND	ND	ND	—	++r,h	—
Large airways	ND	ND	ND	ND	ND	ND	—	+r,h	—

Tissue	α_{1A}	α_{1B}	α_{1D}	α_{2A}	α_{2B}	α_{2C}	β_1	β_2	β_3
Pancreas									
• Islets	ND	ND	ND	+h	+h	+h	ND	++h	ND
• Exocrine	ND	ND	ND	++h	++h	++h	ND	—	ND
Heart									
• Myocardium	ND	ND	ND	—	—	—	+h,gp	+h,gp	ND
• AV node	ND	ND	ND	ND	ND	ND	+h	++h,gp	ND
• S-A node	ND	ND	ND	ND	ND	ND	+h	+h	ND
• Bundle of His	ND	ND	ND	ND	ND	ND	+h	+h	ND
• Interventricular septum	ND	ND	ND	ND	ND	ND	+h	+h	ND
Arteries									
• Endothelial/intimal	—	—	—	—	—	—	—	++h	ND
• Medial layer	++r	+r	+r	+r	—	+r	+h	—	ND
• Adventitia	ND	ND	ND	—	—	—	—	+r,h	ND
Lymphocytes	+h	++h	+h	ND	ND	ND	ND	ND	ND
Adipocytes	ND	ND	ND	ND	ND	ND	++h, rb	+rb	+h,rb

gp, guinea pig; h, human; m, mouse; ND, not determined; r, rat; rb, rabbit; —, not detected; +, low expression; ++, medium expression; +++, high expression.

In another study, α_{1D}-AR mRNA was expressed at high levels in the PVN, primarily in magnocellular cells, and at low levels in parvocellular cells *(9)*. This receptor mRNA is not regulated by glucocorticoids in vivo. In addition, the same group found by *in situ* hybridization that the α_{1B}-AR mRNA was also expressed in CRH-containing, stress-responsive cells of the PVN and was highly sensitive to circulating levels of corticosterone *(10)*, and that the mRNA encoding the α_{1B}-AR subtype was present at moderate levels in parvocellular cells of the rat PVN *(2,3,9)*. Expression of α_{1B}-AR mRNA within the PVN and its dependence on circulating glucocorticoids is consistent with the observation that the promoter region of the gene contains a glucocorticoid response element *(11)*. So, both α_1-AR subtypes may be present in the hypothalamus, but because the RNA may be regulated differently, no conclusions about protein abundance can be justified.

The hippocampus receives major adrenergic input from the locus ceruleus *(12)*, and various ARs are present in various types of cells in the hippocampus, determined through patch-clamping of the principal excitatory neurons *(13)*, interneurons *(14)*, and glial cells *(15)*. Based on mRNA arguments, the α_{1D}-AR is also thought to be the major α_1-AR subtype expressed in hippocampus *(16)*. Other studies suggested that the α_{1A}-AR is dominant, but the α_{1B}-AR message is still present, although at 10-fold lower values *(17)*. The distributions of the α_1-AR subtypes (α_{1A} and α_{1B}) in human and rat hippocampus were analyzed by quantitative receptor autoradiography. α_1-ARs are labeled by [^{3}H]prazosin. The α_{1A}-AR subtype is visualized by [^{3}H]prazosin after irreversible blockade of α_{1B}-ARs with chloroethylclonidine or directly by [^{3}H]5-methylurapidil. The α_{1B}-AR subtype is investigated by [^{3}H]prazosin binding in the presence of the α_{1A}-AR antagonist 5-methylurapidil. Considerable differences in the regional and laminar patterns of α_1-ARs are found between rat and human hippocampi. A low overall density and a rather homogeneous distribution characterize the rat hippocampus. This is in contrast to the human pattern, which shows a much higher overall level of α_1-AR density and a restriction of α_1-ARs to the CA3 region of Ammon's horn and the dentate gyrus. Moreover, α_{1A}- and α_{1B}-ARs of the human hippocampus are differentially distributed, with the α_{1A}-AR subtype concentrated in the hilus and lucidum layer of CA3 and the α_{1B}-AR subtype concentrated in the molecular layer of the dentate gyrus *(18)*. In another study using [^{3}H]5-methylurapidil, suggesting α_{1A}-AR-binding sites, the CA1, CA3, and dentate gyrus were labeled in the rat *(19)*.

In the spinal cord, α_1-AR mRNA was detected at four levels in humans (cervical enlargement, thoracic, lumbar, sacral). α_1-AR mRNA was present in ventral gray matter, anterior horn motor neurons at all levels, dorsal nucleus of Clarke and intermediolateral columns in cervical enlargement, and parasympathetic nucleus in sacral spinal cord. However, although all three α_1-AR subtypes were present throughout human spinal cord, again the α_{1D}-AR mRNA predominated overall *(20)*.

The postnatal development of α_1-ARs was also studied in the rat brain with receptor autoradiography using [I^{125}]HEAT *(21)*. In some regions, such as the globus pallidus, binding sites were present at birth and increased during the first week but then decreased to very low levels by adulthood. In contrast, other regions, such as the olfactory bulb and cerebral cortex, had little binding at birth but showed an increase in receptor density during week 2 that continued to adulthood. Several regions had binding at birth, an increase in binding sites in the first few weeks, and then a small decrease in binding sites as adulthood approached. These studies suggest that α_1-ARs in various brain regions develop at different rates.

The limitations in these studies are that hybridization of the probes is not equal among the α_1-AR subtypes, which may be dependent on the secondary structure of the probes. Therefore, probe intensity cannot be used to quantitate mRNA levels. Another limitation is that the α_{1D}-AR is known to express an abundance of mRNA, but the expression of functional protein is usually the lowest among the α_1-AR subtypes, at least in transfected systems and in some limited mouse tissue-binding studies *(22)*. In the α_{1D}-AR knockout mice of Tanoue et al. *(23)*, the α_{1D}-AR density was only 10% reduced in whole brain, also suggesting poor protein expression of this subtype in the brain.

2.2. Kidney, Urethra, Bladder, and Prostate

In both proximal and distal renal tubules, each of the α_1-AR mRNAs was less abundant in the cytoplasm than in the arteries. In the glomeruli, weak staining was detected in the endothelium, but there was no obvious staining in the veins *(24)*. [^{3}H]Prazosin binding to rat, dog, and human kidney revealed binding to the vasculature, with additional receptors confined to the renal cortex in rat. In the rat kidney, autoradiography showed that binding in the renal cortex was largely in the proximal tubules. In all three species, the autoradiographic studies support a role for α_1-ARs in control of renal blood flow. In the rat, the location of α_1-ARs suggests that they can also have an important influence on fluid and electrolyte balance, gluconeogenesis, and production of prostanoids *(25)*.

α_1-ARs are predominantly located in urethral smooth muscle, indicating their contractile importance in maintaining continence *(26)*. Furthermore, autoradiographic studies showed a heterogeneous distribution of α_1-AR along the longitudinal axis of the urethra within the smooth muscle fibers, with the receptors localized more densely in the proximal than in the distal urethra *(27)*. *In situ* hybridization studies showed no significant differences in the cross-sectional distribution of α_1-AR subtype mRNAs between male and female human urethras. Among the subtypes, intense α_{1A}-AR localization was observed in the smooth muscle of the urethra, but α_{1B} and α_{1D}-AR expression was much less intense *(28)*.

The α_{1A}-AR mRNA was localized in all smooth muscle areas of the rat, monkey, and human urinary bladder and prostate. High levels of α_{1A} mRNA were detected in bladder dome and bladder base urothelium *(29)*. In the prostate, *in situ* hybridization localizes the α_{1A}-AR mRNA predominantly to the stromal compartment *(30)*. By immunohistochemistry, using the low-affinity antibodies, the α_{1A}-AR was also detected in the stroma and not in the glandular epithelium. The α_{1B}-AR was localized predominantly in the epithelium and was weakly present in the stroma. Lower levels of the α_{1B}-AR were detected in the hyperplastic prostatic epithelium. The α_{1D}-AR was detected in areas of stroma and was abundantly present in blood vessels *(31)*. In another study, WB-4101 and SNAP 5272, which are α_{1A}-AR selective, inhibited 100% of the specific [^{125}I]HEAT binding in the stroma, suggesting that all of the stromal α_1-AR population is the α_{1A}-AR subtype. WB-4101 inhibited none of the specific [^{125}I]HEAT binding in the epithelium, suggesting that the α_1-ARs in the epithelium are the α_{1B}-AR subtype *(32)*. In a third study, the α_{1A}-AR subtype was found in both prostate stromal and glandular cells; α_{1B}-AR and α_{1D}-AR subtypes were expressed in glandular cells *(33)*. Therefore, a consensus is that the α_{1A}-AR is prominent in the stroma, and the other subtypes are prominent in the glandular areas.

2.3. Vasculature

In situ hybridization showed that all three α_1-AR subtype mRNAs are localized in the smooth muscle cells of the medial layer of arteries *(34,35)*, and the distribution pattern of all three mRNAs in the main arteries was the same as in the branch arteries. However, the intensity of signals for α_{1D}-AR and α_{1B}-AR probes was lower than that for the α_{1A}-AR probe *(36)*. Expression of all three α_1-AR subtype mRNAs was confirmed in the arteries of the renal cortex (arciform, interlobular, arteriole), but among the three subtypes, the α_{1B}-AR was less apparent *(24)*.

2.4. Lymphocytes

In situ hybridization cytochemistry revealed the presence of all three α_1-AR mRNA in human peripheral blood lymphocytes. Lymphocytes hybridized for the α_{1A}-AR subtype represented approx 30% of total lymphocytes; those hybridized for the α_{1B}- and α_{1D}-AR subtypes averaged 42 and 25% of total lymphocytes, respectively *(37)*.

3. Localization Based on *In Situ* or Autoradiography : α_2-Adrenergic Receptors

3.1. Brain

In early studies, localization of α_2-ARs in the rat brain with [^{3}H]idazoxan binding sites closely paralleled that of [^{3}H]clonidine sites and corresponded to areas of noradrenergic innervation. The α_2-ARs, labeled with [^{3}H]idazoxan, were found mainly in laminae II, III, and X, with moderate densities in lamina IX of the cerebral cortex *(5)*. Densest [^{3}H]idazoxan labeling appeared over anterior olfactory nuclei, fundus striatum, septum, thalamus, hypothalamus, amygdala, entorhinal cortex, central gray, inferior colliculus, dorsal parabrachial nucleus, locus ceruleus, and nucleus of the solitary tract. High-density [^{3}H]rauwolscine labeling appeared over nucleus caudate putamen, nucleus accumbens, olfactory tubercle, islands of Calleja, hippocampus, parasubiculum, basolateral amygdaloid nucleus, and substantia nigra. *(38)*. Since then, some reports have determined the localization of these receptors in rat brain cells by using *in situ* hybridization with oligonucleotides or riboprobes *(39–41)*; however, there are inconsistencies among the several studies similar to the results in the α_1-AR.

α_{2A}-AR mRNA labeling was most pronounced in neurons in layer VI of the cerebral cortex, hypothalamic PVN, reticular thalamic nucleus, pontine nuclei, locus coeruleus, vestibular nuclei, trapezoid nuclei, deep cerebellar nuclei, nucleus tractus solitarii, ventrolateral medullary reticular formation, and the intermediolateral cell column of the thoracic spinal cord. The α_{2B}-AR probe, which primarily labels the kidney, gave only a very light signal in the thalamus in the central nervous system (CNS). α_{2C}-AR mRNA labeling was primarily observed in the olfactory bulb, cerebral cortex, islands of Calleja, striatum, hippocampal formation, cerebellar cortex, and dorsal root ganglia *(41)*. α_{2C}-AR localization via an antibody approach also found labeling in the anterior olfactory nucleus, piriform cortex, septum, diagonal band, pallidum, preoptic areas, supraoptic nucleus, suprachiasmatic nucleus, PVN, amygdala, hippocampus (CA1 and dentate gyrus), substantia nigra, ventral tegmental area, raphe (pontine and medullary), motor trigeminal nucleus, facial nucleus, vestibular nucleus, dorsal motor nucleus of the vagus, and hypoglossal nucleus. Labeling was found in specific laminae throughout the cortex, and a sparse distribution of very darkly labeled cells was observed in the striatum *(42)*. In the human frontal cortex, in addition to binding to the α_{2A}-AR subtype, [^{3}H]RX-821002 bound also to a small portion of α_{2B}- and α_{2C}-AR in layer III. In the hippocampus, both α_{2A}- and non-α_{2A}-ARs were labeled in the dentate gyrus and the CA1 field, together with 5-HT$_{1A}$ receptors *(43)*. Receptor localization was not determined in areas containing principally white matter, but the optical density in those areas was similar to film background, suggesting a very low receptor density. However, low receptor concentrations were also found in areas that do not contain a high percentage of white matter, such as lateral septum and ventromedial hypothalamic nucleus *(44)*.

Although the α_{2A}-AR mRNA is highly expressed in layer VI of the cortex and the locus coeruleus, α_{2B}-AR mRNA is expressed predominantly in the thalamus and in the Purkinje layer of the cerebellum, and α_{2C}-AR mRNA is expressed in the putamen caudate region of the mouse brain. Both α_{2A} and α_{2C}-AR mRNA demonstrate strong expression in the amygdaloid complex, hypothalamus, olfactory system, and the hippocampal formation. A transgenic approach was attempted with 3 kb of the upstream promoter for the α_{2A}-AR gene fused to LacZ as a reporter gene, and expression of β-galactosidase activity was assessed in transgenic offspring. Therefore, this system used the promoter to drive a reporter gene, not the actual receptor. Although the spatial expression of LacZ in the adult brain often overlaps that for the endogenous α_{2A}-AR, both ectopic expression and the absence of appropriate expression were noted, but in contrast, five of the six lines showed temporal expression characteristic of the endogenous α_{2A}-AR gene. The findings from these studies indicated that 3 kb of promoter has imparted faithful temporal but not spatial expression for the α_{2A}-AR gene, suggesting that additional regulatory sequences might be necessary *(45)*.

In an attempt to delineate the regulatory mechanism of the α_{2B}-AR subtype expression in the CNS, Wang et al. *(46)* created another transgenic mouse that regulated transgene (LacZ) expression by the 4.7-kb promoter region of α_{2B}-AR gene. The selective expression of α_{2B}-AR in the brain as indexed by β-galactosidase activity was examined during development. The temporal course of examination was from gestation day 9.5 (E9.5) to postnatal day 28 (P28). Significant expression was detected in the dorsal root ganglion and cranial nerves V and VII at E12.5. By E18.5, expression was noted in the cerebral cortex, anterior olfactory nucleus, hypothalamus, brainstem, and cerebellar Purkinje cells. Reporter expression was detected in the hippocampal dentate gyrus first at P4. The temporal course of expression up to P28 in this area is in accordance with the developmental profiles of granule neurons of dentate gyrus. From P7 on, transgene expression was detected in additional brain areas, including the septum and thalamus. The expression correlates well with the noradrenergic innervations as evidenced by co-localization by using tyrosine hydroxylase or dopamine-β-hydroxylase immunocytochemistry *(46)*. This mouse seemed to correlate better with previous endogenous expression than the α_{2A}-AR promoter mouse earlier studied. In another developmental study, α_{2A}-AR mRNA was strongly increased by E19 and E20. The increased expression was in the cortical plate and intermediate and subventricular zones, corresponding to tiers of migrating and differentiating neurons. This transient upregulation of α_{2A}-ARs was restricted to the lateral neocortex *(47)*.

Strong α_{2A}- and α_{2C}-AR mRNA expression was also found in motor neurons and other cells in the ventral horns of the spinal cord *(48,49)*. In the dorsal horns, strong α_{2A}-AR mRNA expression was found in all layers and in the lateral spinal nucleus, whereas α_{2C}-AR mRNA was weakly expressed. The α_{2B}-AR mRNA signal was only detected in some small cells superficially in the dorsal horn. Regarding axotomy, only a marginal effect was observed for α_{2C}-AR mRNA in the ventral horn, indicating that the α_{2C}-AR-expressing cells are interneurons.

The results suggest that α_2-ARs are involved in both sensory and motor processing *(48,49)*.

3.2. Vasculature

To investigate the hypothesis that differing mRNA levels underlie gender differences in the contractile response of the rat tail artery, α_2-AR mRNA was measured using *in situ* hybridization. RNA for the α_{2A}- and α_{2C}-AR subtypes was localized to the smooth muscle layer. There was no detectable mRNA present for the α_{2B}-AR subtype *(50)*.

3.3. Pancreas and Kidney

All three $_2$-AR subtypes were identified in sections of formalin-fixed, paraffin-embedded human pancreas using riboprobes labeled with digoxigenin. Although some labeling of the three α_2-AR mRNA subtypes was seen in the islets, the labeling was most intense in the exocrine tissue of the pancreas for each receptor subtype *(51)*. Using an antibody to the third intracellular loop of the α_{2B}-AR, the receptor protein was localized in the basolateral membrane of proximal convoluted and straight tubules. No specific immunoreactivity was detected in other nephron segments *(52)*.

4. Localization Based on *In Situ* or Autoradiography: β-Adrenergic Receptors

4.1. Brain

Cells containing β_1-AR mRNA are located in the superficial pineal gland, deep pineal gland, and pineal stalk of the rat *(53)*. By *in situ* hybridization, Northern blot analysis, and reverse transcriptase PCR, a day/night rhythm in β_1-AR mRNA was seen in the rat pineal gland, with elevated levels during the dark period *(54)*, confirming localization. By oligonucleotide probes, labeling for β_1-AR mRNA was found in the anterior olfactory nucleus, cerebral cortex, lateral intermediate septal nucleus, reticular thalamic nucleus, oculomotor complex, vestibular nuclei, deep cerebellar nuclei, trapezoid nucleus, abducens nucleus, ventrolateral pontine and medullary reticular formations, intermediate gray matter of the spinal cord, and pineal gland; β_2-AR mRNA expression was strongest in the olfactory bulb, piriform cortex, hippocampal formation, thalamic intralaminar nuclei, and cerebellar cortex *(55)*. Again, the use of oligonucleotides may not be sensitive enough to be discriminatory. Using [^{125}I]cyanopindolol ([^{125}I]-CYP) and selective antagonists in autoradiography, β_1-AR was highly expressed in the rat cerebral cortex, piriform, amygdaloid, thalamic nuclei, caudate putamen, globus pallidus, substantia nigra, and superior colliculus, and β_2-AR signals were lower in those areas *(56)*. High-level expression of β_2-AR mRNA was also observed in the parietal, frontal, and piriform cortices; the medial septal nuclei;

the olfactory tubercle; and the midbrain. Moderate signals were found in the striatum, the retrosplenial cortex, the hippocampus, and the thalamic nuclei *(57)*.

Dramatic species differences between rats and guinea pigs were observed in the neuroanatomical regional localization of the β-AR subtypes. For example, using [^{125}I]CYP autoradiography in the thalamus, prominent β_1- and β_2-AR populations were identified in the rat; however, the entire thalamus of the guinea pig had few, if any, β-ARs of either subtype. Hippocampal area CA1 had high levels of β_2-ARs in both rats and guinea pigs but was accompanied by a widespread distribution of β_2-ARs only in rats *(58)*.

The localization of β-AR in the rabbit pituitary has also been studied using [^{125}I]CYP for autoradiographic distribution. The displacement curves obtained from optical density of radioautograms demonstrated that β-ARs were mostly of the β_2-AR subtype and highly concentrated in the intermediate lobe. Low concentrations of β_2-ARs were evenly distributed in both the anterior and posterior lobes (59). Rat pituitary autoradiograms showed specific binding sites for [^{125}I]CYP in anterior, intermediate, and posterior lobes, with highest concentrations found in the intermediate lobe and progressively lower concentrations in posterior and anterior lobes, respectively. In another study, autoradiograms of [^{125}I]CYP binding in human pituitary showed a significantly higher concentration of β_2-ARs in the posterior than in the anterior lobe of the pituitary. Therefore, there is a homogeneous distribution of β_2-ARs within each lobe of both rat and human pituitary glands *(60)*.

4.2. Kidney

β-ARs in rat kidney were found to be almost exclusively β_1-ARs. They were located mainly on glomeruli and to a lesser extent on the straight part of the distal tubules and the cortical portion of the collecting ducts. Some β_2-ARs were localized around the corticomedullary junction. Localization was undetectable by autoradiography in the inner medulla and papilla. Glomeruli and distal tubules of the guinea pig kidney also possess only β_1-ARs, but in contrast to the rat, extremely high concentrations of β_2-ARs were associated with the straight part of the proximal tubules in the cortex and possibly with the cortical portion of the collecting duct. Labeling was not detected on the proximal convoluted tubule in either species *(61)*. In another study, autoradiographic analysis demonstrated the presence of β_1-ARs on rat cortical structures such as glomeruli and tubules. β-ARs were present on tubules (minor population), collecting tubules in outer medulla, and the adventitia and adventitial-medial border of intraparenchymal branches of the renal artery *(62)*.

4.3. Lymph and Spleen

The anatomical localization of β_1- and β_2-ARs was studied in rat lymphoid tissues by quantitative autoradiography using [^{125}I]CYP as a ligand. In lymph nodes, a significant density of these receptors was found in the medullary cords and the interfollicular cortex; only low densities were observed in the paracortex. No detectable binding appeared in the remaining areas. In the spleen, these receptors were mainly localized in the capsule, marginal zone of white pulp, and red pulp, and the expression over the white pulp was extremely low. The β_2-AR subtype was predominant in both lymph nodes and spleen. The results suggest that β-ARs are present in mature cells in lymphoid tissues *(63)*.

4.4. Heart

The density and distribution of β_1- and β_2-ARs in the atrioventricular conducting system and interatrial and interventricular septa from human hearts with idiopathic dilated cardiomyopathy and ischemic heart disease was determined by quantitative autoradiography using [^{125}I]CYP, the selective β_1-AR antagonist CGP 20712A, and the selective β_2-AR antagonist ICI 118,551. Both β_1- and β_2-ARs were present in the atrioventricular node, bundle of His, and interatrial and interventricular septa *(64)*. Quantitative autoradiography was also used to determine the location and densities of β_1- and β_2-ARs in guinea pig heart. Both β_1- and β_2-ARs were distributed on myocardium. The atrioventricular conducting system had a higher density of β_2-ARs compared with myocardium *(65)*. Highly localized binding was observed to regions closely associated with the sinoatrial node, atrioventricular node, and bundle of His but was not observed on myocardial, pacemaker, and conducting cells or adipose tissue *(66)*.

4.5. Vasculature

In human arteries, autoradiographic analysis revealed a predominance of β_1-ARs in the medial layer. β_2-ARs were localized primarily in the adventitia, in the adventitial-medial border, and in the intimal layer *(67)*. The distribution of β_1- and β_2-AR subtypes in the human internal mammary artery and saphenous vein showed a high expression of β_2-ARs localized to the endothelium of the internal mammary artery and fewer β_2-ARs on the smooth muscle. Images of [^{125}I]CYP binding to the saphenous vein showed localization of β_2-ARs to the outer smooth muscle and not to the endothelium. This localization was confirmed by relaxation experiments in mammary artery and saphenous vein to (−)-isoprenaline and found to be mediated via β_2-ARs located on the smooth muscle *(68)*.

4.6. Lung

In rat lung tissue using the photoaffinity-labeling, nonselective [^{125}I]cyanopindololazide II, there was strong, specific β-AR binding on alveolar parenchyma and bronchial epithelium of large and small bronchioles, lesser binding to smooth muscle bundles of large airways, and only sparse binding to the smooth muscle of small bronchioles or peripheral branches of pulmonary artery *(69)*. The localization of mRNA encoding the β_2-AR in tissue sections of the human and rat lung was compared with the distribution of β_2-AR binding sites using receptor autoradiography. A similar distribution of β_2-AR mRNA was identified in both species. The highest expression of β_2-AR mRNA was detected in smooth muscle of small airways, airway epithelium, and pulmonary blood vessels. Lower expression of β_2-AR mRNA was identified in smooth muscle of large airways and alveolar epithelium *(70)*. This distribution was confirmed by the studies of Mak et al. *(71)*. Cultured human airway epithelial cells and airway smooth muscle cells expressed only β2-AR mRNA. *In situ* hybridization in human lung revealed a high level of expression of β_1- and β_2-AR mRNAs in the pulmonary blood vessels and high level of expression of β_2-AR mRNA in the alveolar walls, with minor expression of β_1-AR mRNA. There was a moderate expression of β_2-AR but not β_1-AR mRNA in airway epithelium and smooth muscle of peripheral airways and no detectable β_3-AR mRNA in any lung structures *(71)*.

4.7. Adipocytes

The expression and function of human β_3-ARs were investigated in subcutaneous white adipocytes of young healthy women. In these cells, β_3-AR mRNAs represent 20% of total β-AR transcripts and less than half of β_1-AR transcripts *(72)*. Rabbit perirenal adipose tissue expressed all three β-AR mRNAs *(71)*.

4.8. Skeletal Muscle

The total tissue content of β-ARs was greater in the soleus, a muscle consisting almost entirely of slow-twitch (type I) fibers than in superficial white vastus lateralis, a muscle composed of greater than 95% fast-twitch (type IIb) fibers *(73)*.

4.9. Uterus and Testis

The majority of β-ARs were of the β_2-AR subtype not only in the rat myometrium but also in the endometrial and serosal epithelia of the uterus. Specific labeling was also observed in glandular elements *(74)*. It was also shown that the majority of β-ARs were of the β_2-AR subtype in the smooth muscle layers as well as in the epithelium. The latter localization suggests a role for epinephrine or norepinephrine on the oviductal epithelium *(75)*. It was found that most receptors were of the β_2-subtype in rat testis, with the greatest density of receptors found in interstitial cells and some specific labeling over the seminiferous tubules *(76)*.

4.10. Pancreas, Bladder, and Prostate

Hybridization on sections of human pancreas with oligonucleotide probes designed to hybridize with the β_2-AR mRNA showed expression in islet β-cells but not in the exocrine tissue of the pancreas *(51)*. *In situ* hybridization with digoxygenin-labeled oligonucleotide probes revealed the presence of the mRNA of the β_3-AR subtype in the smooth muscle of the urinary bladder *(77,78)*. There was a predominant expression of β_3-AR mRNA in human bladder tissue, with

97% of total β-AR mRNA represented by the β_3-AR. In the prostate, β-ARs of an unknown subtype were present exclusively in the epithelial cells, and no receptors could be detected in the stromal cells *(79)*.

5. In Vivo Localization
Using Fluorescent-Tagged G Protein-Coupled Receptors

Although our system is the first model to use a transgenic mouse fluorescent-tagged G protein-coupled receptor (GPCR) approach, other examples exist in the literature that used steroid hormone receptors fused to green fluorescent protein (GFP) and "knocked-in" to its own promoter regulatory site *(80)*. This system produced viable, functional receptors that fluoresced green when labeled with an antibody to GFP used to determine its expression during thymocyte development. The rhodopsin promoter has also been thoroughly characterized and used in several different transgenic approaches in rats and frogs, some using GFP as a reporter *(81,82)*.

5.1. Promoter

A powerful approach to study regulation of receptor expression in vivo is to use a transgenic mouse model. Such a model would preserve the complex cellular relationships found within each tissue that are required for principal cell-specific gene expression. However, the expense and time required for analysis are minimized by initial in vitro experiments using a cell culture system, ideally from the same species, that retains differentiated features. Therefore, the first characterization that needs to be established is the promoter fragment, which should be long enough to impart cell-type specificity. It should also be cloned from the same species in which the transgene is to be expressed (i.e., isogenic) to maintain the same regulatory elements used in determining cell specificity. For the α_{1B}-AR, we used a 3.4-kb fragment of the mouse α_{1B}-AR promoter and showed in various cell lines that it retained cell-specificity expression and had the same regulation by forskolin and hypoxia *(83)*.

We also showed that the promoter could drive mRNA production to the same domains in the brain as endogenous mRNA localization, and tissue-binding studies confirmed expression in α_{1B}-AR-containing tissue, with no expression in tissues known not to contain the α_{1B}-AR (84). For the α_{1A}-AR, a 4.4-kb fragment of the mouse promoter was active in cardiac myocytes but not in fibroblasts *(85)*. In the α_2-ARs, it was found that a 3-kb promoter fragment was not sufficient to drive selective expression in tissue expressing the endogenous subtype, but a 4.7-kb fragment was sufficient *(45,46)*. We caution that a promoter fragment may not impart 100% fidelity of cell-type specificity; but until high-avidity antibodies are available to verify endogenous expression, promoter analysis remains a viable tool.

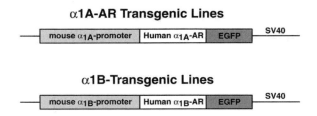

Fig. 1. Transgenic constructs. A map of the transgene constructs used to generate the various lines of mice that resulted in endogenous expression of an EGFP-tagged α_1-AR. To drive endogenous expression, 3.4- and 4.4-kb mouse promoter fragments were used for the α_{1B}- and α_{1A}-AR, respectively. The EGFP, a fluorescent protein, was placed in-frame after the stop codon of the wild-type human α_{1B}-AR and α_{1A}-AR cDNAs. SV40 polyA sequence was used to increase stability of the mRNA.

A novel transgenic system has also been used to study cell-specific expression in frog. One group used a 5.5-kb 5′ upstream fragment from the *Xenopus* principal rod opsin gene *(86)*, controlling expression of GFP to produce numerous independent transgenic *Xenopus*. Rapid production of transgenic tadpoles and the generation of large numbers of independent transgenic lines are achievable and cheaper in this model system. In this study, expression of rhodopsin tagged at the C-tail with GFP in principal rods of *Xenopus laevis* generated tadpoles with green fluorescent eyes *(87)*.

5.2. Construct

The DNA constructs we used for the injection are shown in Fig. 1. It had been previously published that EGFP-tagged α_1-ARs showed normal binding and functional properties *(88)*. Various other colored fluorophores can be used in place of EGFP. Many of the same antibodies that recognize EGFP can also recognize its multicolor variants. The construct should end with a poly A tail such as that from SV40 for stability of the message. Excessive DNA from the vector used in the construction should be digested away as much as possible. Integration also favors blunt ends and promotes the formation of concatamers. However, the length of the construct can be considerable (>20kb) and still integrate well into the mouse genome.

Offspring showed normal phenotype and development at least early in life. This permitted us to mate the heterozygous offspring and to produce homozygous animals in most cases. The homozygous α_{1B}-AR–EGFP mice begin to show neurodegeneration at about 6 mo of age, consistent with previous reports *(84)*. Therefore, localization studies are carried out on mice that are 4 mo old or younger, before they show signs of the disease. The α_{1A}–EGFP does not show evidence of neurodegeneration, at least until 6 mo of age.

6. Transgenic-Based Localization in the Central Nervous System
6.1. Tissue Processing

We began our localization studies in the brain because this organ appears to express the AR subtypes in discreet and recognizable domains, and previous studies using receptor autoradiography or *in situ* hybridization to examine localization in brain had considerable discrepancies. The tissue can be processed either by frozen sectioning or by vibrotome. The fresh tissue processing of the vibrotome method leads to less quenching of the EGFP signal, which is one advantage.

We found that the tissues needed to be treated with an antibody against EGFP to enhance the weak endogenous fluorescence. This primary antibody is then incubated with a secondary antibody coupled to FITC to maintain the same spectral properties as the EGFP protein. Left untreated, some areas in the brain are barely detected based on EGFP fluorescence alone. This low expression of the receptor is not unexpected because the endogenous promoters tend to be similar to housekeeping gene promoters *(89)*. We also discovered through trial and error that the antibody to EGFP needed to be made using the full-length protein. Using fragments of the GFP proteins (i.e., N-terminus peptides) to generate the antibodies does not produce highly specific and avid antibodies that recognize the epitopes of the fused EGFP. This could be because of the specific conformation the EGFP-protein adopts in the cell, possible signaling contacts with the C-tail of the receptor that disrupt EGFP folding, and the effects that the receptor itself may have on the folding properties of the EGFP.

We also found that the mouse brain (as opposed to rat brain) does have a higher degree of autofluorescence, which is the major limitation of doing fluorescence studies. However, we have found that dipping the processed tissue (after antibody treatment) in copper sulfate (1 h in 10 mM CuSO$_4$ in 50 mM NH$_4$ acetate, pH 5.0) reduces the autofluorescence caused by lipofuscin. This technique does not work in other tissues, and the amount of autofluorescence can be quite high.

6.2. The Mouse CNS

The α_{1B}-AR in the mouse brain was expressed predominantly in the neuronal cells of the cerebral cortex (Fig. 2). We confirmed neuronal expression by using an antibody directed against neurons (NEUN) and showed co-localization with the EGFP expression. This is consistent with the *in situ* hybridization data, which predicted that the cerebral cortex was one area of the rat brain that contained a high population of this α_1-AR subtype (Table 1). Expression was evenly distributed through the different laminae of the cortex. For the α_{1A}-AR, expression was also evident in the neuronal cell populations of the cerebral cortex, but a different neuronal cell type was even more pronounced in expression (Fig. 3). Differences in expression between the α_{1A}- and α_{1B}-ARs is not caused by differences in

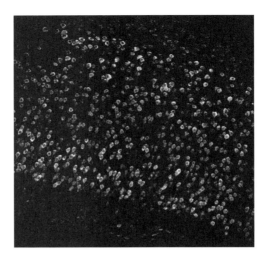

Fig. 2. α_{1B}-AR expression in the mouse cerebral cortex. Confocal image showing that EGFP-expressing cells of the α_{1B}-AR are located in the neurons of various laminae of the mouse cerebral cortex. Neurons were identified using an antibody directed against neurons (NEUN), which showed co-localization with the EGFP expression (data not shown). Original magnification ×20.

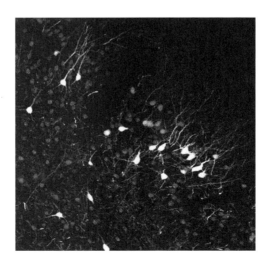

Fig. 3. α_{1A}-AR expression in the mouse cerebral cortex. Confocal image showing that EGFP-expressing cells of the α_{1A}-AR are located in the neurons of the various laminae of the cerebral cortex, just like the α_{1B}-AR. However, there was also a higher expressing subset of neuronal cells, which we are currently trying to identify. Original magnification ×28.

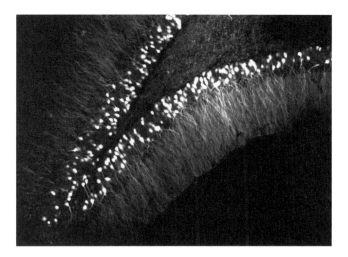

Fig. 4. α_{1A}-AR in the mouse dentate gyrus. Confocal image of cells expressing the α_{1A}-AR subtype in the dentate gyrus of the mouse hippocampus. The α_{1A}-AR is located in the granular layer with neuronal extensions into the strata. The α_{1A}-AR expression in the hippocampus was much more abundant than the expression of the α_{1B}-AR subtype. Original magnification ×10.

transgene integration and copy number because binding and signaling experiments revealed about equal levels of overexpression and signaling in common tissues. We are currently testing to determine the specific neuronal cell type expressing the α_{1A}-AR but speculate that it is an interneuron. However, despite this cell-type difference, it appears that both the α_{1A} and α_{1B}-AR subtypes co-localize to similar neuronal cell types in the cerebral cortex laminae. This result is also consistent with binding studies in murine cerebral cortex, which suggested a two-site mixture of α_{1A}- and α_{1B}-AR of about a 30 to 70% ratio, respectively *(22)*. We cannot be sure whether the same neuron expresses both receptor subtypes until transgenic mice expressing subtypes linked with different fluorophores are crossed.

A dominant region of α_{1A}-AR expression is the hippocampus (Fig. 4), where the α_{1A}-AR is expressed in the granular cell layer of the dentate gyrus and in the pyramidal and granular cell layers of the CA1, CA2, and CA3 regions. This receptor is also expressed in neuronal and interneuronal-like cells in the strata radiatum and oriens. The α_{1B}-AR–EGFP also has expression throughout the regions of the hippocampus *(90)*, although it is minor compared with the α_{1A}-AR. However, based on mRNA abundance the α_{1D}-AR is thought to be the major α_1-AR subtype expressed in hippocampus *(16)*. Because we do not have the corre-

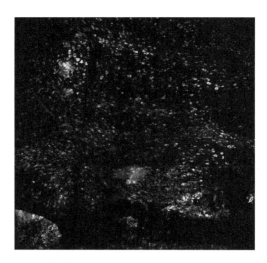

Fig. 5. α_{1B}-AR expression in the mouse medulla. The α_{1B}-AR is expressed in the various neuronal layers of the mouse medulla. Original magnification ×10.

sponding α_{1D}-AR mouse for comparison, we cannot compare the α_{1A}-AR mRNA density to the α_{1D}-AR protein. Using competitive PCR, other studies suggested that the α_{1A}-AR is dominant, but the α_{1B}-AR message is still present, albeit at much lower values *(17)*. The α_{1B}-AR subtype in the rat hippocampus as determined by [³H]prazosin autoradiography in the presence of the α_{1A}-AR antagonist 5-methylurapidil also showed a low overall homogeneous density *(18)*. Our studies are consistent with this low homogeneous distribution of the α_{1B}-AR and stronger expression of the α_{1A}-AR. As noted, the major flaw in using mRNA abundance for localization is that mRNA levels do not equate to protein levels, as appears to be the case for the α_{1D}-AR. This argument was supported by binding studies using the α_{1D}-AR knockout mice, which only lost 10% of its binding sites in the brain *(23)*.

The mouse cerebellum was previously thought not to have much expression of the α_{1B}-AR. We have shown that expression of this subtype is prominent in the molecular, granular, and Purkinje cells layers of the mouse cerebellum *(91)*. However, we also showed high expression of the α_{1A}-AR in mouse cerebellum. Our results are inconsistent with binding studies in mouse cerebellum that supported the presence of one population of binding sites with low affinity for niguldipine and norepinephrine, suggesting a dominance of the α_{1B}-AR binding site *(22)*, but our studies are more consistent with the α_{1B}-AR knockout studies that suggested that about 70% of the receptors in cerebellum are non-α_{1B}-ARs *(92)*. The α_{1B}-AR is also expressed at moderate levels in the medulla (Fig. 5),

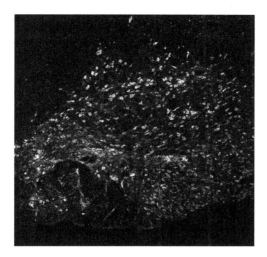

Fig. 6. α_{1B}-AR expression in the mouse spinal cord. The α_{1B}-AR is expressed in the various neuronal layers of the beginning segments of the mouse spinal cord. EGFP-expressing cells are present in the anterior gray, commissure, and anterior and lateral white columns of the spinal cord. Expression extends into the deeper layers of the spinal cord and includes the intermediolateral gray columns. Image is 1/2 spinal cord. Original magnification ×10.

especially in the pons and olive areas, not previously considered to express this receptor subtype. This expression of the α_{1B}-AR is also consistent with our mouse movement disorder phenotype (84), similar to multiple system atrophy, which has Purkinje cell and olivopontine cell loss *(93)*. Consistent with the literature, we also found that the α_{1B}-AR was expressed in mouse spinal cord in areas important for movement control (Fig. 6).

By *in situ* hybridization of mRNA, the α_{1B}-AR is highly expressed throughout the thalamus (Table 1). Although we observed moderate expression levels of the α_{1B}-AR–EGFP protein throughout the thalamic regions, the mRNA expression of this transgene showed high levels of transgenic mRNA in the reticular thalamic nuclei and lower expression in other thalamic nuclei (84). Again, these results suggest that the mRNA method can be deceptive in predicting localization of protein.

An interesting but logical finding is the lack of α_1-AR localization in cerebral blood vessels. The α_1-ARs play a major role in the constriction of peripheral blood vessels, found mostly in the medial smooth muscle layer and regulated through presynaptic α_2-AR release. In brain, however, the lack of α_1-AR on blood vessels may "protect" the smaller arteries in the brain against vasoconstriction caused by sudden stress-induced increases in epinephrine discharge. There is no convincing evidence that neurons in the brain play any important role in regulating cerebral blood flow *(94)*. This makes sense because you do not want to restrict blood flow to the brain when the body needs to respond to stress stimuli. There are many studies that also support the fact that brain vasoconstriction operates through a different mechanism from what takes place in the peripheral vasculature. This mechanism is summarized in ref. *95*, which indicates that there is limited α-AR-mediated contraction in large cerebral vessels that becomes progressively less important with branching. Strongly supporting this hypothesis, we found no localization of either the α_{1A}-AR or the α_{1B}-AR in cerebral blood vessels.

7. Transgenic-Based Localization in Peripheral Tissues

One of the obvious advantages of designing a systemic model of an endogenous GPCR-EGFP transgenic is the potential to study localization in any tissue of choice. The limitation we are experiencing is that the ratio of receptor expression to the autofluorescence in particular tissues must be sufficient to produce a detectable specific signal. We have identified specific signals in liver and prostate tissues.

7.1. Liver

Rat liver has pharmacologically been used as a pure α_{1B}-AR system of expression. However, the liver from other species has mixtures of the α_1-AR subtypes *(96)*. Mouse ligand-binding studies also indicated a pure α_{1B}-AR population *(22)*, as well as 98% loss of the binding sites from the α_{1B}-AR knockout mice *(92)*. In contrast, we found that mouse liver contains both the α_{1A}-AR and α_{1B}-AR. The α_{1A}-AR was only localized to the hepatic blood vessels (Fig. 7) and NK killer cells (lymphocytes) that circulate through the bile ducts (data not shown); and the α_{1B}-AR was localized specifically to heptocytes (Fig. 8). We could not detect the expression of the α_{1B}-AR in liver blood vessels. The interesting result was that the α_{1B}-AR localization varied in individual hepatocytes and was not evenly distributed. Because the α_{1B}-AR can control glycogen stores, we speculate the expression of this receptor may be linked to glycogen content.

7.2. Prostate

Smooth muscle tone, which contributes to the urethral constriction in the prostate gland, appears to be mediated by the α_1-ARs, as indicated by the potency of doxazosin for inhibiting phenylephrine-induced contractions in the prostate *(97)*. RNA and PCR approaches have established localization of the α_1-AR subtypes in the prostate. The α_{1A}-AR subtype was found in both prostate stromal and glandular cells; α_{1B}- and α_{1D}-AR subtypes were expressed only in the glandu-

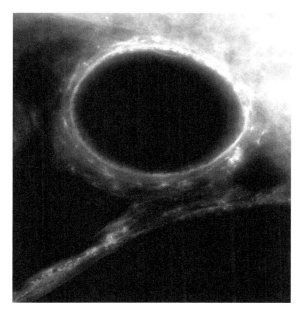

Fig. 7. α_{1A}-AR expression in mouse liver vasculature. The α_{1A}-AR is expressed in the various blood vessels of the mouse liver. The α_{1A} expression was not found in the hepatocyte. Original magnification ×40.

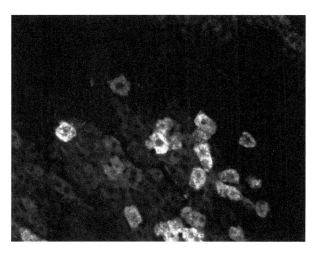

Fig. 8. α_{1B}-AR expression in mouse liver hepatocytes. Expression of the α_{1B}-AR in the mouse liver was localized to hepatocytes. However, expression of the receptor was not evenly distributed. No expression was seen in the blood vessels of the liver. Original magnification ×20.

lar cells *(33)*. A previous report indicated that contraction of the prostate is mediated by a new, uncloned α_1-AR subtype termed the α_{1L} (for low affinity to prazosin), but this was subsequently redefined as a slice variant of the α_{1A}-AR *(98)*. We found that the α_{1B}-AR is localized to both the stroma and glandular epithelial cells (data not shown), although glandular expression was indeed higher. We have not yet looked at the α_{1A}-AR expression in the prostate.

8. Summary

Localization of the adrenergic subtypes has been limited because of the lack of highly specific and avid antibodies. Most characterization of tissue distribution is based on radiolabeled ligand-binding studies but is limited by poor selectivity of available ligands, and low resolution has made subtype and cell-type discrimination still questionable entities. Although *in situ* mRNA localization has provided a good foundation for cell-type discrimination, the equation of mRNA quantity to protein abundance and the transport of mRNA are two issues limiting the interpretation of these studies. Most sympathetic tissues express a combination of most of the AR subtypes. The future opus is to determine their individual or collective roles in function.

We have provided a characterization of a potential model system to demonstrate cell-type localization of ARs using transgenic systemic expression of EGFP-tagged ARs, with the α_1-AR subtypes given as an example. Although expression levels are too low to detect EGFP fluorescence, the availability of high-affinity antibodies against the EGFP protein alleviates this problem. We have shown examples of receptor protein localization of both the α_{1A}- and α_{1B}- AR subtypes in the CNS and in peripheral tissues.

References

1. Jones LS, Gauger LL, Davis JN. Anatomy of brain α_1-adrenergic receptors: in vitro autoradiography with [^{125}I]-heat. J Comp Neurol 1985;231:190–208.
2. McCune SK, Voigt MM, Hill JM. Expression of multiple α-adrenergic receptor subtype messenger RNAs in the adult rat brain. Neuroscience 1993;57:143–151.
3. Pieribone VA, Nicholas A P, Dagerlind A, Hokfelt T. Distribution of α_1-adrenoceptors in rat brain revealed by *in situ* hybridization experiments utilizing subtype-specific probes. J Neurosci 1994;14:4252–4268.
4. Palacios JM, Hoyer D, and Cortes R. α_1-Adrenoceptors in the mammalian brain: similar pharmacology but different distribution in rodents and primates. Brain Res 1987;419:65–75.
5. Giroux N, Rossignol S, Reader TA. Autoradiographic study of α_1- and α_2-noradrenergic and serotonin$_{1A}$ receptors in the spinal cord of normal and chronically transected cats. J Comp Neurol 1999;406:402–414.
6. Domyancic AV, Morilak DA. Distribution of α_{1A} adrenergic receptor mRNA in the rat brain visualized by *in situ* hybridization. J Comp Neurol 1997;386:358–378.

7. Acosta-Martinez M, Fiber JM, Brown RD, Etgen AM. Localization of α_{1B}-adrenergic receptor in female rat brain regions involved in stress and neuroendocrine function. Neurochem Int 1999;35:383–391.

8. Sands SA, Morilak DA. Expression of α_{1D} adrenergic receptor messenger RNA in oxytocin- and corticotropin-releasing hormone-synthesizing neurons in the rat paraventricular nucleus. Neuroscience 1999;91:639–649.

9. Day HEW, Campeau S, Watson SJ, Akil H. Distribution of α_{1a}, α_{1b} and α_{1d} adrenergic receptor mRNAs in the rat brain and spinal cord. J Chem Neuroanat 1997;13: 115–139.

10. Day HE, Campeau S, Watson SJ Jr, Akil H. Expression of α_{1b} adrenoceptor mRNA in corticotropin-releasing hormone-containing cells of the rat hypothalamus and its regulation by corticosterone. J Neurosci 1999;19:10,098–10,106.

11. Gao B, Kunos G. Isolation and characterization of the gene encoding the rat α_{1B} adrenergic receptor. Gene 1993;131:243–247.

12. Moore RY, Bloom FE. Central catecholamine neuron systems: anatomy and physiology of the norepinephrine and epinephrine systems. Annu Rev Neurosci 1979;2: 113–168.

13. Madison DV, Nicoll RA. Noradrenaline blocks accommodation of pyramidal cell discharge in the hippocampus. Nature Lond 1982;299:636–638.

14. Bergles DE, Doze VA, Madison DV, Smith SJ. Excitatory actions of norepinephrine on multiple classes of hippocampal CA1 interneurons. J Neurosci 1996;16: 572–585.

15. Duffy S, Macvicar BA. Adrenergic calcium signaling in astrocyte networks within the hippocampal slice. J Neurosci 1995;15:5535–5550.

16. Williams AM, Nguyen ML, Morilak DA. Co-localization of α_{1D} adrenergic receptor mRNA with mineralocorticoid and glucocorticoid receptor mRNA in rat hippocampus. J Neuroendocrinol 1997;9:113–119.

17. Kreiner G, Sanak M, Zelek-Molik A, Nalepa I. Using reverse transcription and a competitive polymerase chain reaction for quantification of α_{1B}-adrenoceptor mRNA. Pol J Pharmacol 2002;54:401–405.

18. Zilles K, Gross G, Schleicher A, et al. Regional and laminar distributions of α_1-adrenoceptors and their subtypes in human and rat hippocampus. Neuroscience 1991;40:307–320.

19. Laporte AM, Schechter LE, Bolanos FJ, Verge D, Hamon M, Gozlan H. [3H]5-Methyl-urapidil labels 5-HT$_{1A}$ receptors and α_1-adrenoceptors in the rat CNS. In vitro binding and autoradiographic studies. Eur J Pharmacol 1991;198:59–67.

20. Smith MS, Schambra UB, Wilson KH, Page SO, Schwinn DA. α_1-adrenergic receptors in human spinal cord: specific localized expression of mRNA encoding α_1-adrenergic receptor subtypes at four distinct levels. Brain Res Mol Brain Res 1999;63:254–261.

21. Jones LS, Gauger LL, Davis JN, Slotkin TA, Bartolome JV. Postnatal development of brain α_1-adrenergic receptors: in vitro autoradiography with [125I] HEAT in normal rats and rats treated with α-difluoromethylornithine, a specific, irreversible inhibitor of ornithine decarboxylase. Neuroscience 1985;15:1195–1202.

22. Yang M, Verfurth F, Buscher R, Michel MC. Is α_{1D}-adrenoceptor protein detectable in rat tissues? Naunyn Schmiedebergs Arch Pharmacol 1997;355:438–446.

23. Tanoue A, Nasa Y, Koshimizu T, et al. The α_{1D}-adrenergic receptor directly regulates arterial blood pressure via vasoconstriction. J Clin Invest 2002;109:765–775.

24. Kurooka Y, Moriyama N, Nasu K, et al. Distribution of α_1-adrenoceptor subtype mRNAs in human renal cortex. BJU Int 1999;83:299–304.

25. Stephenson JA, Summers RJ. Autoradiographic evidence for a heterogeneous distribution of α_1-adrenoreceptors labelled by [^{3}H] prazosin in rat, dog and human kidney. J Auton Pharmacol 1986;6:109–116.

26. Monneron MC, Gillberg PG, Ohman B, Alberts P. In vitro α-adrenoceptor autoradiography of the urethra and urinary bladder of the female pig, cat, guinea-pig and rat. Scand J Urol Nephrol 2000;34:233–238.

27. Nishi K, Latifpour J, Saito M, Foster HE Jr, Yoshida M, Weiss RM. Characterization, localization and distribution of α_1 adrenoceptor subtype in male rabbit urethra. J Urol 1998;160:196–205.

28. Nasu K, Moriyama N, Fukasawa R, et al. Quantification and distribution of α_1-adrenoceptor subtype mRNAs in human proximal urethra. Br J Pharmacol 1998;123: 1289–1293.

29. Walden PD, Durkin MM, Lepor H, Wetzel JM, Gluchowski C, Gustafson EL. Localization of mRNA and receptor binding sites for the α_{1a}-adrenoceptor subtype in the rat, monkey and human urinary bladder and prostate. J Urol 1997;157:1032–1038.

30. Price DT, Schwinn DA, Lomasney JW, Allen LF, Caron MG, Lefkowitz RJ. Identification, quantification, and localization of mRNA for three distinct α_1 adrenergic receptor subtypes in human prostate. J Urol 1993;150:546–551.

31. Walden PD, Gerardi C, Lepor H. Localization and expression of the α_{1A}-, α_{1B} and α_{1D}-adrenoceptors in hyperplastic and non-hyperplastic human prostate. J Urol 1999;161:635–640.

32. Lepor H, Tang R, Kobayashi S, et al. Localization of the α_{1A}-adrenoceptor in the human prostate. J Urol 1995;154:2096–2069.

33. Tseng-Crank J, Kost T, Goetz A, et al. The α_{1C}-adrenoceptor in human prostate: cloning, functional expression, and localization to specific prostatic cell types. Br J Pharmacol 1995;115:1475–1485.

34. Perez DM, Piascik MT, Malik N, Gaivin R, Graham RM. Cloning, expression, and tissue distribution of the rat homolog of the bovine α_{1C}-adrenergic receptor provide evidence for its classification as the α_{1A} subtype. Mol Pharmacol 1994;46: 823–831.

35. Piascik MT, Smith MS, Soltis EE, Perez DM. Identification of the mRNA for the novel α_{1D}-adrenoceptor and two other α_1-adrenoceptors in vascular smooth muscle. Mol Pharmacol 1994;46:30–40.

36. Moriyama N, Kurooka Y, Nasu K, et al. Distribution of α_1-adrenoceptor subtype mRNA and identification of subtype responsible for renovascular contraction in human renal artery. Life Sci 2000;66:915–926.

37. Tayebati SK, Bronzetti E, Morra Di Cella S, et al. *In situ* hybridization and immunocytochemistry of α_1-adrenoceptors in human peripheral blood lymphocytes. J Auton Pharmacol 2000;20:305–312.

38. Boyajian CL, Loughlin SE, Leslie FM. Anatomical evidence for α_2 adrenoceptor heterogeneity: differential autoradiographic distribution of [^{3}H]rauwolcine and [^{3}H]idaxozan in rat brain. J Pharmacol Exp Ther 1987;241:1079–1091.

39. Scheinin M, Lomasney JW, Hayden-Hixson DM, et al. Distribution of α_2-adrenergic receptor subtype gene expression in rat brain. Mol Brain Res 1994;21: 133–149.

40. Rosin DL, Zeng D, Stornetta RL, et al. Immunohistochemical localization of α_{2A}-adrenergic receptors in catecholaminergic and other brainstem neurons in the rat. Neuroscience 1993;56:139–155.

41. Nicholas AP, Pieribone V, Hokfelt T. Distributions of mRNAs for α_2 adrenergic receptor subtypes in rat brain: an *in situ* hybridization study. J Comp Neurol 1993; 328:575–594.

42. Rosin DL, Talley EM, Lee A, et al. Distribution of α_{2C}-adrenergic receptor-like immunoreactivity in the rat central nervous system. J Comp Neurol 1996;372: 135–165.

43. Grijalba B, Callado LF, Javier Meana J, Garcia-Sevilla JA, Pazos A. α_2-adrenoceptor subtypes in the human brain: a pharmacological delineation of [^{3}H]RX-821002 binding to membranes and tissue sections. Eur J Pharmacol 1996; 310:83–93.

44. Nock B, Johnson AE, Feder HH, McEwen BS. Tritium-sensitive film autoradiography of guinea pig brain α_2-noradrenergic receptors. Brain Res 1985;336: 148–152.

45. Wang R, Macmillan LB, Fremeau RT Jr, Magnuson MA, Lindner J, Limbird LE. Expression of α_2-adrenergic receptor subtypes in the mouse brain: evaluation of spatial and temporal information imparted by 3 kb of 5′ regulatory sequence for the α_{2A} AR-receptor gene in transgenic animals. Neuroscience 1996;74:199–218.

46. Wang GS, Chang NC, Wu SC, Chang AC. Regulated expression of α_{2B} adrenoceptor during development. Dev Dyn 2002;225:142–152.

47. Winzer-Serhan UH, Leslie FM. Expression of α_{2A} adrenoceptors during rat neocortical development. J Neurobiol 1999;38:259–269.

48. Shi TJ, Winzer-Serhan U, Leslie F, Hokfelt T. Distribution of α_2-adrenoceptor mRNAs in the rat lumbar spinal cord in normal and axotomized rats. Neuroreport 1999;10:2835–2839.

49. Stone LS, Broberger C, Vulchanova L, et al. Differential distribution of α_{2A} and α_{2C} adrenergic receptor immunoreactivity in the rat spinal cord. J Neurosci 1998; 18:5928–5937.

50. McNeill AM, Leslie FM, Krause DN, Duckles SP. Gender differences in levels of α_2-adrenoceptor mRNA in the rat tail artery. Eur J Pharmacol 1999;366:233–236.

51. Lacey RJ, Chan SL, Cable HC, et al. Expression of α_2- and β-adrenoceptor subtypes in human islets of Langerhans. J Endocrinol 1996;148:531–543.

52. Huang L, Wei YY, Momose-Hotokezaka A, Dickey J, Okusa MD. α_{2B}-Adrenergic receptors: immunolocalization and regulation by potassium depletion in rat kidney. Am J Physiol 1996;270:F1015–F1026.

53. Moller M, Phansuwan-Pujito P, Morgan KC, Badiu C. Localization and diurnal expression of mRNA encoding the β_1-adrenoceptor in the rat pineal gland: an *in situ* hybridization study. Cell Tissue Res 1997;288:279–284.

54. Pfeffer M, Kuhn R, Krug L, Korf HW, Stehle JH. Rhythmic variation in β_1-adrenergic receptor mRNA levels in the rat pineal gland: circadian and developmental regulation. Eur J Neurosci 1998;10:2896–2904.

55. Nicholas AP, Pieribone VA, Hokfelt T. Cellular localization of messenger RNA for β_1 and β_2 adrenergic receptors in rat brain: an *in situ* hybridization study. Neuroscience 1993;56:1023–1039.

56. Grimm LJ, Blendy JA, Kellar KJ, Perry DC. Chronic reserpine administration selectively up-regulates β_1- and α_{1b}-adrenergic receptors in rat brain: an autoradiographic study. Neuroscience 1992;47:77–86.

57. Asanuma M, Ogawa N, Mizukawa K, Haba K, Hirata H, Mori A. Distribution of the β_2 adrenergic receptor messenger RNA in the rat brain by *in situ* hybridization histochemistry: effects of chronic reserpine treatment. Neurochem Res 1991;16: 1253–1256.

58. Booze RM, Crisostomo EA, Davis JN. Species differences in the localization and number of CNS β-adrenergic receptors: rat vs guinea pig. J Pharmacol Exp Ther 1989;249:911–920.

59. Schimchowitsch S, Williams LM, Pelletier G. Autoradiographic localization of β-adrenergic receptors in the rabbit pituitary. Brain Res Bull 1986;17:705–710.

60. De Souza EB. β_2-Adrenergic receptors in pituitary. Identification, characterization, and autoradiographic localization. Neuroendocrinology 1985;41:289–296.

61. Engel G, Maurer R, Perrot K, Richardson BP. α-Adrenoceptor subtypes in sections of rat and guinea pig kidney. Naunyn Schmiedebergs Arch Pharmacol 1985;328: 354–357.

62. Lakhlani PP, Amenta F, Napoleone P, Felici L, Eikenburg DC. Pharmacological characterization and anatomical localization of prejunctional β-adrenoceptors in the rat kidney. Br J Pharmacol 1994;111:1296–1308.

63. Fernandez-Lopez A, Revilla V, Candelas MA, Aller MI, Soria C, Pazos A. Identification of β-adrenoceptors in rat lymph nodes and spleen: an autoradiographic study. Eur J Pharmacol 1994;262:283–286.

64. Elnatan J, Molenaar P, Rosenfeldt FL, Summers RJ. Autoradiographic localization and quantitation of β_1- and β_2-adrenoceptors in the human atrioventricular conducting system: a comparison of patients with idiopathic dilated cardiomyopathy and ischemic heart disease. J Mol Cell Cardiol 1994;26:313–323.

65. Molenaar P, Russell FD, Shimada T, Summers RJ. Function, characterization and autoradiographic localization and quantitation of β-adrenoceptors in cardiac tissues. Clin Exp Pharmacol Physiol 1989;16:529–533.

66. Molenaar P, Kompa AR, Roberts SJ, Pak HS, Summers RJ. Localization of (−)-[^{125}I]cyanopindolol binding in guinea-pig heart: characteristics of non-β-adrenoceptor related binding in cardiac pacemaker and conducting regions. Neurosci Lett 1992;136:118–122.

67. Amenta F, Coppola L, Gallo P, et al. Autoradiographic localization of β-adrenergic receptors in human large coronary arteries. Circ Res 1991;68:1591–1599.

68. Molenaar P, Malta E, Jones CR, Buxton BF, Summers RJ. Autoradiographic localization and function of β-adrenoceptors on the human internal mammary artery and saphenous vein. Br J Pharmacol 1988;95:225–233.

69. Hesse L, Erdmann G, Eschenhagen T, Wellhoner HH. Improved method for autoradiographic localization of β-adrenoceptors using photoaffinity labelling. Naunyn Schmiedebergs Arch Pharmacol 1993;347:494–499.

70. Hamid QA, Mak JC, Sheppard MN, Corrin B, Venter JC, Barnes PJ. Localization of β_2-adrenoceptor messenger RNA in human and rat lung using *in situ* hybridization: correlation with receptor autoradiography. Eur J Pharmacol 1991;206: 133–138.
71. Mak JC, Nishikawa M, Haddad EB, et al. Localisation and expression of β-adrenoceptor subtype mRNAs in human lung. Eur J Pharmacol 1996;302:215–221.
72. Tavernier G, Barbe P, Galitzky J, et al. Expression of β_3-adrenoceptors with low lipolytic action in human subcutaneous white adipocytes. J Lipid Res 1996;37: 87–97.
73. Martin WH 3rd, Murphree SS, Saffitz JE. β-Adrenergic receptor distribution among muscle fiber types and resistance arterioles of white, red, and intermediate skeletal muscle. Circ Res 1989;64:1096–1105.
74. Tolszczuk M, Pelletier G. Autoradiographic localization of β-adrenoreceptors in rat uterus. J Histochem Cytochem 1988;36:1475–1479.
75. Tolszczuk M, Pelletier G. Autoradiographic localization of β-adrenergic receptors in rat oviduct. Mol Cell Endocrinol 1988;60:95–99.
76. Tolszczuk M, Follea N, Pelletier G. Characterization and localization of β-adrenergic receptors in control and cryptorchidized rat testis by in vitro autoradiography. J Androl 1988;9:172–177.
77. Takeda M, Obara K, Mizusawa T, et al. Evidence for β_3-adrenoceptor subtypes in relaxation of the human urinary bladder detrusor: analysis by molecular biological and pharmacological methods. J Pharmacol Exp Ther 1999;288:1367–1373.
78. Yamaguchi O. β_3-Adrenoceptors in human detrusor muscle. Urology 2002;59: 25–29.
79. Dube D, Poyet P, Pelletier G, Labrie F. Radioautographic localization of β-adrenergic receptors in the rat ventral prostate. J Androl 1986;7:169–174.
80. Brewer JA, Sleckman BP, Swat W, Muglia LJ. Green fluorescent protein–glucocorticoid receptor knockin mice reveal dynamic receptor modulation during thymocyte development. J Immunol 2002;169:1309–1318.
81. Lewin AS, Drenser KA, Hauswirth WW, et al. Ribozyme rescue of photoreceptor cells in a transgenic rat model of autosomal dominant retinitis pigmentosa. Nat Med 1998;4:967–71.
82. Knox BE, Schlueter C, Sanger BM, Green CB, Besharse JC. Transgene expression in Xenopus rods. FEBS Lett 1998;423:117–121.
83. Zuscik MJ, Piascik MT, Perez DM. Cloning, cell-type specificity and regulatory function of the murine α_{1b}-adrenergic receptor promoter. Mol Pharmacol 1999;56: 1288–1297.
84. Zuscik MJ, Sand S, Ross SA, et al. Overexpression of the α_{1b}-adrenergic receptor causes apoptotic neurodegeneration: a multiple system atrophy. Nat Med 2000;6: 1388–1394.
85. O'Connell TD, Rokosh DG, Simpson PC. Cloning and characterization of the mouse $\alpha_{1C/A}$-adrenergic receptor gene and analysis of an α_{1C} promoter in cardiac myocytes: role of an MCAT element that binds transcriptional enhancer factor-1 (TEF-1). Mol Pharmacol 2001;59:1225–1234.
86. Batni S, Scalzetti L, Moody SA, Knox BE. Characterization of the *Xenopus rhodopsin* gene. J Biol Chem 1996;271:3179–3186.

87. Moritz OL, Tam BM, Papermaster DS, Nakayama T. A functional rhodopsin-green fluorescent protein fusion protein localizes correctly in transgenic *Xenopus laevis* retinal rods and is expressed in a time-dependent pattern. J Biol Chem 2001;276:28,242–28,251.

88. Awaji T, Hirasawa A, Kataoka M, et al. Real-time optical monitoring of ligand-mediated internalization of α_{1b}-adrenoceptor with green fluorescent protein. Mol Endocrinol 1998;12:1099–1111.

89. Ramarao CS, Denker JMK, Perez DM, Riek RP, Graham RM. Genomic organization of the human α_{1b}-adrenergic receptor. J Biol Chem 1992;267:21,936–21,945.

90. Yun J, Gaivin RJ, McCune DF, et al. Gene expression profiles of neurodegeneration induced by the α_{1b}-adrenergic receptor: NMDA/$GABA_A$ dysregulation and apoptosis. Brain 2003;126:2667–2681.

91. Papay R, Gaivin R, McCune DF, et al. The α_{1b}-adrenergic receptor is expressed in neurons and NG2 oligodendrocytes. J Comp Neurol. 2004; 248:1-10.

92. Cavalli A, Lattion A-L, Hummler E, et al. Decreased blood pressure response in mice deficient of the α_{1b}-adrenergic receptor. Proc Natl Acad Sci USA 1997;94: 11,589–11,594

93. Papay R, Zuscik MT, Ross SA, et al. Mice expressing the α_{1b}-adrenergic receptor induces a synucleinopathy with excessive tyrosine nitration but decreased phosphorylation. J Neurochem 2002;83:1–12.

94. Heistad DD, Marcus ML. Evidence that neural mechanisms do not have important effects on cerebral blood flow. Circ Res 1978;42:295–302.

95. Bevan JA, Duckworth J, Laher I, Oriowo MA, McPherson GA, Bevan RD. Sympathetic control of cerebral arteries: specialization in receptor type, reserve, affinity, and distribution. FASEB J 1987;1:193–198.

96. Garcia-Sainz JA, Romero-Avila MT, Hernandez RA, Macias-Silva M, Olivares-Reyes A, Gonzalez-Espinosa C. Species heterogeneity of hepatic α_1-adrenoceptors: α_{1A}-, α_{1B}- and α_{1C}-subtypes. Biochem Biophys Res Commun 1992;186: 760–767.

97. Lepor H, Baumann M, Shapiro E. Binding and functional properties of doxazosin in the human prostate adenoma and canine brain. Prostate 1990;16:29–38.

98. Ford AP, Arredondo NF, Blue DR Jr, et al. RS-17053 (N-[2-(2-cyclopropyl-methoxyphenoxy)ethyl]-5-chloro-α, α-dimethyl-1H-indole-3-ethanamine hydrochloride), a selective α_{1A}-adrenoceptor antagonist, displays low affinity for functional α_1-adrenoceptors in human prostate: implications for adrenoceptor classification. Mol Pharmacol 1996;49:209–215.

PART IV
GENETICALLY ALTERED MOUSE MODELS

8

The α_1-Adrenergic Receptors:

Lessons From Knockouts

Paul C. Simpson

Summary

α_1-Adrenergic receptors (ARs) exist in three distinct molecular subtypes: A, B, and D. They are expected to have distinct physiological roles in vivo, but this has been hard to prove because the pharmacological tools to distinguish the subtypes are limited and not always very selective. For this reason, several laboratories have turned to the knockout (KO) approach to dissect the physiological roles of α_1-ARs and α_1-AR subtypes in vivo. The KOs confirm the importance of α_1-ARs in vasoconstriction and blood pressure regulation, but a surprise is the apparently small role of the B in this respect. The D seems limited to a vascular role and probably brain. D-selective antagonists might have an advantage in hypertension treatment if human subtypes are similar to mouse. The B role in glucose metabolism is notable. Perhaps the biggest surprise from the KOs is the essential role of the A or the B in physiological cardiac hypertrophy and cardiac adaptation to stress. The AB KO data provide a plausible mechanism for the adverse effects of nonselective α_1-antagonists in clinical trials and raise further concern about use of these drugs in patients with hypertension or prostate disease.

Key Words: α_1-Adrenergic receptor; blood pressure; cardiac; cardiovascular; hypertrophy; knockout.

1. Introduction

α_1-Adrenergic receptors (ARs) exist in three distinct molecular subtypes: A, B, and D. The A was originally named the C, and this subtype is sometimes called the

From: *The Receptors: The Adrenergic Receptors: In the 21st Century*
Edited by: D. Perez © Humana Press Inc., Totowa, NJ

A/C. They share activation by the endogenous catecholamines norepinephrine (NE) and epinephrine, inhibition by the antagonist prazosin and other piperazinyl quinazolines, and coupling to Gq. However, amino acid sequence is only about one-third identical overall, and the subtypes have distinct tissue distributions, regulation, G and other protein coupling, and signaling. Thus, they are expected to have distinct physiological roles in vivo, but this has been hard to prove because the pharmacological tools to distinguish the subtypes are limited and not always very selective.

For this reason, several laboratories have turned to the knockout (KO) approach to dissect the physiological roles of α_1-ARs and α_1-AR subtypes in vivo. Single KOs of the A, B, and D and double KO of the A and B are published; the other double KOs (AD and BD) and the triple ABD KO are being studied. The KO approach will define the physiological roles of α_1-ARs as a class in the intact animal and distinguish the individual contributions of each subtype. Isolated tissues and cells from KO mice will be a valuable resource for further study of α_1-AR subtype regulation and function. There is always concern about extrapolation from mouse to humans, but mouse KOs are proving to be predictive of drug effects in humans; therefore, results from α_1-AR KO mice should help guide drug development.

This chapter reviews the α_1-AR subtype KOs made and characterized so far. These studies are still in their very early stages, but they highlight the required role of α_1-ARs in cardiac hypertrophy and adaptation, vascular function, metabolism, and behavior.

2. Construction and Validation
of the Three α_1-Adrenergic Receptor Subtype Knockouts
2.1. Construction

All three single-KO models used homologous recombination in embryonic stem cells to disrupt the α_1-AR subtype gene (1–3). Table 1 summarizes the construction and validation. Each α_1-AR gene consists of two exons separated by a large intron of at least 18 kb, inserted between the end of the sixth transmembrane domain and the start of the third extracellular loop (4a). Thus, exon 1 encodes the receptor from the N-terminus through the first six transmembrane domains, and exon 2 encodes the remainder of the protein. The targeting strategy for all KOs replaced a portion of the α_1-AR coding sequence with a deoxyribonucleic acid (DNA) cassette that included the coding sequence for neomycin resistance, driven by the phosphoglycerate kinase promoter, to select for targeted stem cells. A caveat to keep in mind is that these foreign DNA sequences might have unanticipated effects, but this has not been seen so far in KO models (the A KO was engineered with loxP sites to remove this cassette with Cre recombinase). The A and B KOs deleted the entire first exon, whereas the D KO removed the residues coding for approximately the first 61 amino acids of exon 1.

Table 1
Construction and Validation of the Three α_1-Adrenergic Receptor Subtype KOs

	A KO	B KO	D KO
Gene sequences deleted	Exon 1 and 450 bp of intron	Exon 1 and portions of 5' flanking and intron	Exon 1 first 61 amino acids
Replacement cassette	LacZ coding and floxed PGK promoter/Neo coding	PGK promoter/Neo coding	PGK promoter/Neo coding
KO confirmation (mRNA)	Exons 1 and 2 absent	Exons 1 and 2 absent	Exon 1 absent; faint exon 2 present
Changes in other α_1-subtypes	NC B mRNA heart; NC B/D binding heart, brain, kidney	NC mRNAs several tissues	NC mRNAs several tissues
Changes in other ARs		NC α_2-AR binding cerebellum; NC β-AR binding heart	
Initial mouse strains	129SvJ × FVB/N	129Sv × C57Bl/6J	129Sv × C57Bl/6J
Reference	2	1	3

NC, no change; Neo, neomycin resistance; PGK, phosphoglycerate kinase.

In the A KO, the replacement cassette also included the LacZ gene coding for bacterial β-galactosidase (β-gal), which cleaves exogenous substrates to produce a colored reaction product (e.g., blue with X-gal cleavage). The LacZ cassette contained a stop codon and an SV40 polyadenylation signal and was inserted exactly at the start site of the deleted α_1A first exon. Thus, β-gal expression was under precise control by endogenous α_1A gene regulatory elements. Indeed, in the A KO, β-gal expression assayed by blue staining, enzyme activity, and protein level on Western blot was proportional to LacZ copy number (i.e., 0, 1, or 2 in wild type [WT], heterozygote, and KO). Also, in the A KO, β-gal was present in the same tissues and at the same times as endogenous A messenger ribonucleic acid (mRNA) and protein in WT mice. Thus, β-gal could be used as a convenient marker for α_1A-subtype regulation in tissues and cells *(2)*.

2.2. Validation

Confirmation that gene targeting was successful in the three KOs involved assays of subtype mRNAs. In the A and B subtype KOs, mRNAs transcribed from exons 1 and 2 were both absent. The D KO had no exon 1 mRNA but a trace of exon 2 mRNA by reverse transcription polymerase chain reaction; however, it is doubtful that this exon 2 mRNA is translated into protein. All studies evaluated potential compensatory changes in the other subtypes. As summarized in Table 1, the other two subtypes were unchanged when any one was knocked out. In the case of the B KO, there were also no changes in α_2- and β-AR binding. Thus, the single KOs were successful, and there were no compensatory changes in the other subtypes or ARs. A study of binding in B KO liver reports compensation by the A, but mRNA levels were not assayed *(4a)*.

2.3. Double KOs and Triple KO

Following construction of the three single KOs, it became a relatively simple matter to generate all possible remaining KO genotypes by crossbreeding (i.e., the double AB, BD, and AD KOs and the triple ABD KO). The double AB KO is discussed in Sections 4 and 5 *(5,6a)*, and the double BD KO has been characterized recently *(6b)*. The double AD KO and the triple ABD KO are both viable (unpublished data, 2004).

2.4. Genetic Background

Finally, the initial reports of each subtype KO used mice with mixed genetic backgrounds, about equal proportions of 129Sv plus FVB or 129Sv plus C57Bl/6 (Table 1). This is a very important point because mice strains differ in many respects, and thus strain background has an important influence on phenotype. For example, we observed increased kidney weight in AB KO females in a mixed 129 ×C57Bl/6×FVB/N background *(5)* but not in AB KO females congenic in C57Bl/6 (unpublished data, 2004). The A KO has now been backcrossed into C57Bl/6 and FVB for several generations and can be considered congenic in both strains (unpublished data, 2004). The seven KO genotypes being bred in our laboratory (A, B, D, AB, BD, AD, and ABD KOs) are all congenic in C57Bl/6 (unpublished data, 2004 and ref. 5). In the case of the original B KO and the WT strain used as its control, published reports involve separate KO and WT lines originating from the initial mixed strains of 129Sv and C57Bl/6 (1,7–12), and this mixed genetic background might complicate phenotype analysis (e.g., if there were differences between the mixed strains not caused by the presence or absence of the B gene or differences between the mixed strains that modify B function).

3. Radioligand Binding in the α_1-Adrenergic Receptor Knockouts

3.1. Advantage of the KOs

A particular advantage of the KO models is an unequivocal estimate of the proportions of each subtype protein in any tissue as measured by radioligand binding. Typically, subtype proportions are determined by competition binding assays using antagonists with varying degrees of selectivity for the subtypes. It is possible to measure the A subtype, which has high affinity for 5-methylurapidil (5MU), vs the combined B and D subtypes, which have lower affinity for 5MU. Indeed, we found very good agreement between the number of α_1A binding sites in brain, heart, and kidney as determined by 5MU competition and the number of binding sites lost in the A KO (2). On the other hand, it is more difficult to distinguish the B from the D. The D antagonist BMY7378 is used for this purpose, but it has remained a question whether the D is expressed in the mouse at the protein level (13).

3.2. Importance of the Preparation Used for Binding

Table 2 summarizes binding data from the four KOs reported so far (1–3,5). It is first notable that the absolute values for receptor protein, expressed as femtomoles per milligram "membrane" protein, vary widely from lab to lab, especially in the heart (5–48 fmol/mg). The differences in levels can very likely be attributed to differences in membrane preparations used for binding and the value of the protein denominator.

For example, we did experiments measuring binding in sequential fractions prepared from isolated adult rat myocytes (unpublished data, 1989). Myocytes were lysed in a high-sucrose buffer, and no material was discarded. The 1000g pellet contained approx 65% of the absolute total number of specific α_1-AR binding sites measured by ^{3}H-prazosin. A 40,000g pellet made from the 1000g supernatant contained about 15% of the binding sites, and a 100,000g pellet from the 40,000g supernatant contained the remaining 20% of α_1-ARs. Thus, a minority of the receptors (15% of total) was in the 40,000g membrane pellet used most

Table 2
Radioligand Binding in the α_1-Adrenergic Receptor Subtype Knockouts

	A KO		B KO		D KO		AB KO	
	fmol/mg WT	% decrease KO	fmol/mg WT	% decrease KO	fmol/mg WT	% decrease KO	fmol/mg WT	% decrease KO
Heart	14	30	5	74	48	0	13	100
Aorta (thoracic)					47	100		
Kidney	56	58	23	0	30	0	67	100
Liver			39	98			124	100
Brain (whole)	137	55			101	10	108	88
• Cerebral cortex			94	42	247	10–40		
• Cerebellum			77	32				
• Hippocampus						25		
Reference	2		1		3		5 and unpublished data, 2004	

often, with a majority in a lower speed pellet and a number at least equivalent in a higher speed pellet. Similar observations that most receptors are present in a low-speed fraction often discarded and that "refined" membrane preparations can miss important aspects of receptor regulation have been made with respect to β-AR binding (14,15).

3.3. Subtypes in Different Tissues

Despite the variance in absolute femtomoles/milligram protein, there is reasonably good agreement among studies on the proportions of each subtype in a given tissue (Table 2). In heart, total α_1-ARs were reduced by approx 30% in the A KO, approx 75% in the B KO, 0% in the D KO, and 100% in the AB KO. These data indicate that the mouse heart has approx 30% A, approx 70% B, and no detectable D binding, even though D mRNA is present (5). These values agree well with competition analyses in WT mouse (2). As discussed in Section 4.4., D in the heart appears to be in the coronary arteries (16).

The KO models suggest that thoracic aorta contains mostly or entirely D, and the liver contains mostly or entirely B (Table 2). There is some disagreement in kidney, with the A and AB KOs suggesting a mixture of A (~60%) and B (~40%), whereas the B KO study found no B in kidney (Table 2). From Table 2, brain has approx 55% A, 35% B, and 10% D. Brain shows considerable regional variation in subtype expression, but data are so far limited. Among the limited tissues tested so far, the A is predominant in brain and kidney, the B is the main subtype in liver and heart, and the D is expressed at the protein level only in thoracic aorta and brain (Table 2). In summary, the KOs confirmed the distribution of subtypes in the mouse.

4. Vascular Phenotypes in the α_1-Adrenergic Receptor Knockouts

α_1-ARs were discovered through their physiological effect to increase smooth muscle contraction, and α_1-AR antagonist drugs are used very commonly to treat disorders with increased smooth muscle contraction, such as hypertension or prostate enlargement with urinary symptoms. Thus, all single-KO studies focused initially on the vascular phenotype, as summarized in Table 3 (1–3,7,10,17–19). The double AB KO also evaluated some aspects of vascular phenotype (5,16).

4.1. Strain, Sex, and Anesthesia Variables in Analysis of Phenotype

Three key variables in these studies are mouse strain, mouse sex, and technique. Strain was mentioned earlier; sex is indicated in Table 3 and is discussed in Section 7. Technique is a third key variable, whether measurements were made in mice under anesthesia or after some period of recovery from anesthesia, as given in Table 3. For example, anesthesia markedly decreases heart rate (HR), blood pressure (BP), and cardiac contractility and causes left ventricular dilation

Table 3
Vascular Phenotypes in α_1-Adrenergic Receptor Subtype Knockouts

	A KO	B KO	D KO	AB KO
Sex	Male and female (2)	Male (1)	Male (3)	Male and female
Body weight	NC (2)	NC (1)	NC (3)	NC (5)
Blood pressure	DEC (2, ab)	NC (1, c; 10, i)	DEC (3, ad; 19, a); NC (17, a)	NC (5, a)
Heart rate	NC (2, ab)	NC (1, c; 10, i)	NC (3, ad; 19, a)	DEC (5, ah)
Baroreflex	Reset (2, b)			
Sympathetic activity	INC[a] (2, bf)		NC?[b] (3,17)	
Acute α_1-pressor response				
• Increase in BP	Absent (A61603) (2, b); NC (PE 1–100 μg/kg) (2, b)	DEC (PE 8 μg/kg) (1, c); NC (AngII, vasopressin) (1, c)	DEC (PE 1–10 μg/kg) (3, d); NC (PE 300 μg/kg) (3, d); DEC (NE 0.5–10 μg/kg) (3, d); DEC (NE 1 μg/kg/min) (3, e); NC (Ang II, vasopressin) (3, d)	
• Final BP	DEC (PE 100 μg/kg) (2, b)	DEC (PE 8 μg/kg) (1, c); DEC (NE 600 ng/kg) (1, c)	NC (PE 300 μg/kg) (3, d); DEC (NE 10 μg/kg) (3, d)	
Arterial contraction in vitro				
• Thoracic aorta		DEC (PE 0.1–1 μM) (1); NC EC_{50}/max (PE 1 nM–100 μM) (7); NC (serotonin) (1)	INC EC_{50} (PE, NE) (3); NC EC_{50} (serotonin) (3)	
• Carotid		DEC EC_{50}, NC max (PE) (7)		
• Mesenteric		NC EC_{50}/max (PE) (7)	DEC (PE) (3)	
• Tail		NC EC_{50}/max (PE) (7)		
• Coronary arteries (isolated heart)			DEC pressure (PE 100 μM) (18)	NC basal flow (16); DEC flow (PE 10 μM) (16) (BMY7378 blocks)

Table 3 (Continued)
Vascular Phenotypes in α_1-Adrenergic Receptor Subtype Knockouts

	A KO	B KO	D KO	AB KO
Stress responses				
• Nephrectomy and saline			DEC hypertension (17, a) INC survival (17)	
• Intracerebroventricular salt			DEC hypertension/tachycardia (19, j) NC hypertension (AngII)	
• Chronic α_1-agonist infusion		DEC hypertension (NE) (10, i) DEC artery remodeling (NE, PE) (10) NC hypertension (AngII) (10, i)	DEC hypertension (NE) (10, i) DEC artery remodeling (NE, PE) (10) NC hypertension (AngII) (10, i)	
Localization in arteries	No β-gal thoracic aorta/branches (2) β-Gal patchy resistance/dermal (2)			
Artery structure	NC lumen area (2)	NC dissecting and mounting (7)		

AngII, angiotensin II; DEC, decreased vs WT control; INC, increased vs WT control; NC, no change; NE, norepinephrine; PE, phenylephrine. The reference number and the technique are indicated parenthetically in the columns. The techniques are designated as follows: a, tail cuff in conscious mice; b, carotid artery in awake mice 24 h after surgery with isoflurane; c, carotid artery in awake mice 3 h after surgery with halothane; d, carotid artery in awake mice 24 h after surgery with pentobarbital; e, carotid artery in mice under pentobarbital anesthesia; f, telemetry in awake mice 1 wk after surgery with isoflurane; g, echo under anesthesia; h, echo in conscious mice; i, femoral artery telemeter 10 d after ketamine and xylazine anesthesia; j, femoral artery in awake mice 3 d after surgery with pentobarbital.

[a] Decreased sympathetic activity by decreased HR variability and faster HR after parasympathetic blockade with atropine.

[b] Serum catecholamines: no change basal; increased after nephrectomy/saline, although less increase than WT.

(5,20). All of these changes will alter systemic BP, which is directly related to cardiac output (CO) and peripheral vascular resistance. Complete recovery from anesthesia required at least 24 h in experiments on β-AR KOs *(21)*. We found that recovery from anesthesia with ketamine plus xylazine was not complete even after 3 d, whereas recovery from isoflurane was rapid *(20)*.

4.2. Blood Pressure

None of the KOs had altered body weight or grossly abnormal development; thus, all KO mice appeared normal as adults. However, there were significant changes in BP and pressor responses, which varied among the subtypes (Table 3). Resting BP was reduced about 10% in the A KO and by a similar degree in two of three studies of the D KO. Resting BP was unchanged in the B KO (Table 3).

In heterozygous A KOs, with only one of two A gene alleles deleted, there was intermediate hypotension; a cohort of male mice in the 129SvJ × C57Bl/6 background also had a significant approx 10% reduction in BP *(2)*. Evidence supporting chronic hypotension in the A KO was resetting of the baroreflex and increased sympathetic activity *(2)*. Baroreflex resetting meant a lower HR for any degree of hypotension and could explain the fact that HR was only slightly and not significantly faster in the A KO (6–10%). Chronic hypotension would be expected to stimulate a reflex increase in sympathetic activity, and evidence for this in the A KO was reduced HR variability and increased HR after parasympathetic blockade *(2)*.

Interestingly, the D KO, despite hypotension, had no change in basal serum catecholamines. After stress, serum catecholamines increased less than in WT mice *(17)*, raising the possibility that the D somehow regulates brain sympathetic outflow. In any case, studies of sympathetic activity in these KO models will be very interesting because changed sympathetic activity is the most likely compensatory change in all KO models. In summary, there was evidence for lower BP in the A KO and D KO but not the B KO.

The AB KO adds a degree of confusion because this mouse had no change in BP measured by tail cuff *(5)*. Possibly, the AB KO has increased sympathetic activity, causing increased activation of the D, although it is unclear why the same mechanism would not normalize BP in the single A KO. Much more speculative is that the B normally has a hypotensive action, so that A and B deletion have offsetting effects on final BP.

4.3. Pressor Responses

Acute in vivo pressor responses to α_1-agonists were tested for all three KOs (Table 3). Here, a distinction should be made between the *increase* in BP with agonist and the *final* BP after agonist. The A-selective agonist A61603 was a very potent vasopressor in conscious WT mice (0.3 µg/kg EC_{50}) but had no effect on BP in the homozygous A KO, confirming the A-selectivity of A61603 in vivo.

In the heterozygous A KO, A61603 stimulated an increase in BP identical to WT, but the final BP was significantly lower, reflecting the lower resting BP in the heterozygous KO. These results establish the vasoconstrictor role of the A subtype, even when receptor levels are only 50% of WT (as deduced from β-gal expression) *(2)*.

The nonselective α_1-agonist phenylephrine (PE) increased BP in conscious WT mice with an 8 μg/kg EC_{50} *(2)*. In the A KO, the relationship between PE dose and BP increase was unchanged, but the final BP was reduced in the A KO, reflecting the lower resting BP in the A KO *(2)*. In the B and D KOs, PE doses near the EC_{50} increased BP less in both KOs than in WT *(1,3)*. In the D KO, maximum doses of PE (100–300 μg/kg) stimulated BP increases identical to WT, and the final BP was also unchanged *(3)*. In the B KO, maximum PE doses were not tested, and the technique was subject to anesthetic variables *(1)*.

With the nonselective agonist NE in the D KO, the BP increase and final BP were both reduced *(3)*. The D has the highest NE affinity of any subtype. In the B KO, the BP response to a submaximal NE dose was reduced very slightly. NE was not tested in the A KO. In summary, KO of only a single α_1-AR subtype impairs the BP increase with a nonselective α_1-agonist modestly or not at all, with the greatest loss seen with NE in the D KO. The final BP after agonist is related to the resting BP, which was lower in the A and D KOs. These results suggest that other subtypes compensate in the pressor response for deletion of any one. Future studies of double- and triple-KO mice will therefore be very informative.

4.4. Arteries In Vitro

Arterial preparations in vitro provide an additional approach to sort subtype roles in vasoconstriction and were used in the B and D KOs (Table 3). In thoracic aortic rings from the B KO, one group found a decrease in contraction with submaximal PE doses *(1)*, whereas another group found in the B KO no change in PE EC_{50} or maximum response *(7)*. In D KO thoracic aortic rings, the EC_{50}s for PE and NE were shifted markedly to the right (40- to 50-fold), indicating reduced potency of these agonists *(3)*, consistent with the observation that the D is the predominant or only α_1-AR in the thoracic aorta (Table 2).

Mesenteric artery was studied in the B and D KOs (Table 3). The B KO had no change in PE EC_{50} or maximum in rings, whereas the D KO had a decreased pressor response to PE in an isolated mesenteric bed preparation *(3,7)*. This evidence for the D in mesenteric arteries fits binding data in WT mice *(22a)*. Carotid and tail artery rings from the B KO had no change in PE effects, except that the carotid from the B KO was more sensitive to PE *(7)*. Coronary arteries were studied in the D and AB KOs by examining coronary flow or pressure in the isolated perfused heart *(16,18)*. Both studies pointed to a role of the D in coronary vasoconstriction (Table 3). In summary, in vitro studies implicated the D in vaso-constriction but not the B. The possibility of patchy subtype expression in arter-ies, shown for the A (*see* Section 4.6.), needs to be kept in mind when interpreting these types of experiments (2).

4.5. Stress Experiments

An experimental stress can sometimes reveal a phenotype in KO models when one is not apparent in the basal or resting state. Thus, vascular effects after stress were studied in the B and D KOs (Table 3). In the D KO, partial nephrectomy plus chronic salt drinking for 35 d was used to induce hypertension. Hyperten-sion was markedly less in the D KO, and less hypertension was associated with a marked improvement in survival (93% D KO vs 53% WT), although the cause of death was not described (17). Also, in the D KO, 0.67M NaCl was injected acutely into the cerebral ventricles through an indwelling cannula, and the result-ing hypertension and tachycardia were measured in conscious mice by a femoral artery catheter. Hypertension and tachycardia after this acute salt loading were markedly blunted in the D KO, but there was no change in the response to AngII (19). Overall, the stress studies further support a role of the D in vasopressor effects and BP regulation.

Technically demanding experiments were done in the B KO, in which femoral artery telemeters and osmotic minipumps were implanted and BP was measured at intervals in conscious mice over 18-d infusion of hypertensive doses of NE and AngII or a subhypertensive dose of PE (10) (Table 3). NE in WT mice caused a progressive increase in BP beginning after 4 d infusion, and hypertension was eliminated in the B KO. By 18 d in WT mice treated with NE or subhypertensive PE, mesenteric arteries (140–200 μm) exhibited "eutrophic remodeling," with a smaller lumen diameter and a larger media-to-lumen ratio, without changes in cell size or number. In the B KO, mesenteric artery remodeling with NE or PE was eliminated. A recent study of the B KO and D KO also implicates the B subtype in carotid artery remodeling (22b). These results implicate the B in hypertension produced by chronic NE infusion and in a process of vascular remodeling. This vascular process is independent of BP per se because it occurred with a subhyper-tensive dose of PE, but the mechanisms are uncertain.

4.6. Receptor Localization

Detailed localization studies of each subtype in various arteries would go a long way toward supporting subtype functional roles. As noted in Table 2, the D appears to predominate in the thoracic aorta and regulates constriction in thoracic aortic rings (Table 3). However, determining localization in smaller arteries is problem-atic because binding studies are difficult in small mouse vessels; antibodies remain to be validated; and mRNAs do not necessarily predict receptor protein.

In the A KO, in which LacZ replaced the first exon (Table 1), blue staining of β-gal could be used to localize normal sites of receptor expression in the vasculature *(2)*. Interestingly, staining was absent in the thoracic aorta, the major thoracic aortic branches (subclavian, carotid), the proximal pulmonary artery, and the superior and inferior vena cavae, indicating that the A was not expressed in these vessels. β-Gal staining became evident in the lower abdominal aorta and then was prominent in the celiac, renal, mesenteric, hepatic, splenic, gastric, testicular, ovarian, iliac, femoral, and tail arteries. Staining was also prominent in approx 20-μm dermal arterioles near hair follicles. These results suggested that the A was expressed normally in the gut, renal, and skin circulations. A particularly intriguing result was the very patchy, circumferential blue staining, even in arteries with robust expression, raising the possibility that arterial strips for in vitro studies could have markedly varying levels of A expression. Overall, the β-gal reporter provided convincing evidence for A localization in vascular beds with major roles in BP regulation, but not in thoracic vasculature, consistent with the functional data *(2)*.

4.7. Vascular Structure

A role for α_1-ARs in vascular growth is suspected, and thus lifelong absence of receptors might change vascular structure, with a secondary effect on BP. This possibility remains to be studied in detail. The A KO had no change in lumen area of the celiac, mesenteric, renal, or carotid arteries *(2)*. The B KO had no obvious changes in dissecting and mounting strips from the thoracic aorta or carotid, mesenteric, and tail arteries *(7)*. As noted above, the B was involved in a process of vascular remodeling with chronic α_1-agonist infusion or injury, but cell size and number were unchanged *(10,22b)*. In many studies, responses to AngII, vasopressin, and serotonin were unchanged in KO mice or arteries (Table 3), further suggesting normal vascular structure. In addition, none of the single KOs had major changes in heart structure or function, as discussed in Section 5 *(see* Table 4), making unlikely an effect on BP secondary to changes in CO. Taken together, it seems likely that changes in BP in the α_1-AR KOs are secondary to functional reductions in vasoconstriction and peripheral vascular resistance rather than changes in vascular structure or CO.

4.8. Summary of Vascular Phenotypes

The role of α_1-ARs in the vasculature, as revealed by the KO approach, should be considered a work in progress. In particular, further work is required on all KO genotypes in congenic backgrounds. However, the data so far suggest the following generalizations. The A is expressed in resistance arteries that regulate BP, is required to maintain resting BP, and is a potent vasoconstrictor. The B has the least effect on BP and vasoconstriction of any of the three subtypes but might be important for chronic vascular remodeling, which can cause hypertension. The D is the main or only subtype in the thoracic aorta, a conductance artery thought to have little effect on BP. However, the D induces vasoconstriction in mesenteric resistance arteries and is required to maintain resting BP and to induce hypertension in various models. The D might be the main subtype in coronary arteries. Thus, the A and D appear to be the main subtypes involved in vasoconstriction.

5. Cardiac Phenotypes in the α_1-Adrenergic Receptor Knockouts

A surprise in α_1-AR biology has been the suggestion that α_1-ARs have important adaptive roles in the heart, including cardiac hypertrophy, preconditioning, protection from apoptosis, and increased contractility *(5,6a,23,24)*. The KO models provide an excellent approach to validate these functions and identify which subtypes are involved.

5.1. Adverse Clinical Effects With α_1-Antagonists

If α_1-ARs mediate adaptive responses in the heart, then blocking these adaptive effects with α_1-antagonist drugs might have negative side effects on the heart. Indeed, the Antihypertensive and Lipid-Lowering Treatment to Prevent Heart Attack Trial (ALLHAT) in hypertension tested the subtype-nonselective α_1-antagonist doxazosin vs the diuretic chlorthalidone in about 24,000 men and women with hypertension and at least one other cardiac risk factor *(25,26)*. This arm of the trail was stopped prematurely because doxazosin doubled the incidence of heart failure, unlike any other antihypertensive medication *(25–28)*. Similarly, in the Vasodilator-Heart Failure Trials (V-HeFT) of vasodilators in heart failure, the α_1-antagonist prazosin did not improve survival as did other vasodilators and even tended to increase mortality *(29)*. Doxazosin and prazosin are piperazinyl quinazolines, which at high doses can cause apoptosis in heart and other tissues independent of α_1-ARs *(30,31)*. Thus, it has remained controversial whether the adverse results in ALLHAT and V-HeFT were caused by α_1-AR inhibition itself or a nonspecific drug effect. This question has important therapeutic implications given the large number of patients treated with α_1-antagonists for hypertension or prostate disease. Indeed, an editorial suggested that over 7 million American men age 65 yr and older with prostate enlargement would benefit from this type of drug *(32)*.

The following sections review new insights from KO models on cardiac biology of α_1-ARs, as summarized in Table 4 for male mice. The focus is on the double AB KO, highlighting the requirement for α_1-AR signaling in the heart. The KO results suggest that adverse clinical consequences of nonselective α_1-antagonists reflect loss of adaptive α_1-AR functions in the heart.

5.2. Cardiac Growth and Hypertrophy

Cardiac hypertrophy is an increase in the size of the heart. Heart enlargement is typically caused by enlargement of the individual muscle cells because heart muscle cells do not divide to any extent after birth. The most common form of cardiac hypertrophy occurs during normal development as the heart enlarges to maintain CO to the growing organism. This is considered an adaptive or physiological hypertrophy because cardiac function improves. In heart disease, hypertrophy is ubiquitous and is thought to be adaptive initially. However, function deteriorates eventually in the hypertrophy seen in heart disease, resulting in the important clinical syndrome of heart failure; therefore, hypertrophy in disease is called maladaptive or pathological hypertrophy.

5.2.1. Cardiac Growth and Hypertrophy in the AB KO and Single KOs

Because each α_1-AR subtype KO is a germline mutation, the subtype is absent throughout development. None of the subtype KOs was lethal, including the triple ABD KO (unpublished data, 2004), indicating that α_1-ARs are not required for prenatal cardiac development, in contrast with the KOs of NE synthesis, which have a lethal effect (33–35). It is straightforward to detect a KO effect on postnatal physiological developmental hypertrophy by measuring the size of the adult heart, indexed by wet heart weight. Adult heart weight was unchanged in all three single KOs (1–3) (Table 4). Because body weight was also unchanged in all KOs, the ratio of the heart weight to the weight of the body, the usual index of heart size, was also unchanged.

However, in the double AB KO, adult heart weight was reduced significantly by 15% vs WT (5). We studied heart weight over time to determine when growth of the heart was reduced during postnatal development in the AB KO. At weaning (3 wk), heart weight was identical in AB KO and WT mice. However, from weaning to adulthood (14 wk), AB KO heart weight was progressively smaller than WT, with a final 40% reduction in postweaning heart growth. Echocardiography confirmed the small-heart phenotype, revealing significant 20% reductions in LV wall thickness and end-diastolic volume (i.e., the maximum filling volume when fully relaxed). The fundamental cause of the small heart was small myocytes, with a 33% reduction in myocyte cross-sectional area in ventricular sections and a 25% reduction in the volume of isolated myocytes. In addition, the mRNAs for two myocyte-specific genes, myosin heavy chain and ANF, were lower in the AB KO by 13–40% when indexed to the ubiquitous actin mRNA. Binucleate myocytes were identical in AB KO and WT myocytes (~90%), suggesting that terminal differentiation was normal in the AB KO (myocyte postnatal terminal differentiation involves a final round of DNA synthesis and nuclear division without cell division, creating binucleate cells). Thus, during postnatal development the AB KO had a generalized impairment of

Table 4
Cardiac Phenotypes in Male α_1-Adrenergic Receptor Subtype Knockouts

	AB KO	A KO	B KO	D KO
Cardiac growth				
• Heart weight (adult)	DEC (5)	NC (2)	NC (1,10)	NC (3,18)
• Echocardiography	DEC LV walls, volume (5)			NC (3,18)
• Heart sections	DEC myocyte area (5)			
• Isolated myocytes	DEC volume, mRNAs (5) NC binucleation (5)			
Heart function				
• Echocardiography	NC to INC EF (5) DEC SV, CO (5)	NC EF (2)	NC EF (10)	NC EF (3,18)
• Isolated heart	INC submaximal LVDP (6a)			NC HR, LVDP, dP/dt (18)
• RV trabeculae	INC submaximal force (6a) INC Ca^{2+} sensitivity (6a) DEC maximum force (6a)	NC maximum force (42)		
• Signaling	NC pHi, Ca^{2+} (6a) DEC ERK (5) DEC myocyte β-ARs, PKA (U)	NC pHi, Ca^{2+} (42)		NC ERK (18)
β-AR responses				
• Mouse		NC hypotension, tachycardia (2)		NC inotropy, chronotropy (18)
• Isolated heart	DEC maximum force (6)			
• RV trabeculae	DEC β-ARs, cAMP (U)			
• Myocytes	DEC TnI, PLN phosphorylation (6a) INC apoptosis (U)			

Continued on next page

Table 4 (Continued)
Cardiac Phenotypes in Male α_1-Adrenergic Receptor Subtype Knockouts

	AB KO	A KO	B KO	D KO
Stress responses				
• Exercise capacity	DEC running wheel, treadmill (5)			
• TAC	INC mortality, cardiomyopathy(U) INC fibrosis, apoptosis (U) DEC ANF, fetal genes (U) NC hypertrophy (U)		NC mortality, function (10) NC hypertrophy, ANF (10)	
• Renal hypertension[a]				NC hypertrophy (17)
• Chronic α_1-agonist	NC hypertrophy (U)		ABSENT hypertrophy, ANF[b] (10) NC function, HR (PE, NE) (10) NC hypertrophy (AngII) (10)	
Acute α_1-agonist responses				
• Isolated heart	Absent PIE (PE[c]) (16) NIE (PE[c]; BMY7378 blocks) (16)	Absent IE (A61603) (42) NC NIE, Ca^{2+} (PE[c]) (42)		DEC coronary pressure (PE 100 μM)(18)
• RV trabeculae	Absent IE (PE[c]) (6a,16)	NC Ca^{2+} (PE[c]) (42)		
• Signaling	DEC ERK, p90RSK, p70S6K (PE[c]) (5) NC ERK (PMA, ET) (5) NC Akt (insulin) (5)			

cAMP, cyclic adenosine 5′-monophosphate; CO, cardiac output; dP/dt, rate of change of LV pressure; EF, ejection fraction; ET, endothelin; LVDP, left ventricular developed pressure; NIE, negative inotropic effect; PIE, positive inotropic effect; PLN, phospholamban; PMA, phorbol myristate acetate; TAC, transverse aortic constriction; TnI, troponin I; SV, stroke volume.

References are given parenthetically in each column (U, unpublished data, 2004).

[a]Partial nephrectomy plus saline in the drinking water for 35 days.
[b]NE 2.5 mg/kg/d, PE 100 μg/kg/d.
[c]PE plus timolol to block β-ARs.

physiological hypertrophy caused by impaired cardiac myocyte hypertrophy and transcription *(5)*. Heart weight is directly related to BP in most cases, but low BP did not cause the small AB KO heart because BP was unchanged in the AB KO *(5)* (Table 3). Thus, the KO confirms in vivo a direct effect of α_1-ARs on cardiac myocyte hypertrophy, an effect first discovered in 1983 using a neonatal rat myocyte culture model *(36)*.

5.2.2. Model for α_1-ARs in Postweaning Hypertrophy

The appearance of the small AB KO heart phenotype beginning after weaning did coincide with three other events at about the time of weaning: (1) the completion of myocyte DNA synthesis *(37–39)*, (2) the first expression of α_1A mRNA in the mouse heart *(4a)*, and (3) the maturing of cardiac adrenergic innervation *(37)*. Thus, we propose a model in which physiological cardiac myocyte hypertrophy after weaning requires activation of myocyte A and B α_1-ARs by NE released from sympathetic terminals during normal daily life.

Which subtype is most responsible for the small heart, the A or the B? The small heart is not an artifact of mixed strains because we confirmed it in mice congenic in C57Bl/6. The single A KO and the single B KO both had unchanged adult heart size, so one possibility is that the subtypes are redundant, and one can compensate when another is deleted, much as in pressor responses discussed earlier. Against the idea of redundancy is preliminary evidence that the subtypes signal distinctly in myocytes (*see* next section). Alternately or in addition, further study of the single KOs in congenic backgrounds might reveal differences not seen in the initial experiments in mixed strains (Table 4). In any case, the individual roles of the A and the B will be important to sort out.

5.2.3. Hypertrophic Signaling in the AB KO

We studied signaling in the AB KO to test if any known postreceptor growth mechanism was abnormal in the AB KO *(5)*. Interestingly, the level of activated extracellular signal-regulated kinase (ERK) was markedly lower in the AB KO myocardium, only approx 30% of WT, as assayed by phosphorylation of Elk1 in vitro by ERK immunoprecipitated from intact hearts. In isolated myocytes from the AB KO heart, PE did not activate ERK and two downstream kinases, p90RSK and p70S6K, whereas all three kinases were activated by PE in WT myocytes, confirming the link between α_1-ARs and the ERK pathway in myocytes. Phorbol ester and endothelin could still activate ERK and downstream kinases in isolated AB KO myocytes, arguing against some generalized abnormality of the ERK pathway in the AB KO. Taken together, these results establish a requirement for specific α_1-AR activation of ERK in postnatal cardiac growth, even though many other agonists can activate ERK in model systems.

ERK might not be the only α_1-AR-mediated signaling pathway reduced in the AB KO. We have preliminary evidence from the single KOs that the subtypes signal distinctly in myocytes, with the A coupling to protein kinase C δ (PKCδ) and ERK and the B coupling to PKCϵ and PKCα (unpublished data, 2003). PKCϵ is also a known pathway of physiological hypertrophy *(40,41)*. Thus, the subtypes might signal cooperatively in physiological hypertrophy by coupling to different hypertrophic signaling pathways.

5.2.4. Summary of Developmental Hypertrophy in the AB KO

In summary, double KO of the A and the B shows that these subtypes are required for the physiological heart and myocyte hypertrophy of normal post-natal cardiac development, independent of BP. A plausible model is that NE released from sympathetic terminals during normal daily life activates the A and B and downstream hypertrophic signaling, such as the ERK pathway and PKCϵ. The relative roles of the A and the B are not known.

5.3. Cardiac Function in the AB KO

It was critical to ask whether the small AB KO heart functioned normally, that is, whether reduction of postnatal physiological hypertrophy caused problems.

5.3.1. Cardiac Function in the Intact Mouse

Ejection fraction (EF) and fractional shortening (FS) are echocardiographic indices of overall systolic function, how well the left ventricle (LV) empties with each contraction. By echocardiography, each single KO had normal LV systolic function. Although the double AB KO had an EF unchanged or slightly increased vs WT, suggesting normal LV systolic function, CO was decreased *(5)*. CO is the product of HR and stroke volume (SV), the volume of blood pumped with each beat. CO was low in the AB KO because of a slow HR, the cause of which is unknown, and a small SV because of the small LV chamber. Thus, the small AB KO heart *per se* impaired cardiac function without necessarily implying abnormal muscle.

5.3.2. Cardiac Function in the Isolated Perfused Heart and Muscle Strips

In the intact mouse, other inotropic mechanisms might compensate to some extent for abnormal cardiac muscle in the AB KO and produce a normal EF. Therefore, we measured function in isolated, perfused heart and muscle preparations. No α_1-agonist was added in these experiments. Interestingly, we found that submaximal force was increased in the isolated AB KO heart and in AB KO right ventricular (RV) trabeculae (19–65% increase) *(6a,16)*. The effect was not reproduced by acute treatment of WT heart with the nonselective α_1-antagonist prazosin, indicating that the functional changes were caused by long-term consequences of α_1-AR deletion. Detailed study in trabeculae revealed that Ca^{2+} transients were unchanged, and that increased submaximal force in the AB KO was explained by increased Ca^{2+} sensitivity of the myofibrils, producing greater force at any level of cytosolic Ca^{2+}. In turn, increased Ca^{2+} sensitivity of the myofibrils was not explained by changes in intracellular pH (alkaline pH can increase Ca^{2+} sensitivity) but was likely related to decreased phosphorylation of troponin I (TnI), a thin filament regulatory protein *(6a)*.

In contrast to the increase in submaximal force, AB KO trabeculae had a decrease in maximal force with saturating Ca^{2+} or tetanus (~20–40% lower). Ca^{2+} transients were unchanged, indicating that the decreased force was caused by impaired myofilament function. The exact abnormality is unknown, but one possibility is a reduction in amount of myofibrils. The relative contribution of the A and the B to development of normal force generation also is unknown. Maximal force was also reduced in single A KO trabeculae (~20%), although this was not significant statistically *(42)*.

5.3.3. Summary of Cardiac Function in the AB KO

In summary, double KO of the A and the B impaired physiological hypertrophy, producing myocardium with increased submaximal force because of increased myofilament Ca^{2+} sensitivity and decreased maximal contraction caused by impaired myofilament function. These two changes, increased Ca^{2+} sensitivity and decreased maximal contraction, plus β-AR downregulation (discussed in the next section) mimic changes seen in human heart failure (*see* ref. *6a*). The changes in the AB KO were the result of chronic loss of α_1-AR signaling, that is, loss of α_1-AR trophic effects on transcription and translation, because they were not reproduced by acute α_1-adrenergic blockade. The functional consequences of decreased maximal force are not clear because the heart operates normally under conditions of submaximal activation. Possibly, AB KO hearts would function worse under conditions of stress, when contractile reserve is required; indeed, we found just that in studies of β-AR stimulation and the stresses of exercise and aortic constriction (*see* Section 5.6.).

5.4. β-AR Responses in the AB KO

Evidence exists for antagonism between α_1- and β-AR signaling in myocytes *(43,44)*, and thus a surprise in the AB KO was downregulated β-ARs and reduced β-AR signaling and function. This anomaly was first noted in AB KO RV trabeculae, which had a marked 40% reduction in β-AR-stimulated maximal force; β-AR-mediated phosphorylation of TnI was also lower in AB KO myocytes *(6a)*. We found that β-AR binding was reduced by 44% in AB KO isolated myocytes, accompanied by blunted β-AR-mediated cAMP accumulation and phosphorylation of phospholamban at the protein kinase A (PKA) site (unpublished data, 2004). These data indicated reduced β-ARs and PKA signaling in AB KO myocytes. In single-subtype KOs, the few studies on β-AR responses did not reveal abnormalities. Specifically, the A KO mouse had unchanged β-adrenergic-induced hypotension and tachycardia *(2)*, and the D KO isolated heart had unchanged β-adrenergic positive chronotropy and inotropy *(18)*. The mechanism for β-AR downregulation in the AB KO is unknown but is an important question for further study. In theory, reduced β-AR signaling in the sinus node might explain the bradycardia in the AB KO *(5)*.

5.5. Apoptosis in AB KO Cardiac Myocytes

β_1-ARs are known to cause apoptosis in myocytes *(45)*, and one might therefore predict less β-adrenergic apoptosis in AB KO myocytes. Instead, a paradoxical effect in AB KO cultured myocytes was an increase in apoptosis stimulated by the β-agonist isoproterenol (unpublished data, 2004). AB KO myocytes also had increased apoptosis with oxidative stress (H_2O_2) (unpublished data, 2004). Thus, despite β-AR downregulation, AB KO myocytes were predisposed to apoptosis. Myocyte α_1-ARs are well recognized to mediate antiapoptotic signaling, probably by multiple mechanisms, including ERK activation, BAD phosphorylation, and increased glucose metabolism *(23,24)*. It is therefore plausible that the observed sensitivity of AB KO myocytes to apoptotic stimuli reflected loss of acute α_1-AR signaling. Sensitivity to apoptosis might also be caused by chronic changes in gene expression, and DNA arrays support this idea (unpublished data, 2004). In any event, sensitivity to apoptosis could contribute to an adverse outcome after stress.

5.6. Stress Experiments in the AB KO and Single KOs

As previously noted, an experimental stress can sometimes reveal a phenotype in KO models when one is not apparent in the basal or resting state. In the AB KO, cardiac abnormalities became much more evident with the stresses of exercise and aortic constriction.

5.6.1. Exercise in the AB KO

We tested exercise capacity using a running wheel and a motorized treadmill. The running wheel tests voluntary exercise because mice can choose to run. Indeed, WT C57Bl/6 mice ran about 6 km each night over 5 h. In the AB KO, exercise distance, time, and speed were all markedly lower than for WT. To test if behavioral factors played a role in wheel running, we tested forced exercise on a treadmill, and AB KO mice were also markedly impaired. In summary, AB KO mice had reduced exercise capacity by two complementary assays, likely because of blunting of the normal CO increase with exercise.

5.6.2. Pressure Overload in the AB KO

We next tested the response to pressure overload, a common cause of pathological hypertrophy seen in human diseases such as hypertension and aortic valve stenosis. We induced pressure overload by transverse aortic constriction (TAC), using surgery to constrict the aorta between the carotids. The TAC was severe, with a pressure gradient across the stenosis of 100 mmHg (i.e., 200 mmHg proximal and 100 mmHg distal), representing the extra work required to pump blood across the stenosis, a pressure overload on the heart. The AB KO had a highly maladaptive response to TAC.

Survival to 2 wk after TAC was only 55% in the AB KO vs 100% in WT. AB KO mice died at 5–8 d after surgery, and postmortem exams suggested that death was caused by heart failure *(5)*. To determine the cause of death in the AB KO after TAC, we studied mice that survived 2 wk (unpublished data, 2005). Echocardiography in conscious AB KO mice revealed lower EFs and larger LVs than in WT mice, defining a worsened dilated cardiomyopathy in the AB KO, with reduced systolic function and LV dilation. Mechanistically, heart weight and myocyte cross-sectional area increased the same with TAC in AB KO and WT mice, indicating that cardiomyopathy was not caused by a reduction of hypertrophy *per se*. However, overloaded AB KO hearts had increased interstitial fibrosis and apoptosis and failed induction of the classical fetal hypertrophic marker genes (unpublished data, 2005). Thus, deletion of the A and B caused a highly maladaptive response to pressure overload, a worsened pathological hypertrophy. Taken together, the data on exercise and pressure overload showed clearly that α_1-AR signaling is required for the heart to adapt to stress.

5.6.3. Stress Experiments in Single KOs

It is unknown whether loss of the A or the B is more important for the maladaptive response to TAC in the AB KO, but stress studies in single KOs might provide clues. In the B KO, TAC induced ANF normally, one of the classical fetal hypertrophic marker genes, and did not increase mortality or reduce systolic function *(10)*. Each of these end points is opposite to what we observed in the AB KO, thus implicating the A in ANF, survival, and function. On the other hand, TAC was less severe in the B KO (70 mmHg gradient for 7 d in the B KO vs 100 mmHg for 14 d in the AB KO), and the B KO studies were in mice with mixed genetic backgrounds (the AB KO mice were congenic in C57Bl/6).

There were also interesting results in the single B KO with chronic agonist infusion *(10)*. In WT mice, an 18-d infusion of NE or a nonhypertensive dose of PE increased heart size and induced ANF, the hypertrophic marker gene. As in other species with chronic α_1-agonist infusion *(46–49)*, the hypertrophy was physiological because systolic function was normal in the hypertrophied heart *(10)*. In the B KO, chronic α_1-agonist infusion did not increase heart size or induce ANF. This result implicates the B in the α_1-agonist-induced hypertrophy and ANF induction, which might be analogous to developmental hypertrophy.

Stress experiments in the single D KO were intriguing as well. In the D KO, nephrectomy plus saline caused hypertrophy, measured as an increase in heart weight, the same as in WT mice, even though nephrectomy plus saline failed to cause hypertension in the D KO *(17)*. The D KO with nephrectomy plus saline did have increased serum catecholamines as compared with sham control D KO mice, and the increased serum catecholamines might have been the stimulus for hypertrophy. This model therefore seems to be another example of α_1-agonist-induced hypertrophy in the absence of hypertension *(17)*. These results suggest no role for the D in heart size, consistent with the apparent absence of D in myocytes.

5.6.4. Summary of Stress Experiments

Taken together, the studies show that the A and the B are required together for an adaptive response to pressure overload. With pressure overload, the AB KO has worsened dilated cardiomyopathy because of fibrosis, apoptosis, and failed gene induction. Single-KO experiments raise the possibility that the subtypes are involved in different aspects of this complex final phenotype, but much more work is needed in congenic KO mice.

5.7. Acute α_1-AR Contractile Responses

α_1-Agonists cause positive inotropic responses, or increases in force of contraction, in myocardium of many species, including rat, rabbit, guinea pig, hamster, dog, and humans *(50)*. It is therefore surprising that negative inotropic effects (NIEs), or decreases in force of contraction, are observed in mouse myocardium and isolated mouse myocytes *(see ref. 16)*. In most species, the α_1-adrenergic inotropic response is typically triphasic, with phase 1 transient positive inotropic responses, a phase 2 transient NIE, and then a phase 3 sustained positive inotropic effect (PIE). In mouse, inotropy is increased in phase 3 relative to phase 2, but the end result is still an NIE *(42)*.

We studied the α_1-adrenergic inotropic response in RV trabeculae from the single A KO *(42)*. The A KO did not appreciably change the negative inotropic response to PE, suggesting that the B (or D, but *see* next paragraphs) can mediate an NIE. The A KO did eliminate the NIE to A61603, reconfirming the selectivity of this agonist and showing that the A can mediate an NIE in mouse RV trabeculae. The mechanism of the NIE was a transient decrease in the Ca^{2+} transient (in phase 2) and a sustained decrease in Ca^{2+} sensitivity of the myofibrils (in phases 2 and 3). The single A KO did not change these significantly. These results suggest redundancy of the A and B in the α_1-adrenergic inotropic effects, in this case, an NIE in response to activation of the A or the B.

Consistent with this, AB KO RV trabeculae had no significant inotropic response to PE, indicating that the D was not involved in inotropy *(16)*. However, in studies of the AB KO isolated heart, we were surprised to find in the WT mouse heart that PE caused a PIE, the first report of this in the mouse. There was a transient NIE, then a sustained PIE, with an increase almost 20% over control.

It is unknown why mouse heart has a PIE, whereas mouse RV trabeculae and myocytes have an NIE. In any case, the AB KO eliminated the PIE with PE, indicating that the A and/or the B mediate the PIE.

Interestingly, elimination of the PIE in the isolated AB KO heart revealed a NIE in response to PE (−13%). The NIE in the AB KO heart could be correlated with a reduction in coronary flow caused by PE (−14%); BMY7378, the D-selective antagonist, inhibited the flow reduction and NIE caused by PE. In the WT heart, PE caused a similar flow reduction, raising the possibility that the final PIE was somewhat underestimated by a flow-related NIE. Thus, the D appeared to cause vasoconstriction and flow reduction, with a secondary decrease in contraction, in WT or AB KO heart, providing further evidence for the D in coronary arteries.

In summary, α_1-adrenergic inotropic responses in the A KO and AB KO reveal negative contractile effects in RV trabeculae mediated by the A or the B, primarily because of decreases in Ca^{2+} sensitivity of the myofibrils, and positive contractile effects of the A or the B in the isolated heart, with unknown mechanism. The D in coronary arteries mediates flow reductions and secondary negative contractile effects.

5.8. Summary of Cardiac Phenotypes

The KO models confirm the essential adaptive roles of α_1-ARs in the heart, where the A and the B are required for chronic trophic or "nutritional" effects that depend ultimately on anabolic, transcriptional, metabolic, and antiapoptotic processes. The A and the B mediate inotropic effects, which depend on the preparation, and the D causes coronary vasoconstriction. The distinct roles of the A and the B in heart remain to be worked out. Clinically, the results emphasize concern about the use of nonselective α_1-antagonist drugs in patients with hypertension or prostate disease. On the other hand, D-selective antagonists might have advantages.

6. Other Phenotypes in the α_1-Adrenergic Receptor Knockouts

Initial work has begun to explore other α_1-AR physiological effects, primarily involving metabolism and behavior, as summarized in Table 5.

6.1. Metabolism

The D KO had a very interesting increase in daily food and water intake, which might in part have been related to chronic hypotension *(17)*. The B KO had a variety of abnormalities of glucose metabolism, including insulin resistance, increased plasma leptin, increased percentage body fat (with no change in body weight), and glucose intolerance and obesity with a high-fat diet *(12)*. The authors offered an explanation involving increased parasympathetic activity caused by increased hypothalamic neuropeptide Y *(12)*, and certainly further work in this area will be interesting and important. A current clinical paradigm is that α_1-antagonists decrease insulin resistance, the opposite of the B KO.

Table 5
Other Phenotypes in the Male α_1-Adrenergic Receptor Subtype Knockouts

	A KO	B KO	D KO	AB KO
Body temperature		NC (54)		
Lung, liver, and kidney weight	NC (2)			NC (5)
Serum electrolytes and renal function	NC (2)		NC (renal) (17)	
Blood cell counts	NC (2)			
Daily food and water intake			INC (19)	
Metabolism		INC plasma leptin (12) INC % body fat (12) Insulin resistance (12) Glucose intolerance, obesity with fat diet (12) INC liver glycogen (12) DEC muscle glycogen (12)		
Hypothalamic neuropeptide Y and agouti mRNAs		INC (12)		
Brain dopamine levels				
• Prefontal cortex		NC (also NC NE) (11)		
• Nucleus accumbens		NC (11)		
• Nucleus accumbens dialysate		DEC (9)		
• Striatum		NC (11,54)		
Pain resonses			Changed latencies (51a)	
Exploratory behavior		NC, INC, DEC exploration/locomotion (8,11,52)	NC (51b); DEC (51c)	
Responses to addicting drugs		DEC locomotion (9,11,54) DEC sensitization (11) DEC neurodegeneration (54) DEC dopamine release striatum, nucleus accumbens (9,54)		

References are given parenthetically in each column.

6.2. Behavior

The D KO had changes in the latencies of responses to painful stimuli, interpreted to show alterations of spinal reflexes and anxiety components *(51a)*. Other tests of behavior in the D KO gave less-clear results *(51b,51c)*. The B KO had conflicting changes in exploratory behavior, which was unchanged, increased, or decreased in different studies, illustrating the many influences on behavior *(8,11,52)*. The B was required for increased locomotion stimulated by the α_1-agonist modafinil *(53)*. Several studies agreed that the B KO was less responsive to drugs of addiction (i.e., amphetamine, cocaine, and morphine). Several aspects of the responses to these drugs were decreased in the B KO, including locomotion, sensitization to repeated doses, neurodegeneration, and brain dopamine release *(8,9,11,52,54)*. These results might suggest that the B is required for toxic and addictive effects through positive control of dopamine release.

7. Sex as a Key Variable in Phenotype

Appreciation is growing of the key role of sex as a determinant of phenotype in genetically modified mice *(55)*. It is obvious that males and females differ, but there is a tendency to study males only, or to disregard sex, and to assume that findings apply to both. In the AB KO, we found several sex differences, summarized in Table 6 *(5,6a)*. In particular, impaired heart and myocyte hypertrophy during normal postweaning development was seen in males but not in females. In fact, in WT mice, male heart and myocyte size were larger than for the female, and the double AB KO had the overall effect to reduce male heart and myocyte size to that of females. The small heart in the male caused a reduced CO not seen in the female *(5)* (Table 6). Males and females were similar in other respects (Table 6), and some abnormalities were observed in the AB KO female (e.g., bradycardia, abnormal heart muscle function, and reduced exercise capacity). The cause of the sex difference is unknown, but it was not eliminated by ovariectomy, suggesting that female sex hormones are not involved. An attractive hypothesis is that males are more dependent on α_1-ARs because sympathetic activity is normally higher in males *(56,57)*. Thus, the effect of α_1-AR KO would be more marked in males, and females might be relatively protected from heart muscle disease, as is observed clinically. In any case, it is clear that sex differences require recognition and careful study.

8. Summary of Subtype Roles and Future Directions

Table 7 summarizes the main locations and physiological roles of the subtypes as deduced from the KOs. This review has emphasized that much more needs to be done, especially in congenic mice, but the assumption is made that

Table 6
Phenotypes in Male vs Female AB Knockout Mice

	Male	Female
Body weight	NC	NC
BP (tail cuff)	NC	NC
Cardiac growth		
• Heart weight (adult)	DEC	NC
• Myocyte size	DEC	NC
Heart function		
• Echocardiography (awake)	DEC HR	DEC HR
	NC EF	NC EF
	DEC LV size	NC LV size
	DEC SV and CO	NC SV and CO
• Submaximal LVDP in isolated heart	INC	INC
• Maximum force in RV trabeculae	DEC	DEC
Signaling		
• α_1-AR binding in heart	Absent	Absent[a]
• α_1 activation of ERK in myocytes	Absent	Absent[a]
• Insulin activation of Akt in myocytes	NC	NC
Stress responses		
• Exercise capacity	DEC	DEC
• Survival after TAC	DEC	NC
Ovariectomy		NC[b]

Data from refs. 5 and 6a and unpublished data, 2003–2005.

[a] In WT male and female myocytes, α_1 binding and ERK pathway activation were identical.

[b] In female WT and AB KO, ovariectomy at weaning plus isoflavone-free diet reduced uterine weight to 5% of sham at age 12 wk but did not change body weight, tibia length, heart weight, BP, or HR.

Table 7
Subtype Roles Deduced From the Knockouts (2004)

A	Located in heart, brain, kidney, and resistance arteries Maintain resting BP Vasopressor responses Cardiac survival and transcription?
B	Located in heart, brain, kidney, and liver Vascular remodeling with α_1-agonist Cardiac hypertrophy with α_1-agonist Glucose metabolism and insulin sensitivity Brain dopamine release and addictive behavior
D	Located in brain and arteries (aorta, coronary, mesenteric) Maintain resting BP Vasopressor and hypertensive responses Coronary vasoconstriction
A and/or B	Cardiac inotropic responses Physiological cardiac hypertrophy Cardiac adaptation to exercise and pressure overload

a subtype is *required* for a function if that function is lost in the KO. In the future, study of the various double KOs and the triple KO should be very informative. In this regard, it is important to recognize that each double KO will be a mouse expressing only a single subtype (e.g., the AB KO is a D-only mouse). Study of these mice should reveal the sufficiency of any subtype for a response and the corollary of whether any subtype can function in isolation in vivo at physiological levels.

The KOs confirm the importance of α_1-ARs in vasoconstriction and BP regulation, but a surprise is the apparently small role of the B in this respect. The D seems limited to a vascular role and probably brain. D-selective antagonists might have an advantage in hypertension treatment if human subtypes are similar to mouse. The B role in glucose metabolism is notable. Perhaps the biggest surprise from the KOs is the essential role of the A or the B in physiological cardiac hypertrophy and cardiac adaptation to stress. The AB KO data provide a plausible mechanism for the adverse effects of nonselective α_1-antagonists in clinical trials and raise further concern about use of these drugs in patients with hypertension or prostate disease. It will be interesting and important to test if α_1-agonists can be used to treat heart muscle disease.

9. Discrepancies in Genetic Models of α_1-Adrenergic Receptor Function

Genetic models to discover the physiological roles of α_1-AR subtypes include receptor overexpression (transgenics, TGs) and deletion (KOs). TGs are especially common in cardiac research because the α-myosin heavy-chain promoter can be used to target any gene specifically to cardiac myocytes *(58)*. Indeed, a cardiac TG of a constitutively activated B was the first to confirm the role of α_1-ARs in cardiac hypertrophy in vivo *(59)*. TGs are the most convincing approach to study hyperactivity of a specific subtype over a long period of time, as might be seen in heart failure or in diseases associated with genetic mutant G protein-coupled receptors. However, a discrepancy is becoming apparent in that several α_1-AR TGs suggest maladaptive cardiac roles of α_1-ARs *(60–63)*, whereas the KOs reviewed here suggest that α_1-ARs are required for cardiac adaptation. How is this discrepancy explained?

Potential artifacts with the TG approach include unanticipated effects from gene regulatory changes caused by the insertion site of the expression cassette. There is also the concern of nonphysiological levels of receptor overexpression or activity. For example, α_1-AR binding was increased 25- to 300-fold in the TGs overexpressing the WT B subtype *(60,61,63)*. Also, a possibility is that signaling by overexpressed α_1-ARs does not mimic signaling by ligand-activated α_1-ARs. This artifact is documented for β_2-ARs *(64,65)*, and it might be more unlikely that constitutively activated α_1-ARs faithfully mimic ligand-activated endogenous

α_1-ARs. Thus, a main problem with the TG approach might be false positives, and this could explain the discrepancy between the cardiac TGs and KOs.

Potential artifacts with the KO approach also include unanticipated changes from the DNA cassette itself plus insertion site effects *(58)*, although insertion sire artifacts should be minimal in the α_1-AR KOs (Table 1). More notably, each of the α_1-AR KOs is systemic and lifelong, with the possibility that developmental and compensatory changes will mask a phenotype and produce a false negative or cause a secondary effect on phenotype related only indirectly to α_1-AR deletion. For example, it is very likely that any KO (or TG for that matter) that changes cardiac or vascular function will alter sympathetic activity, with secondary effects via other ARs. Indeed, we saw sympathetic activation in the single A KO *(2)*.

It is possible technically to make an α_1-AR KO that is both inducible in time and tissue specific to avoid developmental and systemic effects *(58)*, but the time and effort required would be enormous, and incomplete KO would almost certainly be a factor. Thus, it is useful to note a key advantage of typical germline mouse KOs: They are predictive of drug effects in humans *(66,67)*. It is also pertinent that drug effects take time, particularly in heart disease. For example, the fraction of life with α_1-antagonist exposure in ALLHAT was about 5% (4 yr of an average 75-yr life expectancy) *(25)*. The fraction of life over which pathology developed in the AB KO was similar, about 8% (8 wk of 104-wk life expectancy). In conclusion, it seems reasonable to expect that the KOs will guide development of new drugs to target α_1-ARs.

Acknowledgments

I thank the National Institute of Health and the Department of Veterans Affairs for support and the many colleagues who have made the work possible, in particular Drs. Rokosh, O'Connell, Rodrigo, Swigart, Baker, Grossman, Foster, McCloskey, Turnbull, Ishizaka, Nakamura, Joho, and Deng.

References

1. Cavalli A, Lattion AL, Hummler E, et al. Decreased blood pressure response in mice deficient of the α_{1b}-adrenergic receptor. Proc Natl Acad Sci USA 1997;94: 11,589–11,594.
2. Rokosh DG, Simpson PC. Knockout of the $\alpha_{1A/C}$-adrenergic receptor subtype: the $\alpha_{1A/C}$ is expressed in resistance arteries and is required to maintain arterial blood pressure. Proc Natl Acad Sci USA 2002;99:9474–9479.
3. Tanoue A, Nasa Y, Koshimizu T, et al. The α_{1D}-adrenergic receptor directly regulates arterial blood pressure via vasoconstriction. J Clin Invest 2002;109: 765–775.
4a. O'Connell TD, Rokosh DG, Simpson PC. Cloning and characterization of the mouse $\alpha_{1C/A}$-adrenergic receptor gene and analysis of an α_{1C} promoter in cardiac

myocytes: role of an MCAT element that binds transcriptional enhancer factor-1 (TEF-1). Mol Pharmacol 2001;59:1225–1234.

4b. Deighan C, Woollhead AM, Colston JF, McGrath JC. Hepatocytes from α1B-adrenoceptor knockout mice reveal compensatory adrenoceptor subtype substitution. Br J Pharmacol. 2004;142:1031–1037.

5. O'Connell TD, Ishizaka S, Nakamura A, et al. The $\alpha_{1A/C}$- and α_{1B}-adrenergic receptors are required for physiological cardiac hypertrophy in the double-knockout mouse. J Clin Invest 2003;111:1783–1791.

6a. McCloskey DT, Turnbull L, Swigart P, O'Connell TD, Simpson PC, Baker AJ. Abnormal myocardial contraction in α_{1A}- and α_{1B}-adrenoceptor double-knockout mice. J Mol Cell Cardiol 2003;35:1207–1216.

6b. Hosoda C, Koshimizu TA, Tanoue A, et al. Two α1-adrenergic receptor subtypes regulating the vasopressor response have differential roles in blood pressure regulation. Mol Pharmacol. 2005;67:912–922.

7. Daly CJ, Deighan C, McGee A, et al. A knockout approach indicates a minor vasoconstrictor role for vascular α_{1B}-adrenoceptors in mouse. Physiol Genomics 2002;9:85–91.

8. Spreng M, Cotecchia S, Schenk F. A behavioral study of α_{1b} adrenergic receptor knockout mice: increased reaction to novelty and selectively reduced learning capacities. Neurobiol Learn Mem 2001;75:214–229.

9. Auclair A, Cotecchia S, Glowinski J, Tassin JP. D-Amphetamine fails to increase extracellular dopamine levels in mice lacking α_{1b}-adrenergic receptors: relationship between functional and nonfunctional dopamine release. J Neurosci 2002;22: 9150–9154.

10. Vecchione C, Fratta L, Rizzoni D, et al. Cardiovascular influences of α_{1b}-adrenergic receptor defect in mice. Circulation 2002;105:1700–1707.

11. Drouin C, Darracq L, Trovero F, et al. α_{1b}-Adrenergic receptors control locomotor and rewarding effects of psychostimulants and opiates. J Neurosci 2002;22:2873–2884.

12. Burcelin R, Uldry M, Foretz M, et al. Impaired glucose homeostasis in mice lacking the α_{1b}-adrenergic receptor subtype. J Biol Chem 2004;279:1108–1115; E-pub October 27, 2003.

13. Yang M, Reese J, Cotecchia S, Michel MC. Murine α_1-adrenoceptor subtypes. I. Radioligand binding studies. J Pharmacol Exp Ther 1998;286:841–847.

14. Wolff AA, Hines DK, Karliner JS. Refined membrane preparations mask ischemic fall in myocardial β-receptor density. Am J Physiol 1989;257:H1032–H1036.

15. Muntz KH, Zhao M, Miller JC. Downregulation of myocardial β-adrenergic receptors. Receptor subtype selectivity. Circ Res 1994;74:369–375.

16. Turnbull L, McCloskey DT, O'Connell TD, Simpson PC, Baker AJ. α_1-Adrenergic receptor responses in a1AB-AR knockout mouse hearts suggest the presence of α_{1D}-AR. Am J Physiol Heart Circ Physiol 2003;284:H1104–H1109.

17. Tanoue A, Koba M, Miyawaki S, et al. Role of the α_{1D}-adrenegric receptor in the development of salt-induced hypertension. Hypertension 2002;40:101–106.

18. Chalothorn D, McCune DF, Edelmann SE, et al. Differential cardiovascular regulatory activities of the α_{1B}- and α_{1D}-adrenoceptor subtypes. J Pharmacol Exp Ther 2003;305:1045–1053.

19. Chu CP, Kunitake T, Kato K, et al. The α_{1D}-adrenergic receptor modulates cardiovascular and drinking responses to central salt loading in mice. Neurosci Lett 2004;356:33–36.

20. Ishizaka S, Sievers RE, Zhu BQ, et al. New technique for measurement of left ventricular pressure in conscious mice. Am J Physiol Heart Circ Physiol 2004;286: H1208–H1215.

21. Rohrer DK, Schauble EH, Desai KH, Kobilka BK, Bernstein D. Alterations in dynamic heart rate control in the β_1-adrenergic receptor knockout mouse. Am J Physiol 1998;274:H1184–H1193.

22a. Yamamoto Y, Koike K. α_1-Adrenoceptor subtypes in the mouse mesenteric artery and abdominal aorta. Br J Pharmacol 2001;134:1045–1054.

22b. Zhang H, Cotecchia S, Thomas SA, Tanoue A, Tsujimoto G, Faber JE. Gene deletion of dopamine beta-hydroxylase and alpha1-adrenoceptors demonstrates involvement of catecholamines in vascular remodeling. Am J Physiol Heart Circ Physiol 2004;287:H2106–H2114.

23. Mani K, Ashton AW, Kitsis RN. Taking the BAD out of adrenergic stimulation. J Mol Cell Cardiol 2002;34:709–712.

24. Salvi S. Protecting the myocardium from ischemic injury: a critical role for α_1-adrenoreceptors? Chest 2001;119:1242–1249.

25. ALLHAT CRG. Major cardiovascular events in hypertensive patients randomized to doxazosin vs chlorthalidone: the antihypertensive and lipid-lowering treatment to prevent heart attack trial (ALLHAT). JAMA 2000;283:1967–1975.

26. Diuretic vs α-blocker as first-step antihypertensive therapy: final results from the Antihypertensive and Lipid-Lowering Treatment to Prevent Heart Attack Trial (ALLHAT). Hypertension 2003;42:239–246.

27. Davis BR, Cutler JA, Furberg CD, et al. Relationship of antihypertensive treatment regimens and change in blood pressure to risk for heart failure in hypertensive patients randomly assigned to doxazosin or chlorthalidone: further analyses from the Antihypertensive and Lipid-Lowering treatment to prevent Heart Attack Trial. Ann Intern Med 2002;137:313–320.

28. Piller LB, Davis BR, Cutler JA, et al. Validation of heart failure events in the Antihypertensive and Lipid Lowering Treatment to Prevent Heart Attack Trial (ALLHAT) participants assigned to doxazosin and chlorthalidone. Curr Control Trials Cardiovasc Med 2002;3:10.

29. Cohn JN. The Vasodilator-Heart Failure Trials (V-HeFT). Mechanistic data from the VA Cooperative Studies. Introduction. Circulation 1993;87:VI1–VI4.

30. Anglin IE, Glassman DT, Kyprianou N. Induction of prostate apoptosis by α_1-adrenoceptor antagonists: mechanistic significance of the quinazoline component. Prostate Cancer Prostatic Dis 2002;5:88–95.

31. Gonzalez-Juanatey JR, Iglesias MJ, Alcaide C, Pineiro R, Lago F. Doxazosin induces apoptosis in cardiomyocytes cultured in vitro by a mechanism that is independent of α_1-adrenergic blockade. Circulation 2003;107:127–131.

32. Vaughan ED Jr. Medical management of benign prostatic hyperplasia—are two drugs better than one? N Engl J Med 2003;349:2449–2451.

33. Kobayashi K, Morita S, Sawada H, et al. Targeted disruption of the tyrosine hydroxylase locus results in severe catecholamine depletion and perinatal lethality in mice. J Biol Chem 1995;270:27,235–27,243.
34. Thomas SA, Matsumoto AM, Palmiter RD. Noradrenaline is essential for mouse fetal development. Nature 1995;374:643–646.
35. Zhou QY, Quaife CJ, Palmiter RD. Targeted disruption of the tyrosine hydroxylase gene reveals that catecholamines are required for mouse fetal development. Nature 1995;374:640–643.
36. Simpson P. Norepinephrine-stimulated hypertrophy of cultured rat myocardial cells is an α_1 adrenergic response. J Clin Invest 1983;72:732–738.
37. Rakusan K. Cardiac growth, maturation and aging. In: Zak R, editor. Growth of the Heart in Health and Disease. New York: Raven Press; 1984:131–164.
38. Soonpaa MH, Koh GY, Pajak L, et al. Cyclin D1 overexpression promotes cardiomyocyte DNA synthesis and multinucleation in transgenic mice. J Clin Invest 1997;99:2644–2654.
39. Liao HS, Kang PM, Nagashima H, et al. Cardiac-specific overexpression of cyclin-dependent kinase 2 increases smaller mononuclear cardiomyocytes. Circ Res 2001;88:443–450.
40. Wu G, Toyokawa T, Hahn H, Dorn GW 2nd. Epsilon protein kinase C in pathological myocardial hypertrophy. Analysis by combined transgenic expression of translocation modifiers and Galphaq. J Biol Chem 2000;275:29,927–29,930.
41. Mochly-Rosen D, Wu G, Hahn H, et al. Cardiotrophic effects of protein kinase C e: analysis by in vivo modulation of PKCe translocation. Circ Res 2000;86:1173–1179.
42. McCloskey DT, Rokosh DG, O'Connell TD, Keung EC, Simpson PC, Baker AJ. α_1-Adrenoceptor subtypes mediate negative inotropy in myocardium from $\alpha_{1A/C}$-knockout and wild type mice. J Mol Cell Cardiol 2002;34:1007–1017.
43. Schafer M, Ponicke K, Heinroth-Hoffmann I, Brodde OE, Piper HM, Schluter KD. β-Adrenoceptor stimulation attenuates the hypertrophic effect of α-adrenoceptor stimulation in adult rat ventricular cardiomyocytes. J Am Coll Cardiol 2001;37:300–307.
44. Xiao l, Shen M, Colucci W. β_1-Adrenergic receptor (AR) stimulation inhibits α_1-AR-stimulated hypertrophic signaling in adult rat ventricular myocytes (ARVM) via activation of cyclic AMP-protein kinase A (PKA) cascade [abstract]. Circulation 2002;106:II-48.
45. Zhu WZ, Wang SQ, Chakir K, et al. Linkage of β_1-adrenergic stimulation to apoptotic heart cell death through protein kinase A-independent activation of Ca^{2+}/calmodulin kinase II. J Clin Invest 2003;111:617–625.
46. Laks MM, Morady F, Swan HJ. Myocardial hypertrophy produced by chronic infusion of subhypertensive doses of norepinephrine in the dog. Chest 1973;64:75–78.
47. King BD, Sack D, Kichuk MR, Hintze TH. Absence of hypertension despite chronic marked elevations in plasma norepinephrine in conscious dogs. Hypertension 1987;9:582–590.
48. Marino TA, Cassidy M, Marino DR, Carson NL, Houser S. Norepinephrine-induced cardiac hypertrophy of the cat heart. Anat Rec 1991;229:505–510.

49. Stewart JM, Patel MB, Wang J, et al. Chronic elevation of norepinephrine in conscious dogs produces hypertrophy with no loss of LV reserve. Am J Physiol 1992;262:H331–H339.

50. Li K, He H, Li C, Sirois P, Rouleau JL. Myocardial α_1-adrenoceptor: inotropic effect and physiologic and pathologic implications. Life Sci 1997;60:1305–1318.

51a. Harasawa I, Honda K, Tanoue A, et al. Responses to noxious stimuli in mice lacking α_{1d}-adrenergic receptors. Neuroreport 2003;14:1857–1860.

51b. Mishima K, Tanoue A, Tsuda M, et al. Characteristics of behavioral abnormalities in alpha1d-adrenoceptors deficient mice. Behav Brain Res. 2004;152:365–373.

51c. Sadalge A, Coughlin L, Fu H, et al. Alpha 1d Adrenoceptor signaling is required for stimulus induced locomotor activity. Mol Psychiatry. 2003;8:664–672.

52. Knauber J, Muller WE. Decreased exploratory activity and impaired passive avoidance behaviour in mice deficient for the α_{1b}-adrenoceptor. Eur Neuropsychopharmacol 2000;10:423–427.

53. Stone EA, Cotecchia S, Lin Y, Quartermain D. Role of brain α_{1B}-adrenoceptors in modafinil-induced behavioral activity. Synapse 2002;46:269–270.

54. Battaglia G, Fornai F, Busceti CL, Lembo G, Nicoletti F, De Blasi A. α_{1B} adrenergic receptor knockout mice are protected against methamphetamine toxicity. J Neurochem 2003;86:413–421.

55. Leinwand LA. Spotlight: sex is a potent modifier of the cardiovascular system. J Clin Invest 2003;112:302–307.

56. Hinojosa-Laborde C, Chapa I, Lange D, Haywood JR. Gender differences in sympathetic nervous system regulation. Clin Exp Pharmacol Physiol 1999;26:122–126.

57. Evans JM, Ziegler MG, Patwardhan AR, et al. Gender differences in autonomic cardiovascular regulation: spectral, hormonal, and hemodynamic indexes. J Appl Physiol 2001;91:2611–2618.

58. Robbins J. Genetic modification of the heart: exploring necessity and sufficiency in the past 10 years. J Mol Cell Cardiol 2004;36:643–652.

59. Milano CA, Dolber PC, Rockman HA, et al. Myocardial expression of a constitutively active α_{1B}-adrenergic receptor in transgenic mice induces cardiac hypertrophy. Proc Natl Acad Sci USA 1994;91:10,109–10,113.

60. Lemire I, Ducharme A, Tardif JC, et al. Cardiac-directed overexpression of wild-type α_{1B}-adrenergic receptor induces dilated cardiomyopathy. Am J Physiol Heart Circ Physiol 2001;281:H931–H938.

61. Grupp IL, Lorenz JN, Walsh RA, Boivin GP, Rindt H. Overexpression of α_{1B}-adrenergic receptor induces left ventricular dysfunction in the absence of hypertrophy. Am J Physiol 1998;275:H1338–H1350.

62. Wang BH, Du XJ, Autelitano DJ, Milano CA, Woodcock EA. Adverse effects of constitutively active α_{1B}-adrenergic receptors after pressure overload in mouse hearts. Am J Physiol Heart Circ Physiol 2000;279:H1079–H1086.

63. Akhter SA, Milano CA, Shotwell KF, et al. Transgenic mice with cardiac overexpression of α_{1B}-adrenergic receptors. In vivo α_1-adrenergic receptor-mediated regulation of β-adrenergic signaling. J Biol Chem 1997;272:21,253–21,259.

64. Zhou YY, Cheng H, Song LS, Wang D, Lakatta EG, Xiao RP. Spontaneous β_2-adrenergic signaling fails to modulate L-type Ca^{2+} current in mouse ventricular myocytes. Mol Pharmacol 1999;56:485–493.

65. Xiao RP, Avdonin P, Zhou YY, et al. Coupling of β_2-adrenoceptor to G_i proteins and its physiological relevance in murine cardiac myocytes. Circ Res 1999;84: 43–52.

66. Zambrowicz BP, Sands AT. Knockouts model the 100 best-selling drugs—will they model the next 100? Nat Rev Drug Discov 2003;2:38–51.

67. Zambrowicz BP, Turner CA, Sands AT. Predicting drug efficacy: knockouts model pipeline drugs of the pharmaceutical industry. Curr Opin Pharmacol 2003;3:563–570.

9

The α_2-Adrenergic Receptors

Lessons From Knockouts

Christopher M. Tan and Lee E. Limbird

Summary

The α_2-adrenergic receptors (α_2-ARs) belong to the G protein-coupled receptor superfamily and are responsible for mediating a diverse array of physiological effects in multiple tissues in response to the endogenous catecholamines epinephrine and norepinephrine delivered either by synapses or the circulation. Biochemical, physiological, and pharmacological studies have shown that three α_2-AR subtypes (α_{2A}, α_{2B}, and α_{2C}) are present in many key target cells and tissues, making them attractive in vivo targets amenable to therapeutic intervention. However, the clarification of the precise in vivo roles attributable to a particular receptor subtype has been complex, largely because of the lack of α_2-AR ligands displaying sufficient selectivity among the three α_2-AR subtypes. The generation of mice harboring a mutant α_{2A}-AR with diminished capacities (D79N α_{2A}-AR), or null for each of the individual receptor subtype alleles, has yielded a wealth of information critical for the identification and elucidation of their in vivo roles. Further insights have been derived from the creation of mice with combinations of targeted null alleles, mice heterozygous for the α_{2A}-AR, and mice overexpressing the α_{2C}-AR. Collectively, studies in these animals have clarified our understanding of the roles of each receptor subtype; the information revealed *en toto* exemplifies the power of employing genetically modified mice to elucidate biological functions and reveal effective therapeutic targets.

Key Words: Adrenergic; α_2-AR; G protein; in vivo; knockout mice; physiology; receptor; review.

From: *The Receptors: The Adrenergic Receptors: In the 21st Century*
Edited by: D. Perez © Humana Press Inc., Totowa, NJ

1. Introduction

The α_2-adrenergic receptor (AR) family consists of the α_{2A}-, α_{2B}-, and α_{2C}-receptor subtypes encoded by three distinct, intronless genes *(1)*. In native target cells, agonist binding and α_2-AR activation leads to coupling via inhibitory pertussis toxin-sensitive heterotrimeric guanine nucleotide inhibitory G_i/G_o proteins to a variety of downstream cellular effectors, including inhibition of adenylyl cyclase, suppression of voltage-gated Ca^{2+} channels, activation of receptor-operated inwardly rectifying K^+ channels, and activation of the mitogen-activated protein kinase (MAPK) cascade. Activation of these pathways in response to circulating catecholamines or synthetic ligands is critical for the regulation of physiological events, including the modulation and regulation of key functions such as sympathetic outflow and cardiovascular, psychomotor, sedative, analgesic, and behavioral functions.

Classically, the physiological functions assigned to the individual subtypes have been determined empirically based on the individual responses to synthetic agonists and antagonists; however, the lack of subtype-selective agents has largely hampered the clarification of subtype-specific functions. The introduction of genetically modified mice either overexpressing a particular subtype or null for a receptor subtype (either alone or in combination) has fueled the identification of the roles these receptors play in vivo *(see* Table 1*)*. The strategies employed to generate these animals is reviewed elsewhere *(2)*. This chapter focuses on the elucidation of the individual roles identified for each subtype as a result of the study of genetically engineered animals with altered expression of each of the α_2-ARs. The critical in vivo evaluation of these receptors represents an excellent example of the utility of genetic manipulations in the mouse to substantiate the multiple physiological and pharmacological roles of a particular subtype.

2. Mice Deficient for the α_2-Adrenergic Receptor or Harboring the D79N α_{2A}-AR Mutation Reveal a Role for the α_{2A}-AR Subtype in Multiple Physiological Functions

2.1. The D79N α_{2A}-AR Encodes a Receptor With Diminished Signaling and Cell Surface Residency Time

Studies from our laboratory had revealed that mutation of an aspartate to asparagine (D79N) at a highly conserved residue in the predicted second transmembrane domain of the α_{2A}-AR resulted in a dysfunctional receptor. When examined in vitro, the D79N α_2-AR was selectively uncoupled from activation of K^+ channels *(3)*. As such, generation of a mouse harboring the D79N α_{2A}-AR (α_{2A}-AR$^{D79N/D79N}$) would have been expected to define α_{2A}-AR-dependent in vivo physiological functions that relied on K^+ current activation. Substitution of the

Table 1

Physiological Consequences of Altering α_2-Adrenergic Receptor Subtype Gene Expression in Mice

A. The α_{2A}-Subtype Mediates Most of the Classical Effects of α_2-Adrenergic Receptor Agonists

Physiological Effect	Genetic alterations			
	α_{2A}-D79N	α_{2A}-KO	α_{2B}-KO	α_{2C}-KO
Hypotensive effects of α_2-adrenergic receptor agonist	X	X	↑	—
Bradycardic effects of α_2-adrenergic receptor agonist	↓	↓	—	—
Hypertensive effects of α_2-adrenergic receptor agonist	↓[a]	—	X	—
Cardiovascular effects of imidazoline agonist	X			
Resting heart rate	—	↑	—	—
Resting blood pressure	—	—	—	—
Salt-induced hypertension			X[b]	—
Sedative effects of dexmedetomidine	X	X	—	—
Antinociceptive effects of α_2-adrenergic receptor agonist	X/↓[c]		—	—
Antinociceptive effects of nitrous oxide			X	
Antinociceptive effects of moxonidine	↓			↓
Adrenergic-opioid synergy in spinal antinociception	X			
Anesthetic-sparing effects of dexmedetomidine	X			
Hypothermic effects of dexmedetomidine	X		—	—/↓
Antiepileptogenic effects of endogenous norepinephrine	X			
Presynaptic inhibition of norepinephrine release	—	↓	—	↓[d]
Autoinhibition of locus coeruleus	X			
Embryonic development			↓[e]	
Anxiety in the open field test		↑		
Adrenal gland inhibition of epinephrine release				X

X, abolished; —, no effect; ↑, accentuated; ↓, attenuated; and blank, not studied.

[a] Dependent on site of agonist administration.

[b] Mice were heterozygous (+/–) for α_{2B}-null mutation.

[c] Extent of attenuation depended on test used.

[d] In α_{2AC}-double-KO mice.

[e] Severely attenuated in α_{2ABC}-triple-KO mice.

Table 1
Physiological Consequences of Altering α_2-Adrenergic Receptor Subtype Gene Expression in Mice

B. Effects of Altered α_{2C}-Adrenergic Receptor Subtype Gene Expression on Behavior

Behavior	Genetic alterations	
	α_{2C}-KO	α_{2C}-OE
Startle reflex	↑	—
Prepulse inhibition of startle reflex	↓	↑
Latency to attack after isolation	↓	↑
General aggression	—	—
Locomotor stimulation of D-amphetamine	↑	↓
L-5-Hydroxytryptophan-induced serotonin syndrome	↓	—
L-5-Hydroxytryptophan-induced head twitches	—	—
Performance in T-maze	↓	
Working memory enhancement of α_2-adrenergic receptor agonist in T-maze	—	
Performance in Morris water maze		↓
Forced-swim stress and behavioral despair test	↓	↑
Learning and memory in Morris water maze		—
Anxiety in open field test		—
Stimulus–response learning in passive avoidance test		—
Cortical electroencephalogram (arousal)		—

—, no effect; ↑, accentuated; ↓, attenuated; blank, not studied.

D79N α_{2A}-AR via hit-and-run homologous recombination yielded mice that were viable, fertile, and bred at the expected Mendelian ratios *(4)*.

Surprisingly, radioligand-binding assays on brain homogenate preparations derived from α_{2A}-AR$^{D79N/D79N}$ mice revealed that cell surface expression of the D79N α_{2A}-AR was significantly reduced (~80%) when compared to α_{2A}-AR levels in wild-type mice *(4)*. Electrophysiological assessment of locus ceruleus neurons from α_{2A}-AR$^{D79N/D79N}$ mice revealed a deficiency in receptor-stimulated K$^+$ current activation, consistent with in vitro observations. However, these studies also demonstrated an unexpected loss of coupling to receptor-mediated inhibition of Ca^{2+} currents *(5)*. Biochemically, the D79N mutation in the α_{2A}-AR imparts structural instability, causing enhanced receptor turnover from the cell surface, accounting for its reduced steady-state receptor density *(6,7)*.

Despite in vitro and in vivo evidence suggesting that the α_{2A}-AR$^{D79N/D79N}$ mouse represents a functional knockout, it is important to note that some α_{2A}-AR physiological functions are retained. Presynaptic feedback inhibition of neurotransmitter release in mouse vas deferens preparations from α_{2A}-AR$^{D79N/D79N}$ mice is normal compared to wild-type preparations *(8)*. Of note, these findings suggest that a high degree of receptor spareness exists for presynaptic regulation of catecholamine release, consistent with previous reports *(9)*. It is conceivable that the reduced α_{2A}-AR complement in these animals is sufficient for function (as seen in a setting with high receptor spareness, i.e., presynaptic control), whereas other responses that require higher fractional occupancy are lost. In this mouse model, therefore, it is likely that the decreased numbers of D79N α_{2A}-AR, rather than a select deficit in receptor signaling, accounts for the deficiency in responses in these animals *(10)*. Nonetheless, the α_{2A}-AR$^{D79N/D79N}$ mouse model has served as an exceptionally useful tool in the elucidation of physiological functions that rely on the α_{2A}-AR subtype.

2.2. The α_{2A}-AR in Blood Pressure Regulation in Response to α_2-AR Agonists

Agents acting via α_2-ARs to elicit changes in blood pressure induce a characteristic biphasic hemodynamic profile; an initial, transient hypertensive response (by which peripherally located arterial α_2-ARs constrict vascular smooth muscle) is followed by a longer-lived, centrally mediated attenuation of sympathetic outflow (culminating in a sustained drop in blood pressure). For this reason, α_2-AR agonists are used to treat high blood pressure in some populations of hypertensive patients.

Studies in mice harboring the D79N α_{2A}-AR mutation or deficient in the α_{2A}-AR (α_{2A}-AR$^{-/-}$) have revealed that the α_{2A}-AR subtype is responsible for the long-lasting hypotensive response of α_2-agonists. In contrast, the immediate pressor response has been shown to be mediated by the α_{2B}-AR subtype *(11)* and is discussed in Section 3.1. (*see* Table 1). In assessing the in vivo cardiovascular responses in conscious, freely moving animals, intra-arterial administration of the non-subtype-selective α_2-agonist dexmedetomidine in wild-type mice induced an immediate rise in blood pressure followed by a prolonged hypotensive response, whereas both α_{2A}-AR$^{D79N/D79N}$ and α_{2A}-AR$^{-/-}$ mice displayed a selective attenuation in the hypotensive phase in response to dexmedetomidine and other imidazoline-based structures *(4,8,12,13)*.

The intracerebroventricular injection of α_2-AR agonists into the anterior hypothalamic nuclei of wild-type and α_{2A}-AR$^{D79N/D79N}$ mice confirmed the role of centrally localized α_{2A}-ARs in hypotensive response *(14)*. Resting heart rate in mice devoid of the α_{2A}-AR was significantly elevated compared to wild-type littermates *(8)*. Elevated sympathetic tone in α_{2A}-AR$^{-/-}$ mice is likely caused by the loss of central α_{2A}-AR-mediated sympathoinhibition as well as the loss of α_{2A}-AR-dependent inhibition of norepinephrine release from cardiac nerve terminals, consistent with a key role for the α_{2A}-AR in hemodynamic regulation *(8)*.

Interestingly, resting blood pressure in α_{2A}-AR$^{-/-}$ mice was comparable to wild-type mice, suggesting that the α_{2A}-AR is not critical for the maintenance of cardiovascular blood pressure homeostasis, but that multiple vasomotor mechanisms, including activation of the α_1-, α_{2B}-, β_1-, and β_2-ARs, regulate baseline blood pressure.

Nonetheless, the findings in genetically altered mice confirm that the α_{2A}-AR subtype plays a major role in mediating blood pressure lowering in response to α_2-agonists and suggest that α_{2A}-AR subtype-selective agents represent an attractive therapeutic approach for antihypertensive therapy in hypertension. The issue of how to address the unwanted side effects of α_{2A}-AR-mediated sedation is addressed in the discussion of studies in heterozygous mice that point to the value of therapeutic utilization of partial agonists at α_{2A}-AR in this clinical setting.

2.3. α_{2A}-AR Regulation of Catecholamine Release

Presynaptic α_2-AR autoreceptors (i.e., receptors sensitive to the neuron's own transmitter substance) *(15)* were among the first receptors identified as playing a role in the regulation of neurotransmitter release *(16)*. Multiple pharmacological studies had supported a predominant role for the α_{2A}-AR subtype in this response *(17–20)*. Evaluation of α_{2A}-AR$^{-/-}$ mice has confirmed these observations, indicating that the main presynaptic autoreceptor is α_{2A}-AR. Presynaptic inhibition of catecholamine release induced by α_2-AR agonists such as dexmedetomidine or medetomidine in mice devoid of the α_{2A}-AR was significantly impaired but not abolished, consistent with the interpretation that this subtype is the major, but not exclusive, autoreceptor *(8,21–25)*. Elegant studies employing double-knockout mice for the α_{2A}-AR and α_{2C}-AR (α_{2C}-AR$^{-/-}$) revealed that the α_{2A}-AR inhibits transmitter release at high stimulation frequencies, interpreted as responding to high synaptic norepinephrine concentrations under conditions of maximal sympathetic activation *(21)*. Moreover, the identity of the non-α_{2A}-AR autoreceptor, the α_{2C}-AR, was established by the evaluation of these mice; atrial preparations derived from α_{2AC}-AR$^{-/-}$ mice were completely refractory to agonist stimulation *(21)*, discussed in Section 4.1. (*see* Table 1).

2.4. The α_{2A}-AR in Sedative, Anesthetic-Sparing, and Analgesic Responses in Response to α_2-Agonists

The sedative, anesthetic-sparing, and analgesic properties of α_2-AR agonists are therapeutically attractive components that are exploited frequently in the clinical setting. For example, the sedative properties of α_2-AR agonists are valuable when employed as preanesthetic or anesthetic-sparing agents *(26)* or for the attenuation of opioid withdrawal symptoms *(27,28)*. Study of α_{2A}-AR$^{D79N/D79N}$ mice and α_{2A}-AR$^{-/-}$ mice revealed that the α_{2A}-AR subtype mediates all three of these physiological effects.

The role of the α_{2A}-AR in sedation was revealed in rotarod latency studies, an experimental paradigm that measures the ability of mice to remain on a rotating bar over time; impaired motor skills caused by sedation would be predicted to decrease rotarod latency and thus can be interpreted as a measure of the sedative response when unperturbed locomotor response has been documented independently in non-sedated animals. Dexmedetomidine dose-dependently reduced the ability of wild-type mice to remain on the rotarod, whereas α_{2A}-AR[D79N/D79N] and α_{2A}-AR[-/-] mice were resistant to even supramaximal doses (5,29). Consistent with these observations, α_{2A}-AR[-/-] mice did not sleep, as assessed via loss-of-righting reflex (5). These findings indicate that the α_{2A}-AR subtype is required to mediate the sedative effects of α_2-AR agonists (Table 1).

As indicated above, α_2-AR agonists are attractive preanesthetic agents because of their ability to reduce the dosing requirements of volatile anesthetic agents. Intraperitoneal administration of dexmedetomidine resulted in a dose-dependent decrease in the amount of halothane (a volatile anesthetic) required to cause loss-of-righting reflex in wild-type mice. In contrast, dexmedetomidine did not induce anesthetic-sparing activity in mice harboring the D79N α_{2A}-AR mutation, indicating that this subtype is required for the anesthetic-sparing response for the volatile anesthetic halothane (5). In contrast, the α_{2A}-AR subtype is not involved in the response to the inhaled anesthetic agent nitrous oxide (N$_2$O). The involvement of this subtype was ruled out in studies demonstrating that N$_2$O exposure caused a dose-dependent antinociceptive response in α_{2A}-AR[D79N/D79N] mice comparable to wild-type controls (30). Subsequent studies have implicated a role for the α_{2B}-AR subtype in mediating the anesthetic effect of N$_2$O (Section 3.3.).

Multiple α_2-AR agonists induce antinociception in experimental models of acute and chronic pain (31). Because mice are unable to convey the emotive experience of pain, it is more appropriate to define the analgesic response as antinociceptive. As assessed in the ramped hot plate test (a paradigm that assesses supraspinal pain perception via the measurement of the response time to an injurious insult, e.g., elevated heat), α_{2A}-AR[D79N/D79N] mice were unresponsive to the antinociceptive effects of dexmedetomidine, whereas α_2-AR activation dose-dependently increased the thermal pain threshold in wild-type counterparts (5). Similarly, α_{2A}-AR[D79N/D79N] mice were completely refractory to dexmedetomidine as an antinociceptive agent in the tail immersion test (a paradigm assessing responsiveness to acute thermal pain), whereas dexmedetomidine produced dose-dependent antinociception in α_{2B}-AR[-/-] and α_{2C}-AR[-/-] animals compared to wild-type controls (32). Taken together, the assessment of α_{2A}-AR[D79N/D79N] and α_{2A}-AR[-/-] mice has provided genetic evidence that the α_{2A}-AR subtype is responsible for mediating antinociceptive responses in mice (Table 1).

2.5. The α_{2A}-AR in Cognitive Function

It has been appreciated that α_2-AR activation plays a crucial role in mediating the enhancement of working memory in human beings and nonhuman primates *(33–37)*. These studies have shown that systemic administration of α_2-AR agonists leads to enhanced performance at various tasks. Rigorous studies in α_{2A}-AR[D79N/D79N] mice revealed the role for the α_{2A}-AR in working memory and cognitive enhancement in response to the α_2-AR agonist guanfacine *(36)*. Insights into the mechanisms responsible for these effects suggest that α_2-AR agonists strengthen working memory functions in the prefrontal cortex, a region that has been shown to be dysfunctional in attention deficit/hyperactivity disorder *(38,39)*. These findings suggest that α_{2A}-AR-selective ligands would represent a useful therapeutic intervention for treatment of cognitive deficits.

As alluded to above, the sedative properties of α_2-AR agonists, although valuable in clinical anesthesia, limit their usefulness in enhancing cognitive function. Studies provoked by observing a loss in sedative response to α_2-agonists in mice heterozygous for the α_{2A}-AR suggest that partial agonists at the α_{2A}-AR could achieve enhanced therapeutic benefit, that is, sedation-free enhancement of cognitive function and attentional focus (*see* Section 2.8.).

2.6. The α_{2A}-AR in the Suppression of Epileptogenesis in Kindling Models

Several studies have implicated a role for the α_2-AR signaling system in the development of epilepsy (i.e., *epileptogenesis*, defined as the development of brain dysfunction characterized by the periodic and unpredictable occurrence of seizures) *(40)*. Norepinephrine is believed to play a unique inhibitory role by eliciting significant antiepileptogenic actions *(41)*. Consistent with this, the selective depletion of norepinephrine-containing locus ceruleus neurons facilitates the development of kindling *(42)*. Kindling represents an experimental paradigm modeling epilepsy; in this paradigm, the repeated administration of an initially subthreshold electrical stimulus results in the progressive development of seizures, culminating in tonic–clonic seizures *(43)*. In addition, the α_2-AR has been shown to mediate the antiepileptogenic actions of norepinephrine *(44)*. Assays in amygdala and pyriform cortex preparations derived from kindled mice vs normal mice revealed reduced α_2-AR density as well as decreased receptor responsiveness, suggesting that decreased α_2-AR number or function may be responsible for the facilitation of epileptogenesis in mice *(45,46)*. However, the identity of the α_2-AR subtype in mediating the suppression of epileptogenesis was unknown until the availability of D79N α_2-AR-mutant mice.

Evaluation of α_{2A}-AR[D79N/D79N] mice in the kindling model of epilepsy revealed that these animals exhibited increased epileptogenesis coupled with an enhanced rate of developing seizures relative to wild-type counterparts *(47)*. The number of electrical stimulations required to achieve class 5 behavioral seizures was significantly less in α_{2A}-AR$^{D79N/D79N}$ mice *(47)*. Of significant interest is the observation that wild-type mice that were treated with the non-subtype-selective α_2-AR antagonist idazoxan demonstrated the identical rate of kindling development as observed in α_{2A}-AR$^{D79N/D79N}$ mice, indicating that the α_{2A}-AR is not only necessary, but also sufficient to regulate epileptogenesis in the kindling model in response to endogenous catecholamines (Table 1). These findings that the α_{2A}-AR subtype suppresses norepinephrine-mediated epileptogenesis may suggest that the α_{2A}-AR should be evaluated as a therapeutic target in different forms of epilepsy.

2.7. The α_{2A}-AR in Depressive Behaviors

The efficacy of agents that suppress depressive behaviors can be assessed using the Porsolt forced swim test *(48,49)*. In this paradigm, immobility in the water chamber can be interpreted as behavioral despair. Increased swimming duration (i.e., a decrease in immobility) has been employed as a useful predictor of an antidepressant agent in mice. Mice deficient for the α_{2A}-AR subtype were less active in this paradigm compared to wild type counterparts, which can be interpreted as α_{2A}-AR$^{-/-}$ mice displaying a higher degree of behavioral despair. Further, α_{2A}-AR$^{-/-}$ mice exhibited more anxietylike behavior when examined for rearing behavior or when assessed in the light–dark paradigm (both models for anxiogenic behavior; *50)*. Mice null for the α_{2A}-AR also appeared more vulnerable to environmental stressors and spent less time exhibiting exploratory behavior after introduction into a novel environment *(51)*. Interestingly, chronic psychosocial stress has been shown to decrease α_{2A}-AR function *(52)*. Importantly, α_{2A}-AR$^{-/-}$ mice did not display general hypoactivity, or a lack of mobility, relative to wild-type mice, so the above changes in behavior can be attributed to behavioral changes in these mice. Taken together, findings in α_{2A}-AR$^{-/-}$ mice suggest that the absence of the α_{2A}-AR confers susceptibility to stressful conditions (Table 1).

Porsolt swim tests employing mice null (α_{2C}-AR$^{-/-}$) or overexpressing (α_{2C}-AR$^{+/+OE}$) the α_{2C}-AR have implicated a role for this subtype in provoking a depressive state in mice (Table 1). The α_{2A}-AR$^{-/-}$ mice were more active and swam longer (i.e., measured as less time spent immobile in the water chamber) than wild-type mice, whereas α_{2C}-AR$^{+/+OE}$ mice were less active (i.e., decreased mobility) and displayed cognitive defects compared to their wild-type counterparts *(50,53–55)*. As described above, mice deficient for the α_{2A}-AR subtype were less active in this paradigm compared to wild-type counterparts and were no longer susceptible to the antidepressant desmethylimipramine, suggesting that in wild-type mice the α_{2A}-AR tonically suppresses "depressive behaviors"

(50). Cumulatively, these data suggest that the development of therapeutic agents that are selective toward the α_{2A}-AR subtype, although devoid of effects at the α_{2C}-AR subtype, would be valuable therapeutic agents in reducing stress-related depressive events in human beings.

Chronic subordinate stress can be modeled using male tree shrews. This confrontational paradigm pits two male shrews against each other to establish a dominant–subordinate hierarchy; as a result, the subordinate endures a stress-dependent chronic overdrive in sympathetic activation *(56).* Although the mechanisms are not clear, chronic subordinate stress correlates with decreased levels of α_{2A}-AR messenger ribonucleic acid (mRNA) expression *(57).*

It is interesting to note the parallels observed when assessing the behavioral despair seen in α_{2A}-AR$^{-/-}$ mice with the findings in the male tree shrew subordinate stress model; these collective data suggest that chronic stress may (via an unknown mechanism) reduce beneficial effects of the α_{2A}-AR in depression and stress, leading to behavioral despair, as witnessed in animals deficient for the α_{2A}-AR. Moreover, α_{2A}-AR activation (or protection from downregulation) could offer a protective mechanism to combat stressful or stress-related events.

2.8. The Assessment of Mice Heterozygous for the α_{2A}-AR

As illustrated throughout this chapter, the use of genetically modified mice has been extremely advantageous in the effort to elucidate the in vivo functions of the α_{2A}-AR. In particular, multiple studies employing these animals have illustrated the crucial role of the α_{2A}-AR in mediating α_2-AR agonist-dependent regulation of blood pressure, sedation, anesthetic sparing, analgesia, antinociception, behavioral responses, cognitive function, and epileptogenesis. In all, the α_{2A}-AR subtype appears to mediate many of the physiological responses elicited by α_2-AR agents. Thus, it can be reasoned that subtype-selective agonists alone cannot ensure optimized therapeutic intervention. For example, the sedative properties of α_2-AR agonists, valuable when employed as preanesthetic agents, limit their usefulness in cognitive enhancement, in treating attentional deficits, or in lowering blood pressure *(35,58,59).* However, the examination of mice heterozygous for the α_{2A}-AR *(29)* has provided a unique strategy for the elucidation of pathways that might be selectively activated in an effort to achieve response-specific therapy, namely, developing drugs that elicit less than 50% maximal response even at full receptor occupancy (i.e., develop partial agonists or allosteric enhancers).

As indicated in Section 2.4., mice null for the α_{2A}-AR or carrying the D79N α_{2A}-AR were resistant to supramaximal doses of dexmedetomidine in the rotarod latency test, indicating a role for the α_{2A}-AR subtype in mediating sedative responses to dexmedetomidine. Surprisingly, mice heterozygous for the D79N α_{2A}-AR (α_{2A}-AR$^{D79N/-}$) were resistant to α_2-AR agonist-mediated sedation. A dominant negative effect of the D79N α_{2A}-AR on the wild-type receptor structure was excluded because mice heterozygous for the wild-type α_{2A}-AR (α_{2A}-AR$^{+/-}$) were also resistant to the α_2-AR agonist-mediated sedative response (29). These findings provided genetic evidence that greater than 50% of α_2-AR must be activated to evoke sedation, consistent with previous studies using covalent inactivation of receptors (60) or antisense strategies (61) as approaches to diminish α_{2A}-AR density and affect pathways.

In contrast to the loss of sedative response to α_2-AR agonists in heterozygous mice, α_{2A}-AR$^{+/-}$ mice remained sensitive to dexmedetomidine-elicited hypotension (29). These observations suggest that different α_{2A}-AR-mediated physiological responses involve different fractional α_{2A}-AR activation. A direct consequence of this insight is that desired therapeutic end points (e.g., achieving reductions in blood pressure) without undesired effects (e.g., sedation) could be achieved clinically by developing agents (either partial agonists or allosteric enhancers) that induce or stabilize a receptor conformation that elicits 50% or less maximal receptor response as noted above. The proof of concept that an α_{2A}-AR partial agonist can selectively lower blood pressure without sedation are findings with moxonidine, which lowered blood pressure without eliciting a sedative response in wild-type mice, an effect that absolutely required expression of the α_{2A}-AR subtype (29,62,63).

Thus, agents displaying partial agonism at the α_{2A}-AR (such as moxonidine) represent a therapeutic approach for selectively modulating physiological responses and may provide benefit when undesired sedative effects are observed following α_{2A}-AR activation (e.g., hypotension, enhancement of cognitive function, and treatment of attentional deficits) (35,58,59). Moreover, these findings also highlight the impact of rigorously assessing heterozygous mice as an experimental approach to define physiological functions that may be differentially sensitive to fractional activation.

3. The α_{2B}-Adrenergic Receptor Null Mice Reveal Roles for the α_{2B}-AR Subtype in Hypertension, Antinociception to Nitrous Oxide, and Development

3.1. The α_{2B}-AR in Blood Pressure Regulation

As discussed above, agents acting via α_2-ARs to elicit changes in blood pressure induce a characteristic biphasic hemodynamic profile consisting of a transient hypertensive response followed by the sustained, centrally localized α_2-AR-mediated drop in blood pressure. As with the α_{2A}-AR, mice null for the α_{2B}-AR (α_{2B}-AR$^{-/-}$) have documented the role of the α_{2B}-AR subtype in modulating the pressor, or increased, blood pressure responses following α_2-agonist activation of peripheral mechanisms (11). Control studies demonstrated that α_{2B}-

AR$^{-/-}$ mice were equally responsive to α_1-AR-mediated vasoconstriction relative to wild-type mice, confirming that blood pressure regulation was not the result of generalized perturbation of vasoconstrictor properties of the vasculature (11).

3.2. The α_{2B}-AR in Salt-Sensitive Hypertension

Patients with essential hypertension frequently display an increased salt sensitivity. Although the mechanisms by which salt (i.e., Na$^+$ ions) elevates blood pressure remain unclear, several studies strongly support the influence of a hyperadrenergic state. Intravenous infusion of hypertonic saline is associated with increases in norepinephrine and vasopressin levels and correlates with increased sympathetic drive (64). Hypertonic saline infusion in various brain regions recapitulates these observations (65–67). Collectively, these findings suggest sodium leads to unregulated sympathetic drive, accounting for excessive catecholamine levels and elevated blood pressure.

The α_{2B}-AR$^{-/-}$ mice have provided evidence for this subtype in salt-induced elevations in blood pressure (Table 1). Mice subjected to subtotal nephrectomy followed by a salt-loading regimen (a model for salt-induced hypertension) revealed that mice devoid of the α_{2B}-AR did not develop hypertension as compared to α_{2A}-AR$^{-/-}$ mice, α_{2C}-AR$^{-/-}$ mice, and wild-type controls exposed to the same salt-loading protocol (68,69). Significantly, elevated blood pressure levels were reduced in wild-type mice with established salt-induced hypertension following intracerebroventricular infusion of either an antisense oligonucleotide specific for the α_{2B}-AR or a cytomegalovirus-driven plasmid encoding this oligonucleotide (70,71). Collectively, these findings suggest a predominant role for the α_{2B}-AR subtype in mediating salt-sensitive hypertension and point toward α_{2B}-AR-selective blockade as a useful therapeutic approach in this pathological condition. One hypothesis suggests that the salt-sensitive hypertensive state is via catecholamine activation of (blood pressure-raising) α_{2B}-ARs in parallel with sodium-dependent decreases in (blood pressure-lowering) α_{2A}-AR potency in counteracting the hypertensive drive (68).

However, both the α_{2A}-AR and α_{2B}-AR subtypes are allosterically modulated by monovalent cations in a similar fashion (72), ruling against a role for selective allosteric regulation; further, there is no direct biological evidence that Na$^+$ sensitivity is critical in vivo for the proper function of these receptors (and G protein-coupled receptors in general, as reviewed by Ceresa and Limbird in ref. 73). Nonetheless, these data point to a major role for the α_{2B}-AR subtype in mediating the hypertensive response, under both physiological and pathological (i.e., salt-sensitive hypertension) conditions, and suggest that agents that are partial agonists at the α_{2A}-AR are devoid of agonist activity at the α_{2B}-AR (or α_{2B}-AR-selective antagonists in the case of salt-sensitive hypertension) would enhance the therapeutic repertoire in treating hypertension and other heart diseases.

3.3. The α_{2B}-AR Mediates Antinociception to Nitrous Oxide

Whereas α_2-agonists induce the analgesic and hypnotic–sedative states via activation of the α_{2A}-AR subtype (see above), the α_{2B}-AR subtype appears to mediate the analgesic response to the inhaled anesthetic agent N_2O. Multiple transduction mechanisms appear to be involved; opioid receptor antagonism blocks N_2O antinociception in mice and analgesia in humans (30,74–76). Previous studies have noted functional interactions between opioid and adrenergic receptor systems (77,78). Indeed, these receptors co-localize to proximal dendrites in primary hippocampal neurons, and μ-opioid–α_2-AR complexes can be detected biochemically (79). However, the role of cross regulation in vivo is incompletely understood.

The involvement of the α_2-AR system in N_2O-dependent analgesia was inferred initially from observations demonstrating that intrathecal administration of α_2-AR antagonists could inhibit N_2O-mediated mouse antinociception. Moreover, selective depletion of noradrenergic nuclei via intracerebroventricular application of the toxin saporin (coupled to an antibody that binds dopamine β-hydroxylase, an enzyme specifically located in noradrenergic/adrenergic neurons) blocked N_2O-mediated antinociception in mice (80). Thus, these data implicated adrenergic signaling, in addition to opiate signaling, in this effect. Importantly, studies in mice null for the α_{2B}-AR revealed that this subtype is critical for N_2O antinociception; N_2O-exposed α_{2B}-AR$^{-/-}$ mice displayed decreased latencies (i.e., were hypersensitive) in the hot plate assay (Table 1). In contrast, α_{2A}-AR$^{D79N/D79N}$, α_{2A}-AR$^{-/-}$, and α_{2C}-AR$^{-/-}$ mice exhibited responses identical to their wild-type counterparts under the same experimental conditions (80). Interestingly, sedative responses to N_2O are α_2-AR independent, suggesting that, at least for N_2O, that antinociception and sedation are dissociable events. Clearly, spinal α_{2B}-ARs are responsible for mediating antinociception in mice in response to N_2O exposure.

3.4. The α_{2B}-AR in Embryonic Development

Studies initiated after the derivation of the α_{2B}-AR$^{-/-}$ mice to assess subtype-specific physiological functions had noted fewer α_{2B}-AR$^{-/-}$ offspring than would have been predicted by Mendelian ratios (11) or had observed that α_{2B}-AR null mice displayed breeding difficulties (68). An elegant and fascinating study pursued the perplexing observation that mice lacking this subtype had reduced survival. In contrast to α_{2B}-AR$^{-/-}$ mice, α_{2A}-AR$^{D79N/D79N}$, α_{2A}-AR$^{-/-}$, and α_{2C}-AR$^{-/-}$ mice were produced as would be expected by Mendelian ratios (4,8,81). Double-knockout α_{2AC}-AR$^{-/-}$ mice were born live from heterozygous crossings at the expected ratios and developed normally (21,22). The crossing of α_{2AC}-AR$^{-/-}$ mice with those null for the α_{2B}-AR to yield mice deficient in all three α_2-ARs (α_{2ABC}-AR$^{-/-}$) revealed that α_{2ABC}-AR$^{-/-}$ embryos died between days 9.5 and 11.5; only 1 of 283 mice offspring survived until weaning (82). Histological analysis

.revealed a poorly developed yolk sac and a poorly vascularized placental laby-rinth in α_{2ABC}-AR$^{-/-}$ embryos, suggesting that placental α_{2B}-ARs are critically localized for vascular development at the mother–embryo interface. Heart struc-ture and the levels of L-dopa and catecholamines were normal in triply deficient mice relative to wild-type embryos, suggesting that embryonic lethality in α_{2ABC}-AR$^{-/-}$ mice was the result of a specific decrement in placental development and the placental circulatory system, not to cardiac structure or circulating hormone levels *(82)*. Reverse transcriptase polymerase chain reaction analysis identified mRNA for all three α_2-ARs in the placenta at E10.5, demonstrating that they are present in these tissues.

Strikingly, radioligand-binding assays employing the non-subtype-selective α_2-AR antagonist [^{3}H]RX821002 performed on placental tissue homogenates revealed comparable levels of receptor expression in α_{2AC}-AR$^{-/-}$ placenta relative to wild-type placenta, establishing that the α_{2B}-AR is the predominant α_2-AR subtype in the embryonic part of the placenta *(82)*. To identify signaling compo-nents that would be negatively affected, it was shown that α_2-AR (but not growth factor)-stimulated MAPK activation was dramatically attenuated in yolk sac preparations derived from α_{2ABC}-AR$^{-/-}$ mice. The data suggest that abrogation of yolk sac α_{2B}-AR-mediated MAPK signaling leads to severe placental defects and embryonic lethality as seen in triply deficient animals; indeed, functional conser-vation of upstream molecules leading to MAPK activation is critical for placental and yolk sac development *(83,84)*. These seminal observations provide a pos-sible explanation for the reduced survival of α_{2B}-AR$^{-/-}$ mice and reveal a role for the α_{2B}-AR subtype in embryonic placental circulatory system development.

To our knowledge, the existence or relevance of imidazoline-binding sites *(85,86)* in response to imidazoline-containing ligands (e.g., clonidine) and struc-turally related compounds has not been addressed in α_{2ABC}-AR$^{-/-}$ mice. The complete absence of the α_2-ARs in triply deficient animals provides an oppor-tunity to evaluate the role of these sites (distinct from α_2-ARs) and their potential contribution to regulating physiological functions, such as the regulation of systemic blood pressure in response to peripherally administered drugs *(87,88)*.

4. The α_{2C}-AR-Deficient Mice and α_{2C}-AR-Overexpressing Mice Define Roles of this Subtype in Neuronal Transmission and in Multiple Behaviors

Studies employing genetically modified mice with overexpression of (α_{2C}-AR$^{+/+OE}$) or null for the α_{2C}-AR (α_{2C}-AR$^{-/-}$) have yielded particularly fruitful insights into the roles that this subtype plays in discrete physiological functions (*see* Table 1). The strength of the data is corroborated by the observation of reciprocal changes in responses observed in these genotypically opposite mice. The α_{2C}-AR subtype is found in a number of brain structures (e.g., hippocampus, cerebral cortex, striatum, and caudate and accumbens nuclei; *89*), suggesting a role for this receptor in behavioral and psychomotor functions. Studies employing these animals have supported a role for the α_{2C}-AR subtype in these physiological functions and have revealed novel roles for this receptor.

4.1. The α_{2C}-AR Regulation of Catecholamine Release

Numerous well-documented studies have defined a major role of the α_{2A}-AR subtype in mediating feedback modulation of neurotransmitter release (reviewed above). However, data from several sources employing pharmacological probes have supported the hypothesis that a second autoreceptor contributes to α_2-AR-mediated regulation of neurotransmitter release *(17,18)*. Studies assessing presynaptic α_2-AR inhibition of electrically stimulated contraction showed that vas deferens preparations derived from α_{2A}-AR$^{-/-}$ mice remained partially sensitive to dexmedetomidine, supporting the second autoreceptor hypothesis. As expected, dexmedetomidine dose-dependently blocked contraction in wild-type vas deferens preparations *(8)*. Interestingly, these same observations were seen in mouse brain cortex slices, suggesting that a second autoreceptor mechanism is conserved in other tissues *(22)*. Again, elegant data generated using the α_{2C}-AR$^{-/-}$ mouse have provided conclusive evidence that the second receptor subtype involved in the regulation of synaptic transmission was the α_{2C}-AR *(21,22)*.

In wild-type atrial preparations, increasing concentrations of the nonselective α_2-AR agonist UK-14,304 dose dependently inhibited electrically-stimulated [^{3}H]norepinephrine release *(21)*. Consistent with previous studies, α_{2A}-AR ablation did not completely attenuate the effects of UK-14,304 in suppressing [^{3}H]norepinephrine release. In contrast, atrial preparations derived from α_{2C}-AR$^{-/-}$ mice were completely unresponsive to UK-14,304 in this functional assay. Additional studies revealed that the α_{2A}-AR and α_{2C}-AR subtypes serve distinct roles in the regulation of neurotransmitter release (Table 1). Frequency inhibition studies showed that the α_{2C}-AR is fine-tuned to respond to low-frequency stimulation (i.e., low norepinephrine concentrations), whereas the α_{2A}-AR is geared to respond to high-frequency stimulation (i.e., high norepinephrine concentrations as would be elicited by sympathetic activation).

Biochemically, norepinephrine possesses a higher affinity for the α_{2C}-AR subtype, suggesting that this receptor is able to respond to low-level circulating catecholamines and minute alterations of them. Alternatively, higher concentrations of norepinephrine will occupy the lower affinity α_{2A}-ARs and involve them in regulating neurotransmitter release. The unique properties of these subtypes play a critical role in vivo; α_{2C}-AR$^{-/-}$ mice display significantly elevated plasma norepinephrine levels in contrast to wild-type, α_{2A}-AR$^{-/-}$, α_{2B}-AR$^{-/-}$, and α_{2C}-AR$^{-/-}$ mice. Assessment of hearts from α_{2C}-AR$^{-/-}$ mice at 4 mo of age revealed marked hypertrophy with decreased left ventricular contractility *(21,90)*. Thus, clinical features of heart failure (e.g., abnormal cardiac function, cardiac hypertrophy) are associated with excessive circulating catecholamine levels and sympathetic hyperactivity (by virtue of no negative feedback) *(91)*. Patients harboring a dysfunctional α_{2C}-AR variant had a worse clinical status and decreased cardiac function *(91)*.

These studies underpin the functional relevance of the α_{2C}-AR, in addition to the α_{2A}-AR, in the regulation of neurotransmitter release and circulating levels of catecholamines. Agonists selective for the α_{2C}-AR may represent novel therapeutic agents to attenuate or prevent the development of heart failure or other diseases associated with deregulated catecholamine levels.

4.2. The α_{2C}-AR in Regulation of Adrenal Gland Catecholamine Release

Although the α_{2C}-AR contributes to the regulation of catecholamine release in some tissues, it serves as the main autoregulator in other organs (Table 1). In particular, the α_{2C}-AR regulates epinephrine secretion from the chromaffin cells of the adrenal gland *(92)*. Plasma epinephrine levels (adrenal chromaffin cells represent the primary source of epinephrine, whereas sympathetic neurons release circulating norepinephrine) *(93)* are selectively elevated in α_{2C}-AR$^{-/-}$ mice *(92)*. In line with this observation, Northern blot analysis demonstrated that α_{2C}-AR mRNA (and not mRNA encoding α_{2A}-AR or α_{2B}-AR) is found in isolated mouse adrenal chromaffin cells; further, α_{2C}-AR mRNA predominates in the human adrenal gland *(94,95)*. In an autocrine fashion analogous to sympathetic neuronal activation, the α_{2C}-AR found on chromaffin cells inhibits stimulated epinephrine release *(92)*. Collectively, these data reinforce the role that this receptor subtype plays in regulating catecholamine release from different biological tissues, and as discussed above, agonists selective for the α_{2C}-AR may represent therapeutic agents to attenuate or prevent the development of pathology associated with overactive adrenal gland function.

4.3. The α_{2C}-AR in Behavior and Psychomotor Function

In general, studies evaluating α_{2C}-AR$^{-/-}$ mice in physiological and behavioral paradigms have revealed that this subtype plays an inhibitory role in the processing of sensory information and central nervous system-related motor and emotive processes *(96)*. Mice null for the α_{2C}-AR are more active; α_{2C}-AR$^{-/-}$ mice displayed an increase in locomotor activity over time following injection of the dopamine stimulant agonist D-amphetamine compared to wild-type controls *(97)*. In contrast, α_{2C}-AR$^{+/+OE}$ mice were significantly less active than wild-type counterparts after amphetamine injection. Consistent with this observation, hyperactive α_{2C}-AR$^{-/-}$ mice were refractory to dexmedetomidine-mediated inhibition of locomotor activity *(93)*. These data suggest that the α_{2C}-AR tonically inhibits locomotion, as observed in the overexpressing mice, and that the loss of α_{2C}-AR promotes a hyperlocomotive phenotype (Table 1).

A variety of experimental animal paradigms exist for in vivo assessment of behavioral functions *(98)*. The startle reflex (defined as the animal's response latency following stimulation elicited by an auditory stimulus) can be inhibited by a preceding stimulus (defined as prepulse inhibition) *(99,100)*. The isolation-induced aggression paradigm assesses the animal's response to an intruding animal and reflects the level of hostility *(98)*. The data derived can be extrapolated to human pathophysiology; for example, deficits in prepulse inhibition (PPI) have been observed in patients suffering from schizophrenia *(101)*, and PPI deficiency in rats can be corrected by antipsychotic treatment *(102)*. Therefore, these experimental paradigms can be employed collectively to assess animal behavior. Compared to control animals, α_{2C}-AR$^{-/-}$ mice are hyperreactive to loud noises (i.e., display enhanced startle response) and display a deficit in PPI, whereas opposite findings were identified in α_{2C}-AR$^{+/+OE}$ animals *(103)*. Further, α_{2C}-AR$^{-/-}$ mice are more aggressive and were on average quicker to initiate an attack after a target mouse was introduced to the test cage. These data reveal that the absence of α_{2C}-AR expression is associated with increased startle reflex, decreased PPI, and reduced attack latency (i.e., increased aggression) in addition to increased motor activity in stimulated conditions (Table 1). These findings suggest that α_{2C}-AR-selective activation may provide clinical benefit in conditions for which enhanced startle responses and motor dysfunction predominate, such as schizophrenia, attention deficit disorder and posttraumatic stress disorder.

Collectively, data from studies manipulating α_{2C}-AR expression in mice revealed that loss of α_{2C}-AR function (by virtue of knockout) leads to hyperreactivity and impulsiveness, whereas overactive signaling (by virtue of overexpression) leads to a depressive- and anxiouslike state. Modulation of α_{2C}-AR signaling, via subtype-selective agonists or antagonists depending on the symptomatology, could thus represent a therapeutic avenue in the treatment of a variety of behavioral diseases.

4.4. The α_{2C}-AR Contribution to Moxonidine-Induced Antinociception

The α_{2C}-AR also appears to contribute to antinociception. Moxonidine-induced antinociception following intrathecal administration was impaired but not abolished in α_{2A}-AR$^{D79N/D79N}$ mice relative to wild-type counterparts, whereas clonidine was ineffective in α_{2A}-AR$^{D79N/D79N}$ animals. These findings suggest either that only fractional activation of the α_{2A}-AR is needed for responding to moxonidine-induced antinociception or that an alternate α_2-AR subtype in addition to the α_{2A}-AR was involved in moxonidine-dependent antinociception *(104)*.

Deletion of the α_{2B}-AR did not affect moxonidine-induced spinal antinociception, ruling out a role for this subtype in this effect (Table 1). The use of α_{2C}-AR-deficient and α_{2A}-AR$^{D79N/D79N}$ mice in conjunction with antisense oligodeoxy-nucleotide strategies provided conclusive evidence for the involvement the α_{2C}-AR together with the α_{2A}-AR in mediating moxonidine-dependent antinociception in mice *(105)*. This dual regulation of a single response by both subtypes is yet another example of their coordinated effects, including modulation of neurotransmitter release.

5. Conclusion

A wealth of knowledge has been generated from the study of genetically engineered animals with altered expression of each of the α_2-AR receptors (*see* Table 1). Specifically, studies of mice carrying the D79N α_{2A}-AR, mice that are singly (α_{2A}-AR$^{-/-}$, α_{2B}-AR$^{-/-}$, α_{2C}-AR$^{-/-}$), doubly (α_{2AC}-AR$^{-/-}$), or triply (α_{2ABC}-AR$^{-/-}$) deficient in a particular subtype, or mice overexpressing the α_{2C}-AR (α_{2C}-AR$^{+/+OE}$) have elucidated myriad in vivo physiological and behavioral functions modulated by circulating catecholamines as well as α_2-AR-directed compounds. It is also conceivable that these mice still have yet to reveal additional roles mediated by these receptors, roles that will come to light in future studies of these genetically modified mice. Findings to date, however, can serve as a basis for programs for the identification of subtype-selective ligands (as well as subtype-selective ligands with varying efficacy) directed against these "druggable" targets to achieve response-specific therapeutic intervention for the control of hypertension, heart failure, suppression of pain, enhancement of cognitive function, and anesthesia, to name a few.

References

1. Philipp M, Hein L. Adrenergic receptor knockout mice: distinct functions of 9 receptor subtypes. Pharmacol Ther 2004;101:65–74.
2. Rohrer DK, Kobilka BK. Insights from in vivo modification of adrenergic receptor gene expression. Annu Rev Pharmacol Toxicol 1998;38:351–373.
3. Surprenant A, Horstman DA, Akbarali H, Limbird LE. A point mutation of the α_2-adrenoceptor that blocks coupling to potassium but not calcium currents. Science 1992; 257:977–980.
4. MacMillan LB, Hein L, Smith MS, Piascik MT, Limbird LE. Central hypotensive effects of the α_{2a}-adrenergic receptor subtype. Science 1996;273:801–803.
5. Lakhlani PP, MacMillan LB, Guo TZ, et al. Substitution of a mutant α_{2a}-adrenergic receptor via "hit and run" gene targeting reveals the role of this subtype in sedative, analgesic, and anesthetic-sparing responses in vivo. Proc Natl Acad Sci USA 1997;94:9950–9955.
6. Wilson MH, Limbird LE. Mechanisms regulating the cell surface residence time of the α_{2A}-adrenergic receptor. Biochemistry 2000;39:693–700.

7. Wilson MH, Highfield HA, Limbird LE. The role of a conserved inter-trans-membrane domain interface in regulating α_{2a}-adrenergic receptor conformational stability and cell-surface turnover. Mol Pharmacol 2001;59:929–938.

8. Altman JD, Trendelenburg AU, MacMillan L, et al. Abnormal regulation of the sympathetic nervous system in α_{2A}-adrenergic receptor knockout mice. Mol Pharmacol 1999;56:154–161.

9. Adler CH, Meller E, Goldstein M. Receptor reserve at the α_2 adrenergic receptor in the rat cerebral cortex. J Pharmacol Exp Ther 1987;240:508–515.

10. Philipp M, Brede ME, Hein L. Physiological significance of α_2-adrenergic receptor subtype diversity: one receptor is not enough. Am J Physiol Regul Integr Comp Physiol 2002;283:R287–R295.

11. Link RE, Desai K, Hein L, et al. Cardiovascular regulation in mice lacking α_2-adrenergic receptor subtypes b and c. Science 1996;273:803–805.

12. Zhu QM, Lesnick JD, Jasper JR, et al. α_{2A} Adrenoceptors, not I1-imidazoline receptors, mediate the hypotensive effects of rilmenidine and moxonidine in conscious mice. In vivo and in vitro studies. Ann N Y Acad Sci 1999;881:287–289.

13. Zhu QM, Lesnick JD, Jasper JR, et al. Cardiovascular effects of rilmenidine, moxonidine and clonidine in conscious wild-type and D79N α_{2A}-adrenoceptor transgenic mice. Br J Pharmacol 1999;126:1522–1530.

14. Peng N, Clark JT, Wei CC, Wyss JM. Estrogen depletion increases blood pressure and hypothalamic norepinephrine in middle-aged spontaneously hypertensive rats. Hypertension 2003;41:1164–1167.

15. Carlsson A. Dopaminergic autoreceptors. In Almgren O, Carlsson A, Engel J, editors. Chemical Tools in Catecholamine Research. Amsterdam, The Netherlands: North-Holland; 1975:219–225.

16. Langer SZ. Presynaptic regulation of catecholamine release. Biochem Pharmacol 1974;23:1793–1800.

17. Limberger N, Trendelenburg AU, Starke K. Pharmacological characterization of presynaptic α_2-autoreceptors in rat submaxillary gland and heart atrium. Br J Pharmacol 1992;107:246–255.

18. Trendelenburg AU, Sutej I, Wahl CA, Molderings GJ, Rump LC, Starke K. A reinvestigation of questionable subclassifications of presynaptic α_2-autoreceptors: rat vena cava, rat atria, human kidney and guinea-pig urethra. Naunyn Schmiedebergs Arch Pharmacol 1997;356:721–737.

19. Docherty JR. Subtypes of functional α_1- and α_2-adrenoceptors. Eur J Pharmacol 1998;361:1–15.

20. Feuerstein TJ, Huber B, Vetter J, Aranda H, Van V, Limberger N. Characterization of the α_2-adrenoceptor subtype, which functions as α_2-autoreceptor in human neocortex. J Pharmacol Exp Ther 2000;294:356–362.

21. Hein L, Altman JD, Kobilka BK. Two functionally distinct α_2-adrenergic receptors regulate sympathetic neurotransmission. Nature 1999;402:181–184.

22. Bucheler MM, Hadamek K, Hein L. Two α_2-adrenergic receptor subtypes, α_{2A} and α_{2C}, inhibit transmitter release in the brain of gene-targeted mice. Neuroscience 2002;109:819–826.

23. Scheibner J, Trendelenburg AU, Hein L, Starke K. Stimulation frequency-noradrenaline release relationships examined in α_{2A}-, α_{2B}- and α_{2C}-adrenoceptor-deficient mice. Naunyn Schmiedebergs Arch Pharmacol 2001;364:321–328.

24. Trendelenburg AU, Klebroff W, Hein L, Starke K. A study of presynaptic α_2-autoreceptors in $\alpha_{2A/D}$-, α_{2B}- and α_{2C}-adrenoceptor-deficient mice. Naunyn Schmiedebergs Arch Pharmacol 2001;364:117–130.

25. Ihalainen JA, Tanila H. In vivo regulation of dopamine and noradrenaline release by α_{2A}-adrenoceptors in the mouse prefrontal cortex. Eur J Neurosci 2002;15:1789–1794.

26. Maze M, Segal IS, Bloor BC. Clonidine and other α_2 adrenergic agonists: strategies for the rational use of these novel anesthetic agents. J Clin Anesth 1988;1:146–157.

27. Hayashi Y, Maze M. α_2 Adrenoceptor agonists and anaesthesia. Br J Anaesth 1993;71:108–118.

28. Dehpour AR, Samini M, Arad MA, Namiranian K. Clonidine attenuates naloxone-induced opioid-withdrawal syndrome in cholestatic mice. Pharmacol Toxicol 2001;89:129–132.

29. Tan CM, Wilson MH, MacMillan LB, Kobilka BK, Limbird LE. Heterozygous α_{2A} adrenergic receptor mice unveil unique therapeutic benefits of partial agonists. Proc Natl Acad Sci USA 2002;99:12,471–12,476.

30. Guo TZ, Davies MF, Kingery WS, Patterson AJ, Limbird LE, Maze M. Nitrous oxide produces antinociceptive response via α_{2B} and/or α_{2C} adrenoceptor subtypes in mice. Anesthesiology 1999;90:470–476.

31. Furst S. Transmitters involved in antinociception in the spinal cord. Brain Res Bull 1999;48:129–141.

32. Hunter JC, Fontana DJ, Hedley LR, et al. Assessment of the role of α_2-adrenoceptor subtypes in the antinociceptive, sedative and hypothermic action of dexmedetomidine in transgenic mice. Br J Pharmacol 1997;122:1339–1344.

33. Cohen DJ, Young JG, Nathanson JA, Shaywitz BA. Clonidine in Tourette's syndrome. Lancet 1979;2:551–553.

34. Sorkin EM, Heel RC. Guanfacine. A review of its pharmacodynamic and pharmacokinetic properties, and therapeutic efficacy in the treatment of hypertension. Drugs 1986;31:301–336.

35. Scahill L, Chappell PB, Kim YS, et al. A placebo-controlled study of guanfacine in the treatment of children with tic disorders and attention deficit hyperactivity disorder. Am J Psychiatry 2001;158:1067–1074.

36. Franowicz JS, Kessler LE, Borja CM, Kobilka BK, Limbird LE, Arnsten AF. Mutation of the α_{2A}-adrenoceptor impairs working memory performance and annuls cognitive enhancement by guanfacine. J Neurosci 2002;22:8771–8777.

37. Arnsten AF, Cai JX, Goldman-Rakic PS. The α_2 adrenergic agonist guanfacine improves memory in aged monkeys without sedative or hypotensive side effects: evidence for α_2 receptor subtypes. J Neurosci 1988;8:4287–4298.

38. Avery RA, Franowicz JS, Studholme C, van Dyck CH, Arnsten AF. The α_{2A} adrenoceptor agonist, guanfacine, increases regional cerebral blood flow in dorsolateral prefrontal cortex of monkeys performing a spatial working memory task. Neuropsychopharmacology 2000;23:240–249.

39. Li BM, Mao ZM, Wang M, Mei ZT. α_2 Adrenergic modulation of prefrontal cortical neuronal activity related to spatial working memory in monkeys. Neuropsychopharmacology 1999;21:601–610.

40. McNamara JO. Drugs effective in the therapy of the epilepsies. In Hardman JG, Limbird LE, editors. Goodman and Gilman's the Pharmacological Basis of Therapeutics. New York: McGraw-Hill; 2001:521–547.
41. McNamara JO. Cellular and molecular basis of epilepsy. J Neurosci 1994;14: 3413–3425.
42. Corcoran ME, Mason ST. Role of forebrain catecholamines in amygdaloid kindling. Brain Res 1980;190:473–484.
43. Goddard GV, McIntyre DC, Leech CK. A permanent change in brain function resulting from daily electrical stimulation. Exp Neurol 1969;25:295–330.
44. Gellman RL, Kallianos JA, McNamara JO. α_2 Receptors mediate an endogenous noradrenergic suppression of kindling development. J Pharmacol Exp Ther 1987; 241:891–898.
45. Chen LS, Weingart JB, McNamara JO. Biochemical and radiohistochemical analyses of α_2 adrenergic receptors in the kindling model of epilepsy. J Pharmacol Exp Ther 1990;253:1272–1277.
46. McIntyre DC, Wong RK. Cellular and synaptic properties of amygdala-kindled pyriform cortex in vitro. J Neurophysiol 1986;55:1295–1307.
47. Janumpalli S, Butler LS, MacMillan LB, Limbird LE, McNamara JO. A point mutation (D79N) of the α_{2A} adrenergic receptor abolishes the antiepileptogenic action of endogenous norepinephrine. J Neurosci 1998;18:2004–2008.
48. Porsolt RD, Anton G, Blavet N, Jalfre M. Behavioural despair in rats: a new model sensitive to antidepressant treatments. Eur J Pharmacol 1978;47:379–391.
49. Porsolt RD, Bertin A, Jalfre M. "Behavioural despair" in rats and mice: strain differences and the effects of imipramine. Eur J Pharmacol 1978;51:291–294.
50. Schramm NL, McDonald MP, Limbird LE. The α_{2a}-adrenergic receptor plays a protective role in mouse behavioral models of depression and anxiety. J Neurosci 2001;21:4875–4882.
51. Lahdesmaki J, Sallinen J, MacDonald E, Kobilka BK, Fagerholm V, Scheinin M. Behavioral and neurochemical characterization of α_{2A}-adrenergic receptor knockout mice. Neuroscience 2002;113:289–299.
52. Flugge G. Alterations in the central nervous α_2-adrenoceptor system under chronic psychosocial stress. Neuroscience 1996;75:187–196.
53. Bjorklund M, Sirvio J, Puolivali J, et al. α_{2C} adrenoceptor-overexpressing mice are impaired in executing nonspatial and spatial escape strategies. Mol Pharmacol 1998;54:569–576.
54. Bjorklund M, Sirvio J, Riekkinen M, Sallinen J, Scheinin M, Riekkinen P Jr. Overexpression of α_{2C}-adrenoceptors impairs water maze navigation. Neuroscience 2000;95:481–487.
55. Bjorklund M, Sirvio J, Sallinen J, Scheinin M, Kobilka BK, Riekkinen P Jr. α_{2C} Adrenoceptor overexpression disrupts execution of spatial and non-spatial search patterns. Neuroscience 1999;88:1187–1198.
56. Fuchs E, Kramer M, Hermes B, Netter P, Hiemke C. Psychosocial stress in tree shrews: clomipramine counteracts behavioral and endocrine changes. Pharmacol Biochem Behav 1996;54:219–228.

57. Meyer H, Palchaudhuri M, Scheinin M, Flugge G. Regulation of α_{2A}-adrenoceptor expression by chronic stress in neurons of the brain stem. Brain Res 2000;880:147–158.

58. Correa-Sales C, Rabin BC, Maze M. A hypnotic response to dexmedetomidine, an α_2 agonist, is mediated in the locus coeruleus in rats. Anesthesiology 1992;76: 948–952.

59. Kita T, Kagawa K, Mammoto T, et al. Supraspinal, not spinal, α_2 adrenoceptors are involved in the anesthetic-sparing and hemodynamic-stabilizing effects of systemic clonidine in rats. Anesth Analg 2000;90:722–726.

60. Rabin BC, Reid K, Guo TZ, Gustafsson E, Zhang C, Maze M. Sympatholytic and minimum anesthetic concentration-sparing responses are preserved in rats rendered tolerant to the hypnotic and analgesic action of dexmedetomidine, a selective α_2-adrenergic agonist. Anesthesiology 1996;85:565–573.

61. Mizobe T, Maghsoudi K, Sitwala K, Tianzhi G, Ou J, Maze M. Antisense technology reveals the α_{2A} adrenoceptor to be the subtype mediating the hypnotic response to the highly selective agonist, dexmedetomidine, in the locus coeruleus of the rat. J Clin Invest 1996;98:1076–1080.

62. Urban R, Szabo B, Starke K. Involvement of α_2-adrenoceptors in the cardiovascular effects of moxonidine. Eur J Pharmacol 1995;282:19–28.

63. Urban R, Szabo B, Starke K. Is the sympathoinhibitory effect of rilmenidine mediated by α_2 adrenoceptors or imidazoline receptors? J Pharmacol Exp Ther 1994;270:572–578.

64. Hatzinikolaou P, Gavras H, Brunner HR, Gavras I. Sodium-induced elevation of blood pressure in the anephric state. Science 1980;209:935–936.

65. Benetos A, Bresnahan M, Gavras I, Gavras H. Central catecholamines and α adrenoceptors in acute hypertension induced by intracerebroventricular hypertonic saline. J Hypertens 1987;5:699–704.

66. Gavras H, Bain GT, Bland L, Vlahakos D, Gavras I. Hypertensive response to saline microinjection in the area of the nucleus tractus solitarii of the rat. Brain Res 1985;343:113–119.

67. Vlahakos D, Gavras I, Gavras H. α-Adrenoceptor agonists applied in the area of the nucleus tractus solitarii in the rat: effect of anesthesia on cardiovascular responses. Brain Res 1985;347:372–375.

68. Makaritsis KP, Handy DE, Johns C, Kobilka B, Gavras I, Gavras H. Role of the α_{2B} adrenergic receptor in the development of salt-induced hypertension. Hypertension 1999;33:14–17.

69. Makaritsis KP, Johns C, Gavras I, et al. Sympathoinhibitory function of the α_{2A}-adrenergic receptor subtype. Hypertension 1999;34:403–407.

70. Kintsurashvili E, Johns C, Ignjacev I, Gavras I, Gavras H. Central α_{2B}-adrenergic receptor antisense in plasmid vector prolongs reversal of salt-dependent hypertension. J Hypertens 2003;21:961–967.

71. Kintsurashvili E, Gavras I, Johns C, Gavras H. Effects of antisense oligodeoxynucleotide targeting of the α_{2B}-adrenergic receptor messenger RNA in the central nervous system. Hypertension 2001;38:1075–1080.

72. Wilson AL, Seibert K, Brandon S, Cragoe EJ Jr, Limbird LE. Monovalent cation and amiloride analog modulation of adrenergic ligand binding to the

unglycosylated α_{2B}-adrenergic receptor subtype. Mol Pharmacol 1991;39:481–486.

73. Ceresa BP, Limbird LE. Mutation of an aspartate residue highly conserved among G protein-coupled receptors results in nonreciprocal disruption of α_2-adrenergic receptor-G-protein interactions. A negative charge at amino acid residue 79 forecasts α_{2A}-adrenergic receptor sensitivity to allosteric modulation by monovalent cations and fully effective receptor/G-protein coupling. J Biol Chem 1994; 269:29,557–29,564.

74. Berkowitz BA, Finck AD, Hynes MD, Ngai SH. Tolerance to nitrous oxide analgesia in rats and mice. Anesthesiology 1979;51:309–312.

75. Berkowitz BA, Finck AD, Ngai SH. Nitrous oxide analgesia: reversal by naloxone and development of tolerance. J Pharmacol Exp Ther 1977;203:539–547.

76. Fang F, Guo TZ, Davies MF, Maze M. Opiate receptors in the periaqueductal gray mediate analgesic effect of nitrous oxide in rats. Eur J Pharmacol 1997;336: 137–141.

77. Stone LS, MacMillan LB, Kitto KF, Limbird LE, Wilcox GL. The α_{2a} adrenergic receptor subtype mediates spinal analgesia evoked by α_2 agonists and is necessary for spinal adrenergic-opioid synergy. J Neurosci 1997;17:7157–7165.

78. Drasner K, Fields HL. Synergy between the antinociceptive effects of intrathecal clonidine and systemic morphine in the rat. Pain 1988;32:309–312.

79. Jordan BA, Gomes I, Rios C, Filipovska J, Devi LA. Functional interactions between mu opioid and α_{2A}-adrenergic receptors. Mol Pharmacol 2003;64:1317–1324.

80. Sawamura S, Kingery WS, Davies MF, et al. Antinociceptive action of nitrous oxide is mediated by stimulation of noradrenergic neurons in the brainstem and activation of α_{2B} adrenoceptors. J Neurosci 2000;20:9242–9251.

81. Link RE, Stevens MS, Kulatunga M, Scheinin M, Barsh GS, Kobilka BK. Targeted inactivation of the gene encoding the mouse α_{2c}-adrenoceptor homolog. Mol Pharmacol 1995;48:48–55.

82. Philipp M, Brede ME, Hadamek K, Gessler M, Lohse MJ, Hein L. Placental α_2-adrenoceptors control vascular development at the interface between mother and embryo. Nat Genet 2002;31:311–315.

83. Mikula M, Schreiber M, Husak Z, et al. Embryonic lethality and fetal liver apoptosis in mice lacking the c-raf-1 gene. EMBO J 2001;20:1952–1962.

84. Qian X, Esteban L, Vass WC, et al. The Sos1 and Sos2 Ras-specific exchange factors: differences in placental expression and signaling properties. EMBO J 2000;19:642–654.

85. Bousquet P, Feldman J, Schwartz J. Central cardiovascular effects of α adrenergic drugs: differences between catecholamines and imidazolines. J Pharmacol Exp Ther 1984;230:232–236.

86. Bousquet P, Feldman J. Drugs acting on imidazoline receptors: a review of their pharmacology, their use in blood pressure control and their potential interest in cardioprotection. Drugs 1999;58:799–812.

87. Eglen RM, Hudson, AL, Kendall DA, et al. "Seeing through a glass darkly": casting light on imidazoline "I" sites. Trends Pharmacol Sci 1998;19:381–390.

88. Parini A, Moudanos CG, Pizzinat N, Lanier SM. The elusive family of imidazoline binding sites. Trends Pharmacol Sci 1996;17:13–16.

89. Wang R, MacMillan LB, Fremeau RT Jr, Magnuson MA, Lindner J, Limbird LE. Expression of α_2-adrenergic receptor subtypes in the mouse brain: evaluation of spatial and temporal information imparted by 3 kb of 5' regulatory sequence for the α_{2A} AR-receptor gene in transgenic animals. Neuroscience 1996;74:199–218.

90. Brum PC, Kosek J, Patterson A, Bernstein D, Kobilka B. Abnormal cardiac function associated with sympathetic nervous system hyperactivity in mice. Am J Physiol Heart Circ Physiol 2002;283:H1838–H1845.

91. Brede M, Wiesmann F, Jahns R, et al. Feedback inhibition of catecholamine release by two different α_2-adrenoceptor subtypes prevents progression of heart failure. Circulation 2002;106:2491–2496.

92. Brede M, Nagy G, Philipp M, Sorensen JB, Lohse MJ, Hein L. Differential control of adrenal and sympathetic catecholamine release by α_2-adrenoceptor subtypes. Mol Endocrinol 2003;17:1640–1646.

93. Hoffman BB. Catecholamines, sympathomimetic drugs, and adrenergic receptor antagonists. In Hardman JG, Limbird LE, editors. Goodman and Gilman's the Pharmacological Basis of Therapeutics. New York: McGraw-Hill; 2001:215–268.

94. Berkowitz DE, Price DT, Bello EA, Page SO, Schwinn DA. Localization of messenger RNA for three distinct α_2-adrenergic receptor subtypes in human tissues. Evidence for species heterogeneity and implications for human pharmacology. Anesthesiology1994;81:1235–1244.

95. Perala M, Hirvonen H, Kalimo H, et al. Differential expression of two α_2-adrenergic receptor subtype mRNAs in human tissues. Brain Res Mol Brain Res 1992;16:57–63.

96. Sallinen J, Link RE, Haapalinna A, et al. Genetic alteration of α_{2C}-adrenoceptor expression in mice: influence on locomotor, hypothermic, and neurochemical effects of dexmedetomidine, a subtype-nonselective α_2-adrenoceptor agonist. Mol Pharmacol 1997;51:36–46.

97. Sallinen J, Haapalinna A, Viitamaa T, Kobilka BK, Scheinin M. d-Amphetamine and L-5-hydroxytryptophan-induced behaviours in mice with genetically-altered expression of the α_{2C}-adrenergic receptor subtype. Neuroscience 1998;86:959–965.

98. Scheinin M, Sallinen J, Haapalinna A. Evaluation of the α_{2C}-adrenoceptor as a neuropsychiatric drug target studies in transgenic mouse models. Life Sci 2001;68:2277–2285.

99. Davis M. Neural systems involved in fear-potentiated startle. Ann N Y Acad Sci 1989;563:165–183.

100. Davis M, Gendelman DS, Tischler MD, Gendelman PM. A primary acoustic startle circuit: lesion and stimulation studies. J Neurosci 1982;2:791–805.

101. Braff D, Stone C, Callaway E, Geyer M, Glick I, Bali L. Prestimulus effects on human startle reflex in normals and schizophrenics. Psychophysiology 1978;15:339–343.

102. Swerdlow NR, Braff DL, Taaid N, Geyer MA. Assessing the validity of an animal model of deficient sensorimotor gating in schizophrenic patients. Arch Gen Psychiatry 1994;51:139–154.

103. Sallinen J, Haapalinna A, Viitamaa T, Kobilka BK, Scheinin M. Adrenergic α_{2C} receptors modulate the acoustic startle reflex, prepulse inhibition, and aggression in mice. J Neurosci 1998;18:3035–3042.
104. Fairbanks CA, Wilcox GL. Moxonidine, a selective α_2-adrenergic and imidazolinereceptor agonist, produces spinal antinociception in mice. J Pharmacol Exp Ther 1999;290:403–412.
105. Fairbanks CA, Stone LS, Kitto KF, Nguyen HO, Posthumus IJ, Wilcox GL. α_{2C}-Adrenergic receptors mediate spinal analgesia and adrenergic-opioid synergy. J Pharmacol Exp Ther 2002;300:282–290.

10

The β-Adrenergic Receptors:

Lessons From Knockouts

Yang Xiang and Brian Kobilka

Summary

β-Adrenergic receptors (β-ARs) are members of the superfamily of G protein-coupled receptors that are stimulated by the catecholamines epinephrine and norepinephine *(1)*. As part of the sympathetic nervous system, β-ARs have important roles in cardiovascular, respiratory, metabolic, central nervous system, and reproductive functions. Mice lacking one or more of the three β-AR subtype genes ($β_1$, $β_2$, and $β_3$) have been generated to elucidate the physiological role of individual subtypes. Moreover, cells and tissues extracted from these mice have been utilized as tools to understand the molecular and cellular basis of subtype-specific receptor function. These studies are summarized in this chapter.

Key Words: Adipocyte; β-adrenergic receptors; apoptosis; cardiovascular; caveolae; knockout; metabolite; mitogen-activated protein kinase; myocyte; PDZ domain; protein kinase A anchoring protein.

1. Introduction

β-Adrenergic receptors (β-ARs) are members of the superfamily of G protein-coupled receptors (GPCRs) that are stimulated by the catecholamines epinephrine and norepinephine *(1)*. β-ARs have been shown to play important roles in the regulation of cardiovascular, respiratory, metabolic, central nervous system, and reproductive functions by the sympathetic nervous system. Three distinct subtypes of β-ARs have been identified and cloned: $β_1$, $β_2$, and $β_3$ *(2–4)*. All three β-ARs are believed to signal by coupling to the stimulatory G protein $G_{sα}$, leading

From: *The Receptors: The Adrenergic Receptors: In the 21st Century*
Edited by: D. Perez © Humana Press Inc., Totowa, NJ

to activation of adenylyl cyclase and accumulation of the second messenger cyclic adenosine 5′-monophosphate (cAMP). However, evidence suggests that β-AR signaling is more complex. One interesting example is that β_2-AR can also couple to the inhibitory G protein $G_{i\alpha}$ (5–7). In addition to activating G protein-coupled pathways for stress responses, β-ARs can activate the mitogen-activated protein kinase (MAPK) cascades that regulate cell growth and cardiac remodeling (8–11) and the caspase-mediated signaling pathways that lead to cell death (12,13).

The three β-ARs exhibit subtype-specific as well as overlapping expression patterns. The β_1- and β_2-ARs are expressed at high level in heart and lung, whereas β_3-AR is the major subtype expressed in adipose tissue and gastrointestinal (GI) tract. The in vivo function of β-AR subtypes was originally assigned on the basis of responses to subtype-selective agonists and antagonists. The β_1-AR subtype is often classified as the "cardiac" β-AR because stimulation of these receptors with agonists in vivo increases both cardiac rate and contractility. The β_2-AR mediates smooth muscle relaxation in the respiratory system and peripheral blood vessels. The β_3-AR has been proposed not only as the major subtype controlling lipolysis and thermogenesis in adipocytes (14), but also in regulating smooth muscle in the GI tract (15). However, there is considerable overlap in the tissue distribution and function of the β-AR subtypes. For example, β_2-ARs are also expressed in the heart, and in some species they may influence heart rate and contractility (16,17). In the adult human left ventricle, the ratio of β_1-ARs to β_2-ARs is 80:20 (16,18), whereas in the atria the ratio decreases to 70:30 (16). In addition, the β_2-ARs may play a more substantial role in mediating contractile changes in the noninnervated fetal and neonatal hearts (19). The β_3-ARs are also present in human cardiomyocytes, in which they inhibit cardiac contractility, possibly through a pertussis-sensitive G protein or synthesis of nitric oxide (20,21). However, stimulation of human β_3-AR overexpressed in the hearts of transgenic mice leads to an increase in the strength of contraction (22). Likewise, there is conflicting evidence regarding the role of β_3-AR in regulating cardiac contractility in other species (23–25).

Although most of the current knowledge of β-AR subtype physiology in vivo has been derived from the use of subtype-selective agonists and antagonists, the inferences derived from these studies are limited by the lack of absolute subtype selectivity of the available drugs. The dose of a drug required to block one subtype completely usually has some effect on at least one of the other subtypes. The fact that tissues such as heart, adipose, and blood vessels often express more than one β-AR subtype makes pharmacological isolation of subtype-specific functions a significant challenge. This mixed expression of multiple β-AR subtypes also explains the pleiotropic effects that follow nonspecific β-AR agonist administration. From a clinic standpoint, there are many instances when β-AR subtype-selective stimulation or blockade is desired; therefore, detailed knowledge of subtype-specific functions is necessary.

Targeted gene modification provides a powerful technique that, when coupled with traditional pharmacological approaches, can provide information unobtainable by either means alone. Transgenic approaches have been utilized to drive myocyte-specific overexpression of β_1-, β_2-, and β_3-ARs *(22,26,27)*. Gene knockout (KO) approaches have also been utilized to disrupt expression of the β_1-, β_2-, and β_3-ARs *(14,28,29)*. In addition, mice lacking both β_1- and β_2-ARs *(30)* and mice lacking all three β-ARs *(31)* have been generated though cross-breeding strains with single β-AR subtype gene knockout. The role of each β-AR subtype in regulating in vivo physiological function has then been determined using standard physiological techniques adapted to the murine model *(14,31–33)*. Furthermore, cells or tissues isolated from these gene-deficient animals have been utilized as model systems to examine the molecular and cellular basis of β-AR subtype-specific function in differentiated cells. In this chapter, we review studies focusing on cardiovascular and metabolic functions.

2. Effect of β-Adrenergic Receptor Gene Disruption on Development and Viability

Given the important role of β-ARs in mediating cardiac contractile function and cardiac growth, as well as the documented cardiac teratogenicity of β-AR antagonists *(34)*, it might have been anticipated that mice lacking β-ARs would not survive to birth. Surprisingly, mice lacking the β_2-AR are viable and fertile, and they display normal resting heart rates and blood pressures *(29)*. The β_3-AR null mice generated on an FVB inbred background are viable and fertile. β_3-AR-KO animals display normal resting heart rates and blood pressures, yet tend to have a modest increase in body fat, with the effect greater in females *(14)*.

In contrast, mice lacking the β_1-AR (β_1-AR-KO) have an increase in prenatal lethality between embryonic days 11 and 18.5, a time when cardiogenesis is complete and after initiation of the heartbeat *(28)*. However, the penetrance of lethality in the β_1-AR-KO mice is strain dependent; approx 90% of mice homozygous for the β_1-AR disruption die *in utero* between embryonic days 10.5 and 18.5, when the disruption is present on a 129-Sv congenic background. The mortality is still evident but reduced (~70%) when the disruption is present on outbred backgrounds. Surviving β_1-AR-KO mice have structurally normal hearts.

To eliminate the possibility that the β_2-AR provides sufficient redundancy to mitigate the loss of β_1-ARs, mice were bred with deletions of both receptors (β_1-/β_2-AR-KO) on a mixed genetic background. Interestingly, there was no increase in prenatal lethality in these double knockouts *(30)*. When $\beta_1^{+/-}\beta_2^{+/-}$ mice were crossbred, expected Mendelian ratios were observed for β_1/β_2-AR-KO. This suggests that prenatal lethality of β_1-AR gene disruption may be caused by an

Table 1
Cardiovascular Function of Knockout Strains
Relative to Wild-Type Controls

	β_1-AR-KO	β_2-AR-KO	$\beta_1\beta_2$-AR-KO
Viability	~10–30% [a]	Normal	Normal [b]
Basal cardiovascular			
• Resting heart rate	Normal	Normal	Normal
• Blood Pressure	Normal	Normal	Normal
• Cardiac output	Normal	Normal	Normal
Response to isoproterenol			
• Heart rate increase	50%	Normal	10%
• Blood pressure change	80%	70%	30%
• dF/dt (right ventricle)	50%	Nd	1%
Exercise at 20 m/min			
• Heart rate increase	23%	Normal	65%
• Blood pressure	Normal	110%	Normal
• Distance	Normal	123.5%	Normal
• VO_2	Normal	Increased [c]	Reduced
• VCO_2	Normal	Normal	Reduced
• RER	Normal	Reduced	Normal

The percentages reflect the ratios between the experimental data of knockout animal and the wild-type controls.

Nd, indicates not determined.

[a] Viability dependent on strain background.

[b] Litter sizes are small relative to wild-type controls with the same genetic background.

[c] This increase is a trend that did not reach statistical significance *(28–30,36)*.

imbalance of β_2-AR and β_1-AR signaling rather than disruption of the β_1-AR gene alone. When the β_1/β_2-AR-KO mice were bred with the β_3-AR-KO mice to generate mice lacking all three receptor subtypes on a mixed genetic background, no increase in prenatal lethality was observed *(31)*.

3. Role of β-Adrenergic Receptor Subtypes in Regulating Cardiac Function

3.1. Basal Cardiovascular Function

Targeted deletion of β_1-, β_2-, and both β_1- and β_2-ARs in mice has no significant impact on resting heart rate, blood pressure, or cardiac output *(28–30,35)* (Table 1) (data from mice lacking all three β-ARs is not available yet). These results suggest that β_1- and β_2-ARs are not required for maintaining normal resting heart rate and blood pressure or for baseline contractile function in the mouse. They differ somewhat from experiments using antagonists to disrupt β-AR function acutely, suggesting some compensation occurs with the disruption of β-AR genes. For example, downregulation of cardiac muscarinic receptors observed in β_1/β_2-AR-KO mice may counterbalance the lack of adrenergic stimulation in maintaining the resting heart rate *(30)*.

3.2. Chronotropic and Inotropic Response to Sympathetic Stimulation

The relative role of β-AR subtypes in modulation of cardiac chronotropy was tested with the nonselective β-AR agonist isoproterenol administered to β-AR-KO mice. Wild-type mice show a robust 200 beats per min increase in heart rate associated with an approx 30 mmHg drop in mean blood pressure. In β_1-AR-KO mice, the heart rate response is attenuated by approx 50% *(28)*. This residual response is not mediated directly by cardiac β_2-ARs but by β_2-AR-mediated vasodilation. The hypotensive effect of activating vascular β_2-ARs leads to a baroreflex-mediated withdrawal of vagal tone. The chronotropic response to isoproterenol in β_1-AR-KO mice can be blocked by atropine, a muscarinic receptor antagonist *(35)*.

The lack of β_2-AR involvement in cardiac chronotropy is further evidenced by the normal heart rate response to isoproterenol in β_2-AR-KO mice *(29)*. In β_1/β_2-AR-KO mice, the heart rate response to isoproterenol is even more severely attenuated because these mice have diminished peripheral vasodilation and hence a smaller baroreflex response than do β_1-AR-KO mice *(30)*. The remaining small baroreflex component in β_1/β_2-AR-KO mice is caused by an enhanced β_3-AR-mediated peripheral vasodilation *(30)*. These results are in agreement with experiments using isolated, spontaneously beating atria *(30)* and cultured neonatal myocytes isolated from each of these knockout strains *(24)*. Together, these data suggest that the β_1-AR is the primary receptor responsible for sympathetic regulation of cardiac chronotropy in adult mice.

Isolated right ventricular tissues were used to measure the contribution of β-AR signaling to contractility. Cardiac inotropy was monitored in isolated, paced right ventricular muscle strips. Preparations from β_1-AR-KO mice failed to show any responsiveness to isoproterenol administration, while wild-type preparations showed robust inotropic responses *(28)*. This lack of contractile response is not caused by generalized hyporesponsiveness of the contractile apparatus because β_1-AR-KO ventricles responded normally to activators of adenylyl cyclase such as forskolin. Surprisingly, disruption of both β_1- and β_2-ARs has only modest effects on resting left ventricular contractility in vivo. When contractility was assessed with a micromanometer-tipped catheter, +dP/dt was reduced by 20% and –dP/dt was reduced by 12% in β_1/β_2-AR-KO mice compared to wild-type mice *(30)*.

$_\alpha$These results are consistent with the ineffectual stimulation of cardiac adenylyl cyclase by β_2-ARs in β_1-AR-KO mice. This observation is somewhat surprising, however, given the fact that, in both native human myocardium and heterologous expression systems, the β_2-AR appears to couple more efficiently to adenylyl cyclase stimulation than does the β_1-AR. One possible explanation is that activation of adenylyl cyclase by the β_2-AR in murine hearts is inhibited by β_2-AR coupling to G_i. Indeed, β_2-AR-selective agonist-mediated inotropic effects on isolated adult ventricular myocytes are greatly enhanced when G_i/G_o proteins are inactivated by pertussis toxin treatment *(6)*. Of interest, transgenic mice with cardiac overexpression of β_2-AR exhibit enhanced contractility and elevated adenylyl cyclase activity *(27)*. Thus, β_2-AR coupling to cardiac ionotropy can occur in murine heart when the appropriate cellular or tissue context is provided.

3.3. Role of β-AR Subtypes
in the Cardiovascular and Metabolic Response to Exercise

Maximal exercise is associated with near maximal sympathetic nervous system activity and dramatic changes in heart rate, contractility, and vascular tone. Surprisingly, even though β_1-ARs are essential for catecholamine stimulation of chronotropy and inotropy, β_1-AR-KO mice exhibited the same exercise capacity as wild-type controls *(32,36)*. The heart rate response to exercise in β_1-AR-KO mice was markedly reduced compared to wild-type mice; yet, there were no differences between β_1-AR-KO mice and wild-type mice in VO_2 and VCO_2 over the entire range of workloads, suggesting no difference in metabolic response to exercise and no difference in O_2 extraction. Thus, β_1-AR-KO mice must compensate for their slower heart rates with greater increases in stroke volume, presumably through preload-dependent mechanisms *(36)*.

Using the same graded treadmill protocol, β_2-AR-KO mice exercised for a longer duration than did wild-type mice *(29)*. Heart rate responses to exercise were similar; however, β_2-AR-KO mice became hypertensive relative to wild-type mice, probably a result of unopposed α_1-AR-mediated peripheral vasoconstriction. At any given workload, VO_2 tended to be slightly higher in the knockout mice, resulting in a lower respiratory exchange ratio (RER; the ratio of $VCO_2:VO_2$). RER is one indicator of substrate utilization, and this difference suggests an alteration in energy metabolism caused by the absence of β_2-ARs. Normally, activation of β_2-ARs enhances glycogenolysis during exercise. Therefore, β_2-AR-KO mice might preferentially metabolize fat, resulting in a higher VO_2. Interestingly, the body fat content is decreased in β_2-AR-KO mice compared with wild-type mice *(29)*.

Similar to β_1-AR-KO mice, β_1/β_2-AR-KO mice are able to achieve exercise capacities equal to those of wild-type mice. Their heart rate response, like those of β_1-AR-KO mice, is blunted. However, in contrast to both of the β_1-AR-KO and β_2-AR-KO mice, the β_1/β_2-AR-KO mice have lower levels of VO_2 at all exercise workloads *(30)*. This metabolic deficit results only from the combined deficiency of both β_1- and β_2-ARs and could be secondary to an inability to mobilize metabolic fuels or to downstream effects that alter metabolic demands—for example, at the level of adenylyl cyclase, Na/K-adenosine triphosphatase, or the calcium channel. Collectively, these results suggest that β_1- and β_2-ARs serve both separate and redundant metabolic functions during exercise, and that both receptors must be ablated before significant metabolic abnormalities are encountered. Despite these deficits and significant deficits in inotropy and chronotropy, β_1/β_2-AR-KO mice were still able to achieve normal exercise capacity, which emphasizes the importance of preload in the response to exercise.

3.4. Role of β-AR Subtypes in the Pathogenesis of Heart Failure

Studies outlined above as well as studies using pharmacological methods showed that the β_1-AR is the dominant subtype regulating cardiac performance. Of interest, the β_1-AR has also been implicated in the pathogenesis of heart failure. It has been shown that the β_1-AR is selectively downregulated in cardiomyopathy *(37)*. Some evidence suggests that β-AR downregulation plays a role in the decrease in cardiac function in heart failure. However, more compelling is evidence that chronic β_1-AR activation contributes to the pathogenesis of heart failure. Chronic exposure to β-agonists leads to myocyte apoptosis, fibrosis, and dysfunction *(13,38)*. Moreover, inhibiting β-ARs with antagonists has been clinically beneficial in patients with cardiomyopathy *(18)*. Transgenic mice with overexpressed β_1-AR develop a cardiomyopathy similar to that seen with chronic catecholamine infusion *(26,39)*. In contrast, overexpressing the human β_2-AR in mouse hearts can significantly increase baseline cardiac contractility *(27)*. Deleterious effects of β_2-AR are observed only at very high levels of cardiac expression *(40)*. In fact, physiological levels of β_2-AR signaling in the heart may be protective. When isoproterenol was administered to mice over 2 wk by isometric infusion pump, β_2-AR-KO mice had higher mortality and more myocyte apoptosis than did wild-type mice *(41)*.

4. Role of β-Adrenergic Receptors in the Regulation of Smooth Muscle Tone

4.1. Regulation of Vascular Tone

In addition to their prominent function in heart, β-ARs are located on vascular smooth muscle cells, where they mediate vasodilating effects of catecholamines. The β_2-AR has been proposed to play a dominant role in catecholamine-induced vasodilation in both pulmonary and peripheral vasculature. Surprisingly, isometric myographic studies on various blood vessels from β-AR-KO mice revealed that the β_1-AR plays a much more prominent role in vasodilation than previously thought *(42)*. The β_1-AR is responsible for vasodilation in femoral and pulmonary arteries. However, in aortic and carotid arteries and in portal veins, the vasodilating effect of isoproterenol was reduced in mice lacking either the β_1- or the β_2-AR, and the effect was abolished in the β_1/β_2-AR-KO mice. Similar contributions of the β_1- and β_2-ARs to isoproterenol-induced vasorelaxation were found when vessels from wild-type mice were treated with isoproterenol in the presence of subtype-selective β-AR antagonists. Thus, the β_1-AR plays a dominant role in adrenergic vasodilation in large to medium-size vessels in the murine vascular system *(42)*. However, the β_2-AR-KO has greater effect on isoproterenol-induced hypotension than does the β_1-AR-KO, suggesting that the β_2-AR plays a more important role in vasodilation of the small arterioles that contribute the most to peripheral vascular resistance *(29)*.

4.2. Regulation of Airway Resistance

In the lung, activation of β-ARs leads to relaxation of airway smooth muscle. Many, if not most, of the different cell types within the lung have been shown to express β_2-AR on the cell surface. There is also significant β_1-AR expression, constituting about 20% of total β-AR in human lung; but no β_3-AR is detectable. β_2-ARs have thus been implicated in the regulation of many aspects of lung function *(43)*. Clinically, β-agonists have been used for treating patients with asthma; however, chronic treatment with β-agonists also leads to increased sensitivity to airway constriction (hyperactivity) drugs, such as muscarinuc receptor agonists. Unexpectedly, mice lacking both β_1- and β_2-ARs had markedly decreased bronchoconstrictive responses to the muscarinic receptor agonist methacholine and other G_q-coupled receptor agonists *(44)*. Moreover, the lack of β-AR signaling leads to increased expression of phospholipase C-β_1, a downstream component of G_q-coupled receptor signaling pathways and low inositol accumulation induced by G_q-coupled receptors. Thus, β-AR antithetically enhances constrictive signals, affecting bronchomotor tone/reactivity by additional means other than direct smooth muscle dilation *(44)*. Future studies with mice lacking individual β-AR subtypes will help clarify the cellular signaling involved in the short-term airway smooth muscle relaxation as well as the exacerbations under chronic β-agonist treatment.

4.3. Regulation of GI Motility

Pharmacological evidence, obtained predominantly using selective agonists, has suggested that β_3-AR causes relaxation in GI tract of rodents in vivo *(45,46)*. After administration of the β_3-AR-selective agonist CL316243, wild-type mice exhibited a significant decrease in the extent of GI motility, indicated by radiotracer in the stomach and intestines *(47)*. In contrast, the decrease in the GI motility induced by CL316243 was absent in the β_3-AR-KO mice, confirming the important role of β_3-AR in regulation of GI motility. However, there is no difference in the decrease in GI motility induced by isoproterenol between the β_3-AR-KO and wild-type mice. Pharmacological studies suggest that an upregulated β_1-AR function compensates for the lack of β_3-AR in regulation of GI motility, an observation similar to that in adipocytes *(14,47)*. These data were further supported by increased β_1-AR messenger ribonucleic acid level in GI tissue from the β_3-AR-KO mice.

5. Role of β-Adrenergic Receptors in the Regulation of Fat Metabolism

The sympathetic nervous system can regulate body temperature through β-ARs in adipose tissue. Pharmacological treatment with β-AR-selective agonists showed that all three β-ARs may play a role in sympathetically driven thermogenesis; however, the relative importance of each is unknown. Stimulating β_1-, β_2-, and β_3-ARs all lead to activation of $G_{s\alpha}$ and protein kinase A (PKA) and subsequent stimulation of lipolysis in white adipocytes and thermogenesis in brown adipocytes *(48)*. The β_3-AR is expressed primarily on white and brown adipocytes in rodents and on brown adipocytes in humans. Pharmacological activation of β_3-ARs results in marked stimulation of energy expenditure. Thus, β_3-ARs have been proposed to play an important role in the regulation of lipolysis, thermogenesis, and energy balance *(49,54)*.

Two independent groups have succeeded in targeted inactivation of the mouse β_3-AR gene *(14,50)*. β_3-AR-KO mice demonstrated a modest increase in body fat and a normal response to cold exposure. The normal response to acute treatment with β_3-selective agonists, including increased serum free fatty acids and insulin levels, increased whole body energy expenditure, and decreased food intake *(51,52)*, are absent in β_3-AR-KO mice *(14)*. Correspondingly, the nonselective β-agonist isoproterenol-stimulated adenylate cyclase activity was markedly impaired in adipocyte membranes derived from β_3-AR-deficient mice (by 80% in isolated white adipocyte membranes and 70% in brown adipose tissue membranes), confirming the predominant contribution of β_3-AR in adrenergic signaling in these tissues. Despite the impaired adenylate cyclase activities in the β_3-AR-KO mice, the isoproterenol-induced increases in serum free fatty acids and glycerol levels and increases in thermogenesis were almost normal, suggesting a compensatory effect of β_1- or β_2-ARs to the loss of β_3-AR for lipolysis and thermogenesis *(14)*. However, the β_1- or β_2-AR-mediated stimulation of lipolysis is extremely sensitive to inhibition of adenylate cyclase by activation of G_i-coupled adenosine receptor *(14)*. These data suggest a minor role of β_1-AR or β_2-ARs in adipocytes in wild-type mice, but their activities are enough to maintain the normal lipolysis in animals when β_3-AR is absent.

Pharmacological studies suggested that upregulation of β_1-AR function can compensate the lack of β_3-AR in regulation of white and brown adipocytes, which was further supported by increased β_1-AR messenger ribonucleic acid levels in these tissues in the β_3-AR-KO mice *(14)*. These compensatory mechanisms operate to maintain brown fat function, thus limiting the development of obesity. The regulatory pathways that mediate compensatory increases in β_1-AR gene expression in β_3-AR-KO mice remain to be determined.

Mice that lack all three β-ARs ($\beta_1\beta_2\beta_3$-AR-KO mice) have been created by cross-breeding β_3-AR-KO mice with $\beta_1\beta_2$-AR-KO mice *(31)*. $\beta_1\beta_2\beta_3$-AR-KO mice are viable and have normal body weight. However, brown adipocytes in these animals are thermogenically inactive, as indicated by the presence of large, unilocular lipid droplets; reduced expression of uncoupling protein 1 (UCP1), a protein expressed at a high level in brown adipose tissue; and complete resistance to cold exposure-induced increases in UCP1 protein and type II thyroxine deiodinase activity. Addition of isoproterenol to isolated brown adipocytes failed to increase oxygen consumption.

When fed a standard chow diet, $\beta_1\beta_2\beta_3$-AR-KO mice had a small increase in fat stores when compared with wild-type mice. However, a calorically dense diet, high in fat and sucrose, induced massive obesity in $\beta_1\beta_2\beta_3$-AR-KO mice. The observed weight gain of 25 g in 8 wk represents the development of extreme obesity and is similar to that observed in leptin-deficient ob/ob mice. The marked obesity observed in high calorie-fed $\beta_1\beta_2\beta_3$-AR-KO mice is caused entirely by a defect in diet-induced thermogenesis *(31)*. These findings establish that β-ARs are required for diet-induced thermogenesis, and that this pathway plays a critical role in the body's defenses against diet-induced obesity. The target tissue mediating sympathetically driven diet-induced thermogenesis is unknown. Although brown adipose has been proposed as the primary target, data from mice lacking UCP1 strongly argue against this. In brown adipose, UCP1 is a downstream component in the generation of heat following sympathetic nerve activity; however, UCP1 knockout mice do not display diet-induced obesity. These data suggest that either different UCP proteins or other sympathetic nerve innervated tissues are responsible for diet-induced thermogenesis, such as skeletal muscle, liver, and white adipose tissue *(53,54)*. It is clear that characterization of the discrepancy between $\beta_1\beta_2\beta_3$-AR-KO mice and UCP1-KO mice, with respect to diet-induced thermogenesis, will result in new insights regarding regulation of body weight.

6. Subtype-Specific β-Adrenergic Receptor Signaling in Cultured Cardiac Myocytes

Gene disruption studies have revealed much about the functional roles of specific β-AR subtypes in vivo; however, the cellular and molecular mechanisms underlying the subtype-specific behavior cannot be determined from whole animal experiments. Tissues and cells extracted from these animals provide valuable model systems to further study the cellular and biochemical properties of these receptors *(24,55)*. This strategy possesses several advantages over more traditional in vitro studies, which are commonly carried out on immortalized cell lines. Primary cultures from wild-type mice can be used to analyze the properties of receptors expressed at physiological levels in the context of a differentiated cell. Cultures from knockout provide ideal controls. This approach is particularly beneficial in analyzing highly homologous receptor subtypes, such as β_1- and β_2-AR, for which the limited subtype selectivity of agonists and antagonists often prevents complete pharmacological isolation of a specific receptor subtype. Moreover, many subtype-selective β-AR agonists are actually partial agonists. Primary cultures from knockout mice also provide model systems for expressing mutated forms of the disrupted gene. This allows structure–function analysis of receptors in differentiated cells without having to account for endogenously expressed wild-type proteins. Together, these advantages have greatly facilitated functional analyses of β-ARs in cardiac myocytes and will likely be extended to studies of other systems regulated by ARs *(56,57)*.

Over the past 5 yr, neonatal and adult myocytes have been successfully cultured from β-AR-KO animals *(24,55)*, and recombinant adenoviruses have been successfully used to express wild-type and mutated receptors in both cultures. Wild-type β-ARs expressed by recombinant adenovirus exhibit functional properties equivalent to those of the endogenous receptors in regulating myocyte contraction rate and contractility, and adenovirus-expressed β_2-AR can rescue the I_{ca} response to β_2-AR agonist stimulation in the adult β_1/β_2-AR-KO myocytes *(24,55)*. One caveat regarding the use of adenovirus with cardiac myocytes is that a relatively high level of expression of the exogenous receptors (above the endogenous levels) is required to achieve functional properties equivalent to those of the endogenous receptors *(24)*.

6.1. Subtype Differences in Basal Activity

One interesting observation from the exogenous expression of β-ARs in adult cardiac myocytes is that β_2-ARs but not β_1-ARs display spontaneous activity *(55)*. The spontaneous activity of β_2-ARs leads to increased basal cAMP levels in cardiac myocytes, which can be inhibited by the β_2-AR-selective inverse agonist ICI118522. The same β_2-AR activity also induces increased myocyte contractility that can be blocked by the nonselective β-AR antagonist propranolol or the inverse agonist ICI118522 *(55)*. These results are consistent with in vivo studies in transgenic mice, in which cardiac-specific overexpression of the β_2-AR leads to an agonist-independent enhancement in both baseline adenylyl cyclase activity and myocardial contractility *(27)*.

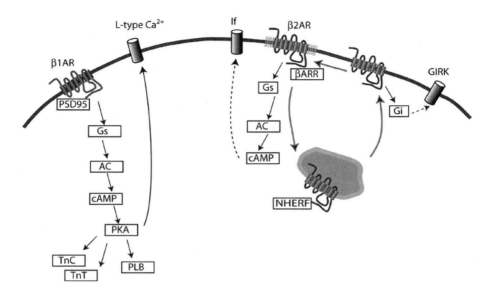

Fig. 1. β-AR subtype-specific signaling in cardiac myocytes. Cav, caveolae; GIRK, G protein coupled inwardly rectifying potassium channel; If, nonselective cation channel; NHERF, indicates NHERF/EBP50 (Na⁺/H⁺ exchange regulatory factor) or a related protein; PLB, phospholamban; PSD-95, indicates PSD-95 or a related protein; TnC, troponin C; TnT, troponin T. Dashed lines indicate postulated signaling pathways that have not been verified experimentally.

6.2 β-AR Stimulation of Myocyte Contraction

β_1-ARs couple to the stimulatory G_s protein in both adult and neonatal myocytes, which leads to activation of adenylyl cyclase and production of cAMP (Fig. 1). In adult myocytes, the cAMP-dependent PKA phosphorylates various substrates, including the L-type Ca^{2+} channel, which increases Ca^{2+} entry into cells. PKA-mediated phosphorylation of phospholamban accelerates Ca^{2+} sequestration into the sarcoplasmic reticulum, resulting in accelerated cardiac relaxation *(17)*. PKA-mediated phosphorylation of troponin I and C proteins reduces myofilament sensitivity to Ca^{2+} *(17)*. The ryanodine receptor is also a substrate for PKA; ryanodine receptor hyperphosphorylation has been observed in the failing human heart and in animal models of heart failure *(58,59)*. Both in vivo and in vitro assays showed that the β_1-AR plays the predominant role in modulating the rate and force of myocyte contraction in the mouse *(24,30,55)*.

In contrast, activated β_2-ARs can couple to both G_s and G_i in animal hearts, including human and murine hearts *(57,60)*, and in the isolated murine cardiac myocytes *(17,24,61)* (Fig. 1). In adult mouse cardiac myocytes, stimulation of the β_2-AR selectively modulates the activity of adjacent L-type Ca^{2+} channels *(17)*. However, in myocytes treated with pertussis toxin to disrupt G_i function, stimulation of β_2-ARs leads to a more generalized global activation of L-type Ca^{2+} channels and a robust increase in phospholamban phosphorylation, similar to that observed following stimulation of the β_1-AR, which accelerates the cardiac relaxation rate *(17,62)*. In mouse neonatal cardiac myocytes, activated β_2-ARs sequentially couple to both G_s and G_i, which induces a small increase followed by a sustained decrease in myocyte contraction rate *(24)*. β_2-AR stimulation leads to smaller cAMP accumulation than observed for β_1-AR stimulation. Surprisingly, inhibition of PKA does not affect the magnitude of neonatal myocyte contraction rate increase or decrease following stimulation of β_2-ARs *(24)*. Similar to observations in adult myocytes, inhibiting G_i results in a more robust β_2-AR mediated increase in contraction rate in neonatal myocytes. The effectors downstream of G_s and G_i in the β_2-AR regulation of neonatal myocyte contraction rate have not been determined. The cAMP-sensitive, nonselective cation channel (I_f) may mediate contraction rate increase, and the $G_{\beta\gamma}$-activated potassium channel my mediate the G_i-dependent decrease in contraction rate.

β_3-AR have been detected in both human and murine hearts, although at lower levels than β_1- and β_2-ARs, and the physiological role of β_3-AR in regulating cardiac function is poorly understood. Stimulation of β_3-ARs in human ventricular muscle reduces the strength of myocyte contraction by a G_i-dependent mechanism *(20)*. Similarly, stimulation of β_3-ARs results in a G_i-dependent decrease in the spontaneous contraction rate of cultured neonatal cardiac myocytes from β_1/β_2-AR-KO mice *(24)*. However, stimulation of human β_3-AR overexpressed in hearts of transgenic mice leads to an increase in the strength of contraction *(22)*. Because β_3-ARs can efficiently couple to G_s signaling in many native cells, the observed result in transgenic mice may in part be because of a loss of signaling fidelity when human β_3-ARs are overexpressed.

6.3. Subtype-Specific Regulation of Myocyte Growth and Apoptosis

Studies have revealed consequences of β-AR stimulation beyond regulating the rate and strength of myocyte contraction. Chronic stimulation of the β_1-AR induces myocyte apoptosis, although the signaling pathway is controversial *(12,63,64)*. In vitro studies suggest that this process requires PKA-independent activation of intracellular Ca^{2+} through L-type Ca^{2+} channels, which leads to Ca^{2+} release from sarcoplasmic reticulum and subsequent activation of calmodulin kinase II in adult cardiac myocytes *(65)*. However, this β_1-AR-stimulated proapoptotic effect appears to be blocked by PKA inhibition in adult rat myocytes *(63)*. In contrast, activation of β_2-ARs has an antiapoptotic effect, which is mediated by the $\beta\gamma$-subunits of G_i in both rat and mouse adult cardiac myocytes

(12,66). In the case of mouse myocytes, it seems that G_{i2} is responsible for the β_2-AR-mediated protective effect *(62)*. The role of specific downstream effectors in G_i signaling is less clear. Studies in adult mouse cardiac myocytes suggested that phosphatidylinositide-3 kinase can be activated by the $\beta\gamma$-subunits of G_i, which leads to activation of the protein kinase B (Akt) pathway that confers the G_i-mediated protection against apoptosis *(12)*. In contrast, studies of rat myocytes showed that stimulation of β_2-AR leads to activation of the p38 MAPK, which is dependent on $G_{i\alpha}$ and $G_{\beta\gamma}$. The activated p38 MAPK plays a role in mediating the antiapoptotic effect of β_2-AR stimulation *(66)*. However, the results from rat myocyte studies are contradictory to those from in vivo activation of p38 MAPK using transgenic overexpression of activated mutants of upstream kinases MKK3bE and MKK6bE in mice *(67)*. Nevertheless, inhibiting the G_i pathway turns β_2-AR signaling from antiapoptotic into proapoptotic in adult mouse cardiac myocytes, suggesting that β_2-AR signaling through G_s can cause myocyte apoptosis when β_2-AR coupling to G_i is inhibited *(12)*. Interestingly, β_2-AR can also activate p38 MAPK through a PKA-dependent pathway in adult mouse cardiac myocytes. The observed differences in the effect of β_2-AR activation on myocyte apoptosis can in part be attributed to differences experimental conditions as well as differences in the species studied.

Stimulation of ARs plays a significant role in the regulation of cardiac growth *(68)*. In neonatal rat cardiomyocytes, both α- and β-AR stimulation increase assembly of myosin light chain-2 into sarcomeric units *(69)*. In vivo, β-AR activation leads to skeletal α-actin gene expression, acting both directly on myocytes and indirectly on cardiac fibroblasts through the elaboration of peptide growth factors *(70)*. The mechanism of β-AR activation of myocyte hypertrophy is less well understood. Activation of G_s by β_1- and β_2-ARs and G_i by β_2-ARs may both be involved *(71)*. In vitro, stimulation of the β-ARs leads to activation of the MAPKs extracellular signal-regulated kinase (ERK)1 and ERK2, which can be mediated by either G_s/PKA pathway or $\beta\gamma$-subunit-dependent Src activation in G_i pathway *(5,72)*. Stimulation of the β-ARs can also lead to assembly of a protein complex containing c-Src and β-arrestin, followed by activation of the MAPKs ERK1 and ERK2 *(73)*. Thus, binding of β-arrestin to the β-AR, normally a step in receptor desensitization, is also the initial step in a mitogenic signaling pathway.

7. Differentiated Localization and Trafficking of β-Adrenergic Receptors Determines Their Signaling in Cardiac Myocyte

7.1. β_2-AR Localization in Caveolae

There is a growing body of evidence that subtype-specific signaling of β-ARs in cardiac myocytes involves the spatial segregation of the β_1-AR and β_2-AR on the cell surface of cardiac myocytes *(74)*. Studies also support that GPCRs function in the context of plasma membrane signaling compartments such as lipid rafts *(75,76)*. These compartments may facilitate the interaction between receptors and specific downstream signaling components while restricting access to other signaling molecules. Caveolae, a flask-shaped membrane domain enriched with caveolins, flotilins, and stomatins, are perhaps the best-characterized lipid rafts. A number of studies have demonstrated that caveolae are enriched in G proteins, GPCRs, and effector molecules *(75,76)*. Therefore, caveolae may act as scaffolds promoting the interaction of specific signaling molecules. However, there is also evidence that caveolins may act to inhibit the function of several signaling molecules, including G proteins and tyrosine kinases *(77)*. Membrane fractionation studies showed that the β_2-ARs, but not the β_1-AR, are found predominantly in a caveolin-enriched membrane fraction from both mouse and rat neonatal myocytes *(78,79)*. The association between β_2-AR and caveolae was further supported by the coimmunoprecipitation of the β_2-AR and caveolin-3 and co-localization between epitope-tagged β_2-AR and endogenous caveolin-3 in mouse neonatal cardiac myocytes isolated from β_1/β_2-AR-KO mice. Moreover, caveolar localization is required for physiological signaling by β_2-AR but not the β_1-AR in neonatal cardiac myocytes. The β_2-AR-stimulated increase in the myocyte contraction rate is increased by approximately twofold and markedly prolonged by filipin, an agent that disrupts lipid rafts, such as caveolae *(79)*. Filipin also significantly reduces coimmunoprecipitation of β_2-AR and caveolin-3 and comigration of β_2-AR with caveolin-3-enriched membranes. In contrast, filipin has no effect on β_1-AR signaling *(79)*. The increase of β_2-AR-stimulated signaling by filipin treatment is consistent with the proposed inhibitory role of caveolins on G proteins. By disrupting the caveolar structure, the β_2-ARs may have enhanced mobility in the plasma membrane, increasing the probability of interacting with both G_s and G_i.

The apparent association of the β_2-AR with caveolin-enriched membrane fraction is disrupted following agonist stimulation in rat neonatal cardiac myocytes *(78)*. Interestingly, stimulated β_2-ARs also undergo significant internalization in mouse cardiac myocytes. This internalization of the β_2-AR is necessary for the sequential coupling to both G_s and G_i, which results in a biphasic effect on contraction rate, with an initial small increase followed by a sustained decrease *(24)*. Blocking the β_2-AR internalization prevents the receptor coupling to G_i, resulting a monophasic increase in contraction rate, presumably from G_s coupling alone. Therefore, the internalization may serve as a mechanism to free the β_2-ARs from the inhibitory environment and hence enhance the opportunity for β_2-AR to couple to G_i. Many other GPCRs, including thyrotropin receptor, endothelin B receptor, and adenosine receptor A_1, undergo the activation-dependent translocation out of caveolae in different cell cultures *(80–82)*, but the role of caveolin/rafts in signaling of these GPCRs is not well understood. In contrast, some activated GPCRs, such as angiotensin and bradykinin receptors, do not move relative to caveolae in membrane fractionation studies *(83,84)*, whereas others, such as the m2 muscarinic acetylcholine receptor, migrate to the caveolae/raft after stimulation *(85)*. The association of a GPCR with caveolin could either facilitate or inhibit the receptor coupling to G proteins; in the latter case, the interaction may serve as part of the mechanism to turn off the receptor signaling.

7.2. β_1-AR Subtype-Specific Signaling and Trafficking Is Regulated by PDZ Domain-Containing Proteins

Evidence shows that GPCRs can form complexes with downstream effectors to facilitate signaling specificity and efficiency. GPCRs can be recruited into the signaling complexes through carboxyl-terminal PDZ domain-binding motifs, which directly interact with PDZ domain-containing scaffolding proteins. A PDZ domain-binding motif on the C-terminus of the β_1-AR selectively binds to a set of PDZ domain-containing proteins, including PSD-95, GIPC, and membrane-associated guanylate kinase inverted-2 (MAGI-2) *(86–88)*. Coexpressing PSD-95 with β_1-AR in HEK-293 cells inhibits the receptor internalization but has no significant effect on β_1-AR-stimulated cAMP accumulation or desensitization *(86)*. Phosphorylation of the β_1-AR by GRK5 reduces receptor binding to PSD-95 *(89)*. In contrast, coexpression of MAGI-2 with the β_1-AR enhances agonist-induced internalization of the receptor *(87)*. The association between β_1-AR and MAGI-2 can be further enhanced by agonist stimulation; however, whether this regulation is mediated by GPCR kinase phosphorylation on the receptor is currently not known *(87)*. Like PSD-95, MAGI-2 has no significant effect on either desensitization of β_1-AR- or β_1-AR-stimulated cAMP accumulation. Coexpressing GIPC with the β_1-AR enhances receptor-mediated ERK activation by β_1-AR while having no significant effect on either receptor internalization or receptor-mediated cAMP accumulation *(88)*. It is currently unknown which, if any, of these PDZ domain-containing proteins regulates β_1-AR signaling in cardiac myocytes. However, a similar interaction between mouse β_1-AR and one or more PDZ domain-containing proteins is necessary to maintain the selective coupling of the β_1-AR to G_s in neonatal mouse cardiac myocytes. Disruption of the β_1-AR PDZ motif leads to promiscuous coupling to both G_s and G_i and to significant agonist-induced internalization in neonatal cardiac myocytes *(90)*. Therefore, the β_1-AR PDZ-mediated interactions with PDZ domain-containing proteins, presumably by a homologue of PSD-95, restricts receptor trafficking and signaling.

7.3. Regulation of β_2-AR Signaling by PDZ Domain-Containing Proteins in Cardiac Myocytes

An interaction between the carboxyl terminal PDZ motif of the β_2-AR and EBP50 (also known as the Na^+/H^+ exchanger regulatory factor, NHERF) has been demonstrated in HEK-293 cells. This interaction is involved in recycling of internalized β_2-ARs and in receptor-mediated activation of Na$^+$/H$^+$ exchanger *(91,92)*. Disruption of the PDZ motif on the mouse β_2-AR has no significant effect on the agonist-stimulated receptor internalization but dramatically reduces the receptor recycling in neonatal cardiac myocytes *(93)*. Interestingly, disruption of the β_2-AR PDZ-binding motif also prevents β_2-AR coupling to G$_i$ protein in cardiac myocytes, resulting monophasic contraction rate increase after agonist stimulation *(93)*. Thus, the PDZ motif is necessary for both the receptor recycling and the receptor coupling to G$_i$, although whether these events are interdependent remains to be determined. The human β_2-AR PDZ motif for binding EBP50/ NHERF also binds to *N*-ethylmaleimide-sensitive factor (NSF) *(94)*. NSF is involved in membrane fusion between vesicles and targeted membrane, a process required for protein trafficking. Disruption of NSF binding also reduces the human β_2-AR recycling in HEK-293 cells *(94)*. The specific roles played by NSF and EBP50/NHERF proteins in recycling of the human β_2-AR are not clear. It is noteworthy that a key residue (leucine 410) in human β_2-AR necessary for NSF binding is not conserved in the mouse β_2-AR. Therefore, NSF may not play a role in regulating the function of the mouse β_2-AR *(93)*.

It is interesting to note that mutating the β_2-AR PDZ-binding motif inhibits receptor coupling to G$_i$; mutation of the β_1-AR PDZ-binding motif promotes coupling to G$_i$ in the neonatal myocytes *(90)*. The ability of these receptors to couple to G$_i$ correlates with their propensity to undergo agonist-induced internalization and recycle back to the plasma membrane. The wild-type β_1-AR does not undergo agonist-induced internalization, and the PDZ motif-mutated β_2-AR cannot recycle back to the cell surface following internalization. In contrast, both wild-type β_2-AR and the PDZ motif-mutated β_1-AR undergo agonist-induced internalization and efficient recycling to the plasma membrane *(90)*. Together, these data show that the β-AR PDZ motif-mediated interactions play critical roles in the receptor subcellular location and trafficking, which in turn dictates subtype-specific signaling in cardiac myocytes.

7.4. A Kinase Anchoring Protein-Mediated Interactions

The β_2-AR has been shown to associate with A kinase anchoring protein 79 (AKAP79) and gravin in vitro and in transfected HEK-293 cells *(95,96)*. Both AKAP79 and gravin are AKAPs that scaffold the β_2-AR to PKA, protein kinase C, PP2A, or L-type Ca^{2+} channels to orchestrate signaling at the plasma membrane *(95,97,98)*. Supporting the concept of β-AR signaling complexes in cardiac myocytes, studies showed that β-AR-mediated cAMP accumulation is concentrated in a striated pattern in rat neonatal cardiac myocytes *(99)*. This local accumulation of cAMP is in part mediated by phosphodiesterase (PDE) activities in myocytes because the striated pattern of cAMP accumulation is disrupted by IBMX, a nonselective PDE inhibitor *(99)*. Thus, PKA activities are restricted to focal compartments in myocytes, possibly by a PDE activity associated with β-ARs. Interestingly, activation of $β_2$-AR can recruit PDE4D to the membrane in both 293 cells and rat neonatal myocytes *(100)*. Although this PDE4D recruitment has been shown to depend on β-arrestin, it remains to be determined if AKAP proteins are involved *(100)*. Coincidently, a muscle-specific AKAP can scaffold PKA and PDE4D together in a complex associated with the sarcomere plasma membrane, suggesting tight regulation of cAMP-dependent PKA action on its targets *(101)*. Together, these data strongly suggest that AKAPs serve as scaffolds for β-AR signaling complexes in cardiac myocytes; however, the functional role of the AKAP-mediated signaling complexes remains to be determined.

8. Conclusions

Targeted disruption of the murine β-AR genes has helped to clarify the role of specific β-AR subtypes in development and in regulating cardiovascular and metabolic functions in vivo *(54,102–104)*. Surprisingly, disruption of the genes for receptors that play such important roles in autonomic regulation of cardiovascular and metabolic functions are relatively well tolerated. This may be partly caused by compensatory mechanisms that are activated when a specific receptor gene is disrupted from the time of conception, such as upregulation of $β_1$-AR signaling in adipocytes of $β_3$-AR-deficient mice. However, when the cardiovascular system is maximally stressed, such as during exercise, more striking differences between the knockout mice and their wild-type littermates can be discerned. For some physiological functions, such as heart rate and contractile function, the dominant role of a single β-AR subtype can be defined. For others, such as vasoregulation, the roles of the three subtypes are additive and integrated. For still others, such as fat metabolism, β-AR actions appear to be partly redundant, and deficits do not become readily apparent until at least two or all subtypes are ablated.

Although the β-AR-KO animals have been extremely useful experimental tools for defining the roles of specific receptor subtypes in normal physiology, their value in predicting subtype-specific function in humans may be limited. The pattern of expression and the physiological role of each receptor subtype may be species specific *(105,106)*, and extrapolation of results to humans must be made very carefully. Nevertheless, the disruption of GPCR genes in mice will continue to provide insight into their physiological function and the potential therapeutic value of drugs that selectively target these receptors.

References

1. Strader CD, Fong TM, Graziano MP, Tota MR. The family of G-protein-coupled receptors. FASEB J 1995;9:745–754.

2. Frielle T, Collins S, Daniel KW, Caron MG, Lefkowitz RJ, Kobilka BK. Cloning of the cDNA for the human β₁-adrenergic receptor. Proc Natl Acad Sci USA 1987; 84:7920–7924.
3. Dixon RA, Kobilka BK, Strader DJ, et al. Cloning of the gene and cDNA for mammalian β-adrenergic receptor and homology with rhodopsin. Nature 1986; 321:75–79.
4. Emorine LJ, Marullo S, Briend-Sutren MM, et al. Molecular characterization of the human β₃-adrenergic receptor. Science 1989;245:1118–1121.
5. Daaka Y, Luttrell LM, Lefkowitz RJ. Switching of the coupling of the β₂-adrenergic receptor to different G proteins by protein kinase A. Nature 1997;390:88–91.
6. Xiao RP, Ji X, Lakatta EG. Functional coupling of the β₂-adrenoceptor to a pertussis toxin-sensitive G protein in cardiac myocytes. Mol Pharmacol 1995;47:322–329.
7. Xiao RP, Avdonin P, Zhou YY, et al. Coupling of β₂-adrenoceptor to Gᵢ proteins and its physiological relevance in murine cardiac myocytes. Circ Res 1999;84:43–52.
8. Luttrell LM, van Biesen T, Hawes BE, et al. G-protein-coupled receptors and their regulation: activation of the MAP kinase signaling pathway by G-protein-coupled receptors. Adv Second Messenger Phosphoprotein Res 1997;31:263–277.
9. Post GR, Goldstein D, Thuerauf DJ, Glembotski CC, Brown JH. Dissociation of p44 and p42 mitogen-activated protein kinase activation from receptor-induced hypertrophy in neonatal rat ventricular myocytes. J Biol Chem 1996;271:8452–8457.
10. McDonald PH, Chow CW, Miller WE, et al. β-Arrestin 2: a receptor-regulated MAPK scaffold for the activation of JNK3. Science 2000;290:1574–1577.
11. Daaka Y, Luttrell LM, Ahn S, et al. Essential role for G protein-coupled receptor endocytosis in the activation of mitogen-activated protein kinase. J Biol Chem 1998;273:685–688.
12. Zhu WZ, Zheng M, Koch WJ, Lefkowitz RJ, Kobilka BK, Xiao RP. Dual modulation of cell survival and cell death by β₂-adrenergic signaling in adult mouse cardiac myocytes. Proc Natl Acad Sci USA 2001;98:1607–1612.
13. Communal C, Singh K, Sawyer DB, Colucci WS. Opposing effects of β₁- and β₂-adrenergic receptors on cardiac myocyte apoptosis: role of a pertussis toxin-sensitive G protein. *Circulation* 1999;100:2210–2212.
14. Susulic VS, Frederich RC, Lawitts J, et al. Targeted disruption of the β₃-adrenergic receptor gene. J Biol Chem 1995;270:29,483–29,492.
15. Croci T, Cecchi R, Tarantino A, et al. Inhibition of rat colon motility by stimulation of atypical β-adrenoceptors with new gut-specific agents. Pharmacol Res Commun 1988;20:147–151.
16. Brodde O. β₁ and β₂-adrenoceptors in the human heart: properties, function, and alterations in chronic heart failure. Pharmacol Rev 1991;43:203–242.
17. Xiao RP. Cell logic for dual coupling of a single class of receptors to Gₛ and Gᵢ proteins. Circ Res 2000;87:635–637.
18. Bristow MR, Gilbert EM, Abraham WT, et al. Carvedilol produces dose-related improvements in left ventricular function and survival in subjects with chronic heart failure. MOCHA Investigators. Circulation 1996;94:2807–2816.

19. Kuznetsov V, Pak E, Robinson RB, Steinberg SF. β_2-Adrenergic receptor actions in neonatal and adult rat ventricular myocytes. Circ Res 1995;76:40–52

20. Gauthier C, Tavernier G, Charpentier F, Langin D, Le Marec H. Functional β_3-adrenoceptor in the human heart. J Clin Invest 1996;98:556–562.

21. Gauthier C, Langin D, Balligand JL. β_3-Adrenoceptors in the cardiovascular system. Trends Pharmacol Sci 2000;21:426–431.

22. Kohout TA, Takaoka H, McDonald PH, et al. Augmentation of cardiac contractility mediated by the human β_3-adrenergic receptor overexpressed in the hearts of transgenic mice. Circulation 2001;104:2485–2491.

23. Cheng HJ, Zhang ZS, Onishi K, Ukai T, Sane DC, Cheng CP. Upregulation of functional β_3-adrenergic receptor in the failing canine myocardium. Circ Res 2001; 89:599–606.

24. Devic E, Xiang Y, Gould D, Kobilka B. β-Adrenergic receptor subtype-specific signaling in cardiac myocytes from β_1 and β_2 adrenoceptor knockout mice. Mol Pharmacol 2001;60:577–583.

25. Oostendorp J, Kaumann AJ. Pertussis toxin suppresses carbachol-evoked cardiodepression but does not modify cardiostimulation mediated through β_1- and putative β_4-adrenoceptors in mouse left atria: no evidence for β_2- and β_3-adrenoreceptor function. Naunyn Schmiedebergs Arch Pharmacol 2000;361: 134–145.

26. Bisognano JD, Weinberger HD, Bohlmeyer TJ, et al. Myocardial-directed overexpression of the human β_1-adrenergic receptor in transgenic mice. J Mol Cell Cardiol 2000;32:817–830.

27. Milano C, Allen L, Rockman H, et al. Enhanced myocardial function in transgenic mice overexpressing the β_2-adrenergic receptor. Science 1994;264: 582–586.

28. Rohrer DK, Desai KH, Jasper JR, et al. Targeted disruption of the mouse β_1-adrenergic receptor gene: developmental and cardiovascular effects. Proc Natl Acad Sci USA 1996;93:7375–7380.

29. Chruscinski AJ, Rohrer DK, Schauble E, Desai KH, Bernstein D, Kobilka BK. Targeted disruption of the β_2 adrenergic receptor gene. J Biol Chem 1999;274: 16,694–16,700.

30. Rohrer DK, Chruscinski A, Schauble EH, Bernstein D, Kobilka BK. Cardiovascular and metabolic alterations in mice lacking both β_1- and β_2-adrenergic receptors. J Biol Chem 1999;274:16,701–16,708.

31. Bachman ES, Dhillon H, Zhang CY, et al. βAR signaling required for diet-induced thermogenesis and obesity resistance. Science 2002;297:843–845.

32. Desai KH, Sato R, Schauble E, Barsh GS, Kobilka BK, Bernstein D. Cardiovascular indexes in the mouse at rest and with exercise: new tools to study models of cardiac disease. Am J Physiol 1997;272:H1053–H1061.

33. Hoit B, Khoury S, Kranias E, Ball N, Walsh R. In vivo echocardiographic detection of enhanced left ventricular function in gene-targeted mice with phospholamban deficiency. Circ Res 1995;77:632–637.

34. Klug S, Thiel R, Schwabe R, Merker HJ, Neubert D. Toxicity of β-blockers in a rat whole embryo culture: concentration–response relationships and tissue concentrations. Arch Toxicol 1994;68:375–384.

35. Rohrer DK, Bernstein D, Chruscinski A, Desai KH, Schauble E, Kobilka BK. The developmental and physiological consequences of disrupting genes encoding β_1 and β_2 adrenoceptors. Adv Pharmacol 1998;42:499–501.
36. Rohrer DK, Schauble EH, Desai KH, Kobilka BK, Bernstein D. Alterations in dynamic heart rate control in the β_1-adrenergic receptor knockout mouse. Am J Physiol 1998;274:H1184–H1193.
37. Bristow M, Ginsburg R, Umans V, et al. β_1- and β_2-adrenergic-receptor subpopulations in nonfailing and failing human ventricular myocardium: coupling of both receptor subtypes to muscle contraction and selective β_1-receptor down-regulation in heart failure. Circ Res 1986;59:297–309.
38. Rona G. Catecholamine cardiotoxicity. J Mol Cell Cardiol 1985;17:291–306.
39. Engelhardt S, Hein L, Wiesmann F, Lohse MJ. Progressive hypertrophy and heart failure in β_1-adrenergic receptor transgenic mice. Proc Natl Acad Sci USA 1999; 96:7059–7064.
40. Liggett SB, Tepe NM, Lorenz JN, et al. Early and delayed consequences of β_2-adrenergic receptor overexpression in mouse hearts: critical role for expression level. Circulation 2000;101:1707–1714.
41. Patterson AJ, Zhu W, Chow A, et al. Protecting the myocardium: a role for the β_2 adrenergic receptor in the heart. Crit Care Med 2004;32:1041–1048.
42. Chruscinski A, Brede ME, Meinel L, Lohse MJ, Kobilka BK, Hein L. Differential distribution of β-adrenergic receptor subtypes in blood vessels of knockout mice lacking β_1- or β_2-adrenergic receptors. Mol Pharmacol 2001;60:955–962.
43. Mak JC, Nishikawa M, Haddad EB, et al. Localisation and expression of β-adrenoceptor subtype mRNAs in human lung. Eur J Pharmacol 1996;302:215–221.
44. McGraw DW, Almoosa KF, Paul RJ, Kobilka BK, Liggett SB. Antithetic regulation by β-adrenergic receptors of G_q receptor signaling via phospholipase C underlies the airway β-agonist paradox. J Clin Invest 2003;112:619–626.
45. Thollander M, Svensson TH, Hellstrom PM. Stimulation of β-adrenoceptors with isoprenaline inhibits small intestinal activity fronts and induces a postprandial-like motility pattern in humans. Gut 1997;40:376–380.
46. Manara L, Croci T, Landi M. β_3-Adrenoceptors and intestinal motility. Fundam Clin Pharmacol 1995;9:332–342.
47. Fletcher DS, Candelore MR, Grujic D, et al. β_3 Adrenergic receptor agonists cause an increase in gastrointestinal transit time in wild-type mice, but not in mice lacking the β_3 adrenergic receptor. J Pharmacol Exp Ther 1998;287:720–724.
48. Rolfe DF, Brown GC. Cellular energy utilization and molecular origin of standard metabolic rate in mammals. Physiol Rev 1997;77:731–758.
49. Strosberg AD. Structure and function of the beta 3-adrenergic receptor. Annu Rev Pharmacol Toxicol 1997;37:421–450.
50. Revelli JP, Preitner F, Samec S, et al. Targeted gene disruption reveals a leptin-independent role for the mouse β_3-adrenoceptor in the regulation of body composition. J Clin Invest 1997;100:1098–1106.
51. Yoshida T. The antidiabetic β_3-adrenoceptor agonist BRL 26830A works by release of endogenous insulin. Am J Clin Nutr 1992;55:237S–241S.

52. Himms-Hagen J, Cui J, Danforth E Jr, et al. Effect of CL-316,243, a thermogenic β_3-agonist, on energy balance and brown and white adipose tissues in rats. Am J Physiol 1994;266:R1371–R1382.

53. Enerback S, Jacobsson A, Simpson EM, et al. Mice lacking mitochondrial uncoupling protein are cold-sensitive but not obese. Nature 1997;387:90–94.

54. Lowell BB, Bachman ES. β-Adrenergic receptors, diet-induced thermogenesis, and obesity. J Biol Chem 2003;278:29,385–29,388.

55. Zhou YY, Wang SQ, Zhu WZ, et al. Culture and adenoviral infection of adult mouse cardiac myocytes: methods for cellular genetic physiology. Am J Physiol Heart Circ Physiol 2000;279:H429–H436.

56. Xiang Y, Kobilka BK. Myocyte adrenoceptor signaling pathways. Science 2003; 300:1530–1532.

57. Xiao RP. β-Adrenergic signaling in the heart: dual coupling of the β_2-adrenergic receptor to Gs and Gi proteins. Sci STKE 2001;RE15.

58. Marks AR, Reiken S, Marx SO. Progression of heart failure: is protein kinase a hyperphosphorylation of the ryanodine receptor a contributing factor? Circulation 2002;105:272–275.

59. Reiken S, Gaburjakova M, Guatimosim S, et al. Protein kinase A phosphorylation of the cardiac calcium release channel (ryanodine receptor) in normal and failing hearts. Role of phosphatases and response to isoproterenol. J Biol Chem 2003;278:444–453.

60. Hasseldine AR, Harper EA, Black JW. Cardiac-specific overexpression of human β_2 adrenoceptors in mice exposes coupling to both Gs and Gi proteins. Br J Pharmacol 2003;138:1358–1366.

61. Kilts JD, Gerhardt MA, Richardson MD, et al. β_2-Adrenergic and several other G protein-coupled receptors in human atrial membranes activate both G_s and G_i. *Circ Res* 2000;87:705–709.

62. Foerster K, Groner F, Matthes J, Koch WJ, Birnbaumer L, Herzig S. Cardioprotection specific for the G protein G_{i2} in chronic adrenergic signaling through β_2-adrenoceptors. Proc Natl Acad Sci USA 2003;100:14,475–14,480.

63. Communal C, Singh K, Pimentel DR, Colucci WS. Norepinephrine stimulates apoptosis in adult rat ventricular myocytes by activation of the β-adrenergic pathway. Circulation 1998;98:1329–1334.

64. Iwai-Kanai E, Hasegawa K, Araki M, Kakita T, Morimoto T, Sasayama S. α- and β-adrenergic pathways differentially regulate cell type- specific apoptosis in rat cardiac myocytes. Circulation 1999;100:305–311.

65. Zhu WZ, Wang SQ, Chakir K, et al. 2003. Linkage of β_1-adrenergic stimulation to apoptotic heart cell death through protein kinase A-independent activation of Ca^{2+}/calmodulin kinase II. J Clin Invest 2003;111:617–625.

66. Singh K, Xiao L, Remondino A, Sawyer DB, Colucci WS. Adrenergic regulation of cardiac myocyte apoptosis. J Cell Physiol 2001;189:257–265.

67. Liao P, Georgakopoulos D, Kovacs A, et al. The in vivo role of p38 MAP kinases in cardiac remodeling and restrictive cardiomyopathy. Proc Natl Acad Sci USA 2001;98:12,283–12,288.

68. Simpson P, Kariya K, Karns L, Long C, Karliner J. Adrenergic hormones and control of cardiac myocyte growth. Mol Cell Biochem 1991;104:35–43.

69. Iwaki K, Sukhatme V, Shubeita H, Chien K. α and β-adrenergic stimulation induced distinct patterns of immediate early gene expression in neonatal rat myocardial cells. J Biol Chem 1990;265:13,809 13,817.

70. Bishopric N, Sato B, Webster K. β-Adrenergic regulation of a myocardial actin gene via a cyclic AMP-independent pathway. J Biol Chem 1992;267:20,932–20,936.

71. Adams JW, Brown JH. G-proteins in growth and apoptosis: lessons from the heart. Oncogene 2001;20:1626–34.

72. Friedman J, Babu B, Clark RB. $β_2$-Adrenergic receptor lacking the cyclic AMP-dependent protein kinase consensus sites fully activates extracellular signal-regulated kinase 1/2 in human embryonic kidney 293 cells: lack of evidence for G_s/G_i switching. Mol Pharmacol 2002;62:1094–1102.

73. Luttrell LM, Ferguson SS, Daaka Y, et al. β-arrestin-dependent formation of $β_2$ adrenergic receptor-Src protein kinase complexes. Science 1999;283:655–661.

74. Steinberg SF, Brunton LL. Compartmentation of G protein-coupled signaling pathways in cardiac myocytes. Annu Rev Pharmacol Toxicol 2001;41:751–773.

75. Oh P, Schnitzer JE. Segregation of heterotrimeric G proteins in cell surface microdomains. G_q binds caveolin to concentrate in caveolae, whereas G_i and G_s target lipid rafts by default. Mol Biol Cell 2001;12:685–698.

76. Galbiati F, Razani B, Lisanti MP. Emerging themes in lipid rafts and caveolae. Cell 2001;106:403–411.

77. Razani B, Lisanti MP. Caveolins and caveolae: molecular and functional relationships. Exp Cell Res 2001;271:36–44.

78. Rybin VO, Xu X, Lisanti MP, Steinberg SF. Differential targeting of β-adrenergic receptor subtypes and adenylyl cyclase to cardiomyocyte caveolae. A mechanism to functionally regulate the cAMP signaling pathway. J Biol Chem 2000;275:41,447–41,457.

79. Xiang Y, Rybin VO, Steinberg SF, Kobilka B. Caveolar localization dictates physiologic signaling of $β_2$-adrenoceptors in neonatal cardiac myocytes. J Biol Chem 2002;277:34,280–34,286.

80. Latif R, Ando T, Daniel S, Davies TF. Localization and regulation of thyrotropin receptors within lipid rafts. Endocrinology 2003;144:4725–4728.

81. Yamaguchi T, Murata Y, Fujiyoshi Y, Doi T. Regulated interaction of endothelin B receptor with caveolin-1. Eur J Biochem 2003;270:1816–1827.

82. Lasley RD, Narayan P, Uittenbogaard A, Smart EJ. Activated cardiac adenosine A1 receptors translocate out of caveolae. J Biol Chem 2000;275:4417–4421.

83. Leclerc PC, Auger-Messier M, Lanctot PM, Escher E, Leduc R, Guillemette G. A polyaromatic caveolin-binding-like motif in the cytoplasmic tail of the type 1 receptor for angiotensin II plays an important role in receptor trafficking and signaling. Endocrinology 2002;143:4702–4710.

84. Lamb ME, Zhang C, Shea T, Kyle DJ, Leeb-Lundberg LM. Human B1 and B2 bradykinin receptors and their agonists target caveolae-related lipid rafts to different degrees in HEK293 cells. Biochemistry 2002;41:14,340 14,347.

85. Feron O, Smith TW, Michel T, Kelly RA. Dynamic targeting of the agonist-stimulated m2 muscarinic acetylcholine receptor to caveolae in cardiac myocytes. J Biol Chem 1997;272:17,744–17,748.

86. Hu LA, Tang Y, Miller WE, et al. β_1-Adrenergic receptor association with PSD-95. Inhibition of receptor internalization and facilitation of β_1-adrenergic receptor interaction with N-methyl-D-aspartate receptors. J Biol Chem 2000;275:38,659–38,666.

87. Xu J, Paquet M, Lau AG, Wood JD, Ross CA, Hall RA. β_1-Adrenergic receptor association with the synaptic scaffolding protein membrane-associated guanylate kinase inverted-2 (MAGI-2). Differential regulation of receptor internalization by MAGI-2 and PSD-95. J Biol Chem 2001;276:41,310–41,317.

88. Hu LA, Chen W, Martin NP, Whalen EJ, Premont RT, Lefkowitz RJ. GIPC interacts with the β_1-adrenergic receptor and regulates β_1-adrenergic receptor-mediated ERK activation. J Biol Chem 2003;278:26,295–26,301.

89. Hu LA, Chen W, Premont RT, Cong M, Lefkowitz RJ. G protein-coupled receptor kinase 5 regulates β_1-adrenergic receptor association with PSD-95. J Biol Chem 2002;277:1607–1613.

90. Xiang Y, Devic E, Kobilka B. The PDZ binding motif of the β_1 adrenergic receptor modulates receptor trafficking and signaling in cardiac myocytes. J Biol Chem 2002;277:33,783–33,790.

91. Hall RA, Premont RT, Chow CW, et al. The β_2-adrenergic receptor interacts with the Na^+/H^+-exchanger regulatory factor to control Na^+/H^+ exchange. Nature 1998; 392:626–630.

92. Cao TT, Deacon HW, Reczek D, Bretscher A, von Zastrow M. A kinase-regulated PDZ-domain interaction controls endocytic sorting of the β_2-adrenergic receptor. Nature 1999;401:286–290.

93. Xiang Y, Kobilka B. The PDZ-binding motif of the β_2-adrenoceptor is essential for physiologic signaling and trafficking in cardiac myocytes. Proc Natl Acad Sci USA 2003;100:10,776–10,781.

94. Cong M, Perry SJ, Hu LA, Hanson PI, Claing A, Lefkowitz RJ. Binding of the β_2 adrenergic receptor to N-ethylmaleimide-sensitive factor regulates receptor recycling. J Biol Chem 2001;276:45,145–45,152.

95. Fraser ID, Cong M, Kim J, et al. Assembly of an A kinase-anchoring protein-β_2-adrenergic receptor complex facilitates receptor phosphorylation and signaling. Curr Biol 2000;10:409–412.

96. Shih M, Lin F, Scott JD, Wang HY, Malbon CC. Dynamic complexes of β_2-adrenergic receptors with protein kinases and phosphatases and the role of gravin. J Biol Chem 1999;274:1588–1595.

97. Davare MA, Avdonin V, Hall DD, et al. A β_2 adrenergic receptor signaling complex assembled with the Ca^{2+} channel Cav1.2. Science 2001;293:98–101.

98. Lin F, Wang H, Malbon CC. Gravin-mediated formation of signaling complexes in β_2-adrenergic receptor desensitization and resensitization. J Biol Chem 2000; 275:19,025–19,034.

99. Zaccolo M, Pozzan T. Discrete microdomains with high concentration of cAMP in stimulated rat neonatal cardiac myocytes. Science 2002;295:1711–1715.

100. Perry SJ, Baillie GS, Kohout TA, et al. Targeting of cyclic AMP degradation to β_2-adrenergic receptors by β-arrestins. Science 2002;298:834–836.

101. Dodge KL, Khouangsathiene S, Kapiloff MS, et al. mAKAP assembles a protein kinase A/PDE4 phosphodiesterase cAMP signaling module. EMBO J 2001;20: 1921–1930.

102. Bernstein D. Cardiovascular and metabolic alterations in mice lacking β_1- and β_2-adrenergic receptors. Trends Cardiovasc Med 2002;12:287–294.
103. Rohrer DK. Physiological consequences of β-adrenergic receptor disruption. J Mol Med 1998;76:764–772.
104. Rohrer DK. Targeted disruption of adrenergic receptor genes. Methods Mol Biol 2000;126:259–277.
105. Sabri A, Muske G, Zhang H, et al. Signaling properties and functions of two distinct cardiomyocyte protease-activated receptors. Circ Res 2000;86:1054–1061.
106. Steinberg SF. The molecular basis for distinct β-adrenergic receptor subtype actions in cardiomyocytes. Circ Res 1999;85:1101–1111.

11

Lessons From Overexpressed Mouse Models

*Cinzia Perrino, Liza Barki-Harrington,
and Howard A. Rockman*

Summary

Adrenergic receptors (ARs) belong to the largest known family of trans-membrane receptors, G protein-coupled receptors (GPCRs). Two subtypes, α and β, have been described, and even though they both respond to norepinephrine and epinephrine, the cellular responses they mediate differ significantly. Many human diseases, such as heart failure, are characterized by alterations in adrenergic signaling. The generation of genetically modified mice with altered expression of one of the AR subtypes has been useful for characterization of the mechanisms of receptor activation, as well as the ensuing in vivo phenotype. The availability of numerous genetically targeted mouse models has been an important tool for the study of AR function and the identification of potential novel therapeutic strategies for a wide range of diseases.

Key Words: Adrenergic receptors; G protein-coupled receptors; gene-targeted mice; transgenic mice.

1. Introduction

Adrenergic receptors (ARs) are the interface between the sympathetic nervous system and the cardiovascular system. ARs include two major subtypes, α and β, based on their pharmacological properties and molecular structure. The α-ARs consist of three α_1-AR subtypes and three α_2-ARs. β-ARs are also classified into three well-characterized subtypes: β_1, β_2, and β_3. Although they respond to the same hormones (norepinephrine and epinephrine), α- and β-ARs differ significantly in the types of cellular responses they mediate.

From: *The Receptors: The Adrenergic Receptors: In the 21st Century*
Edited by: D. Perez © Humana Press Inc., Totowa, NJ

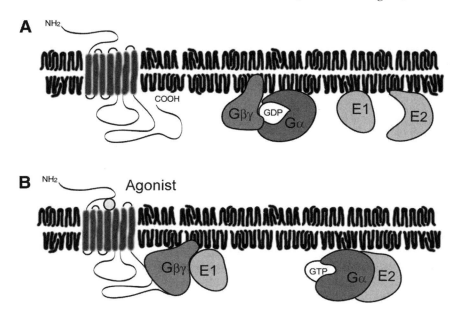

Fig. 1. Classical AR signaling. (**A**) In the absence of agonist, ARs are in the low-affinity state, and G proteins form a heterotrimeric complex bound to guanosine 5′-diphosphate (GDP). Ligand binding allows the formation of a transient complex of activated receptor and G protein. GDP is released from G proteins and is replaced by guanosine 5′-triphosphate (GTP). (**B**) This leads to dissociation of G proteins into G_α- and $G_{\beta\gamma}$-subunits and activation. Both subunits are able to activate different effectors. (*See* Color Plate 2 following p. 148.)

Activation of all types of ARs results in G protein-mediated generation of second messengers or activation of ion channels. By inducing conformational changes in the receptor, agonist stimulation allows interaction with the cognate heterotrimeric G proteins, promoting dissociation of G proteins into G_α- and $G_{\beta\gamma}$-subunits (Fig. 1; *see* Color Plate 2 following p. 148.) and activation.

Both G_α-subunits and $G_{\beta\gamma}$ amplify and propagate signals intracellularly by activating one or more effector molecules (Fig. 1). Examples of effector molecules are adenylyl cyclases (ACs), phospholipases, and ion channels, which in turn generate different second messengers *(1)*. Given the biological relevance of these receptors, it is not surprising that they have evolutionarily developed a highly regulated mechanism to turn off the signal *(1)*. The most well-established mechanism of regulation of ARs is desensitization; a slow instrument for receptor desensitization (hours or days) is receptor downregulation *(1)*, which is the net loss of cell surface receptors *(2,3)*.

Rapid waning of receptor responsiveness (within seconds or minutes) is usually dependent on receptor phosphorylation and uncoupling from its signal-transducing G protein. Phosphorylation can be mediated by second messenger kinases (e.g., protein kinase A [PKA] or protein kinase C [PKC]) which induce non agonist/heterologous desensitization or by a family of G protein-coupled receptors kinases (GRKs) that phosphorylate only agonist-occupied receptors, thereby triggering agonist-specific or homologous desensitization *(1,4)*. The β-adrenergic receptor kinase-1 (β-ARK1), also known as GRK2, is the most abundant GRK expressed in the heart *(5,6)*.

Binding of cytosolic β-ARK to $G_{\beta\gamma}$-subunit of the heterotrimeric G protein facilitates its translocation to the plasma membrane, where it then phosphorylates the agonist-bound receptor *(7)*. GRK-mediated phosphorylation of agonist-occupied GPCRs enhances the affinity of the receptor for interaction with cytosolic proteins known as β-arrestins. Once bound to the receptor, β-arrestins not only interdict further G protein coupling and target the activated receptor for endocytosis *(8)*, but also act as a scaffold, assembling complex cascades, like mitogen-activated protein kinase (MAPK) pathways *(9,10)*.

An important consequence of agonist-mediated receptor phosphorylation is the subsequent endocytosis of agonist-bound receptors into intracellular compartments *(11)*. There is now growing evidence that phosphatidyl-inositol phospholipids play an important role in receptor endocytosis. It has been demonstrated that β-ARK1 and phosphatidylinositol-3 kinase (PI3K) form a cytosolic complex *(12)*. On agonist binding to the receptor and release of $G_{\beta\gamma}$-subunits, β-ARK1 translocates to the membrane and mediates the translocation of PI3K to the receptor complex, where it generates D-3 phosphoinositides that regulate receptor internalization (Fig. 2; *see* Color Plate 3 following p. 148.) *(12)*. Disruption of β-ARK1/PI3K complex prevents translocation of endogenous PI3K and markedly attenuates β_2-AR endocytosis *(13)*, demonstrating that production of phosphatidil-inositol-3,4,5-triphosphate at the receptor complex is necessary for efficient receptor endocytosis.

Many human diseases are characterized by alterations in adrenergic signaling. The ability to manipulate gene expression in vivo has been proven to be the most powerful tool to analyze GPCR function (Tables 1–3). Overexpression of nonmutated ARs in transgenic mice has been useful to characterize the mechanisms of receptor activation and the functional consequences of receptor overexpression. The creation of transgenic animals bearing engineered mutations or naturally occurring polymorphisms of ARs can be also used to elucidate the role of specific domains or residues in terms of receptor function. More important, overexpression mouse models, as well as knockout studies, have been invaluable to determine the role of specific AR subtypes and to identify potential novel therapeutic strategies.

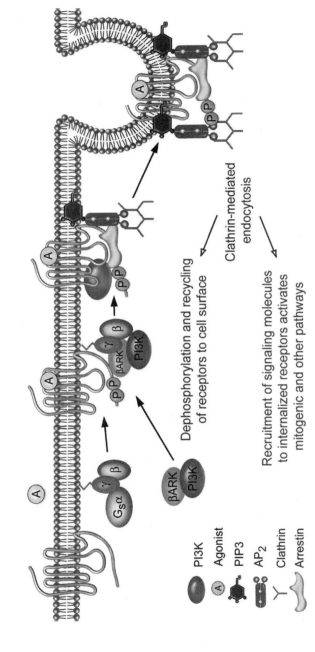

Fig. 2. Major mechanisms involved in β-AR desensitization and internalization. AP2, adaptor protein 2; β-ARK, β-adrenergic receptor kinase; PI3K, phosphatidylinositol-3 kinase; PIP₃, phosphatidyl-inositol-3,4,5-triphosphate. (*See* Color Plate 3 following p. 148.)

Table 1

Physiological Effects of Altering α_1-Adrenergic Receptor Gene Expression In Vivo

| Gene | Transgenic overexpression | | Knockout |
	Promoter/Receptor	Phenotype	Phenotype
α_{1A}	αMHC, WT	↑ Cardiac contractility (29)	↓ Resting blood pressure (43) ↓ Pressor response to catecholamines (43)
α_{1B}	αMHC, CA	Cardiac hypertrophy (35)	↓ Pressor response to catecholamines (34) ↓ Memory and activity (120)
	αMHC, WT Isogenic promoter	Cardiac dysfunction (37) Cardiac hypertrophy (39) ↓ Catecholamines levels (39) Hypotension (39) Autonomic failure (47) Neurodegeneration (47)	
α_{1D}			Modest resting hypotension (44) ↓ Pressor response to catecholamines (44) ↓ Arterial contractility (44) ↓ Hypertension after nephrectomy and salt loading (121) ↓ Nociception (122)

CA, constitutively active; αMHC, α-myosin heavy chain; WT, wild-type receptor. Isogenic promoter: constructs including 5′ flanking regions of the endogenous gene were used.

Table 2
Physiological Effects of Altering α_2-Adrenergic Receptor Gene Expression In Vivo

Gene	Transgenic overexpression		Knockout
	Promoter/Receptor	Phenotype	Phenotype
α_{2A}	αMHC, α_{2A}-D79N	↓ Pressor and bradycardic response to α_2-agonists (51) ↓ Sedation and analgesia (66,67) ↑ Development of seizures (65)	↓ Pressor and bradycardic response to α_2-agonists (58) Resting tachycardia (58) ↓ β-AR density (58) ↓ Tissue NE (58)
α_{2B}			Abolished hypertensive response to α_2-agonists (60) ↓ Hypertension after nephrectomy and salt loading (62)
α_{2C}	Isogenic promoter	Impaired escape strategies (71,72) ↓ Dopamine and homovanillic acid levels (68) ↓ Locomotor activity (69)	Normal hypotensive, hypertensive, and bradycardic response to α_2-agonists (59) ↑ Dopamine and homovanillic acid levels (68) ↑ Locomotor activity (69)
α_{2A} and α_{2C}			Cardiac hypertrophy (61) ↓ Cardiac contractility (61) ↑ Plasma catecholamine levels (61)

αMHC, α-myosin heavy chain; NE, norepinephrine. Isogenic promoter: constructs including 5′ flanking regions of the endogenous gene were used.

Table 3
Physiological Effects of Altering β-Adrenergic Receptor Gene Expression In Vivo

Gene	Transgenic overexpression		Knockout
	Promoter/Receptor (Fold overexpression)	Phenotype	Phenotype
β_1	αMHC, WT	Cardiac hypertrophy (94,95) ↑ Cardiac fibrosis (94,95) and apoptosis (95) Cardiac dysfunction (94,95)	↑ Intrauterine mortality (75) ↓ Inotropic and chronotropic response to ISO (75)
β_2	αMHC, WT (>350) αMHC, WT (>60) αMHC, WT (>60, >100, >150, 300)	Baseline maximal β-AR signaling activation (98) Fibrotic dilated cardiomyopathy (99) ↑ Baseline AC activity and contractility (99) ↑ NaF/Forskolin induced AC activity (99)	↓ Hypotensive response to ISO (78) ↑ Hypertension during exercise (78)
β_1/β_2			↓↓ Chronotropic response to ISO (123) ↓↓ Hypotensive response to ISO (123) Downregulation of muscarinic receptors (123)
β_3	αMHC, WT Downregulation of β₁-ARs (118) Upregulation of β₁-ARs (79)	↑ AC activity and contractility on β₃ stimulation (118) ↑ Fat stores on high-fat diet (80)	↑ Fat stores (79)

AC, adenylyl cyclase; ISO, isoproterenol; αMHC, α-myosin heavy chain; WT, wild-type receptor.

2. α_1-Adrenergic Receptors

The α_1-ARs are expressed in many tissues and play a major role in a variety of physiological processes, including blood pressure regulation, myocardial inotropy/chronotropy, and neuronal function. Three different genes, corresponding to three α_1-AR subtypes, have been cloned so far (α_{1A}-, α_{1B}-, and α_{1D}-ARs). α_{1A}-ARs are abundantly expressed in human liver, heart, cerebellum, cerebral cortex, and prostate *(14–16)*. α_{1B}-AR messenger ribonucleic acid (mRNA) is present at high levels in human spleen and kidney; α_{1D}-AR mRNA is abundant in human aorta *(17)*. Stimulation of α_1-ARs activates multiple signaling pathways. All three cloned α_1-AR subtypes are capable of activating calcium signaling by interacting with G proteins of the G_q family, leading to the activation of phospholipase C *(18)* and the hydrolysis of membrane-bound phosphoinositol 4,5-biphosphate, generating diacylglycerol (DAG) and inositol-1,4,5-triphosphate. Although DAG is a potent activator of protein kinase C, inositol-1,4,5-triphosphate stimulates the release of calcium from intracellular stores. In addition to mobilizing intracellular calcium, α_1-ARs have been shown to activate calcium influx via voltage-dependent and -independent calcium channels *(19)*. In addition, α_1-ARs stimulation activates a number of calcium- and calmodulin-sensitive kinases *(20)*, as well as phospholipase D *(21)*. There is also evidence that pertussis toxin (PTX)-sensitive G proteins (G_i) mediate α_1-adrenergic actions *(22)*.

In addition to modulating calcium movements and smooth muscle contraction, the α_1-ARs are also involved in cell growth and hypertrophy. Stimulation of α_1-ARs in cardiac myocytes induces protein synthesis, expression of immediate-early genes, and reactivation of embryonic genes *(23,24)*. The three α_1-AR subtypes also seem to differently activate enzymes of the MAPK family *(25)*. Because of the lack of subtype-selective drugs, the functional implications of α_1-AR heterogeneity remain largely unknown. To address this issue, several mouse strains with genetic alterations of α-ARs have been reported.

2.1. α_1-ARs and Cardiac Function

In the heart, all three α_1-AR subtypes have been identified at the mRNA level, but only α_{1A} and α_{1B} appear to be translated and functional *(26)*. A large body of evidence indicates that α_{1A}-ARs are very important in the hypertrophic growth response in vitro *(27,28)*. An important possible role for α_1-ARs in the heart is as an alternate source of inotropic reserve in pathophysiological conditions in which the β-adrenergic system is desensitized. Transgenic overexpression of the wild-type (WT) α_{1A}-AR under the α-myosin heavy chain (αMHC) promoter induced marked enhancement of cardiac contractility (Fig. 3A) that could be completely reversed by acute α_{1A}-AR blockade but not β-AR blockade (Fig. 3B) *(29)*. Surprisingly, despite the change in cardiac contractility, the α_{1A} transgenic mice did not display any morphological, histological, or echocardiographic signs

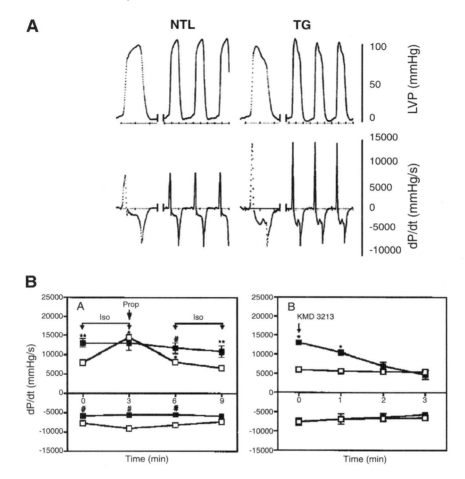

Fig. 3. α_{1A}-AR overexpression induces enhanced contractility but not cardiac hypertrophy. **(A)** Representative left ventricular pressure (LVP) and dP/dT tracings from transgenic animals (TG) and nontransgenic littermates (NTL). A slower recording speed is shown at the beginning. **(B)** In vivo effects of ISO administration before and after complete β-AR blockade with propanolol (left panel) in NTL (open square) and TG (closed square) mice. Effects of selective α_{1A}-AR blocker KMD3213 on +dP/dT and −dP/dT are shown in the right panel. (From ref. *29*; © 2001 Lippincott Williams & Wilkins.)

of cardiac hypertrophy *(29)*, and expression of hypertrophy-associated genes was unchanged *(29)*. The dissociation of inotropy and hypertrophy of these mice is quite surprising and contrasts with the marked hypertrophy observed in mice with cardiac overexpression of G_q *(30)* and other G_q-coupled receptors, like angiotensin II receptors *(31)* or with the blunted hypertrophy in mice lacking G_q

signaling *(32)*. Indeed, although α_{1A}- or α_{1B}-AR single-knockout mice did not show changes in cardiac phenotype, double-mutant mice lacking both ARs displayed smaller myocyte and heart sizes *(33)*, indicating that α_{1A}- and α_{1B}-ARs are required for normal postnatal growth of cardiac myocytes.

Stronger evidence for a role of α_{1B}-ARs in cardiac function has been obtained in studies with transgenic mice because the α_{1B}-AR single knockout did not show any remarkable changes in cardiac development or function *(34)*. Mice that overexpressed a constitutively active form of the α_{1B}-AR exhibited a phenotype consistent with cardiac hypertrophy, with increased heart/body weight ratios, myocyte cross-sectional area, and atrial natriuretic factor (ANF) mRNA levels *(35)*. After pressure overload, enhanced activity of α_{1B}-ARs in the heart exerted detrimental effects and accelerated the progression toward heart failure *(36)*. Surprisingly, cardiac hypertrophy was not observed in mice overexpressing the WT form of α_{1B}-ARs, despite an increase in basal myocardial DAG content and ANF expression *(37)*. On the contrary, these mice showed left ventricular dysfunction *(38)* and reduced response to βAR agonist isoproterenol (ISO) in physiology studies *(37)*. Also, significantly attenuated AC activity was observed in membranes from the same animals, both in basal conditions and on ISO stimulation *(37)*. Interestingly, these abnormalities were reversed by PTX treatment, indicating that very high levels of α_{1B}-ARs can lead to coupling to PTX-sensitive G proteins, like G_i *(37)*.

The reasons for these unexpected results are still poorly understood. One possible explanation is that the agonist-independent signaling through the constitutively active α_{1B}-AR differs from the enhanced signaling through over-expressed WT receptors. This was confirmed in transgenic mice overexpressing either the WT or the constitutively active mutant of the α_{1B}-AR gene under control of the isogenic promoter *(39)*. The systemic overexpression of constitutively active α_{1B}-ARs led to left ventricular hypertrophy, cardiac dysfunction, hypotension, and decreased pressor response *(39)*. Plasma epinephrine and norepinephrine were also reduced in these mice, suggesting that the hypotensive and bradycardic phenotype may be a manifestation of the autonomic failure that typically occurs in this model.

2.2. α_1-ARs and Blood Pressure Regulation

All α_1-AR RNA and proteins are expressed on peripheral arteries from humans *(40)*, and α_1-blockers have been used for many years in the treatment of arterial hypertension. Data from isolated vessels have shown that there is considerable diversity in the vascular tree regarding the α_1-subtypes that regulate smooth muscle cells contractions. Although there is little evidence supporting a role for α_{1B}-ARs as mediators of vascular contraction, α_{1A}-ARs have been shown to regulate both renal and caudal arteries *(41,42)*, and α_{1D}-ARs have been implicated in the contraction of the aorta, femoral, iliac, and superior mesenteric arteries *(41,42)*. The gene knockout approach has been used to test the role of individual α_1-AR subtypes in blood pressure regulation and the functional redundancy among receptor subtypes. Mice with a deletion of the α_{1A}-, α_{1B}-, or α_{1D}-AR gene have been generated *(34,43,44)*, as well as double-knockout mice for α_{1A} and α_{1B} *(33)* (for details on knockouts studies, *see* chapter 10). Knockout of the α_{1A}-receptor caused reduced blood pressure at rest and following infusion of catecholamines *(43)*, and similar findings were shown in the mouse model lacking the α_{1D}-ARs *(44)*.

Although α_{1B}-knockout mice showed significantly reduced blood pressure, they displayed reduced, instead of increased, systemic arterial blood pressure compared to WT *(39)* and a normal contractile response of mesenteric segments to α_1-agonists *(39)*. The mechanism of the hypotension is likely the autonomic failure that characterizes the α_{1B}-transgenic mice, indicating that α_{1B}-ARs are not significant players in vasoconstriction.

2.3. α_1-ARs and Neurological Function

Although localization of each α_1-AR subtype has been described in rat, mouse, and human central nervous systems by different techniques *(16,17)*, little is known about the functional roles of the distinct α_1-ARs subtypes in the central nervous system. Pharmacological studies have shown that α_1-ARs play a functional role in the control of motor activity *(45)* and cognitive functions *(46)*. Interestingly, isogenic overexpression of the α_{1B}-subtype induced a neurodegenerative phenotype with symptoms and histology similar to the parkinsonian degenerative disease called multiple system atrophy *(47)*. These mice also displayed a grand mal seizure disorder that is not typically seen in multiple system atrophy and might actually be a species-related manifestation of the disease *(47)*. The neurodegenerative phenotype could be partially rescued by the α_1-AR antagonist terazosin, suggesting that α_1-ARs antagonists might have a potential therapeutic role in the treatment of neurodegenerative disorders *(47)*.

3. α_2-Adrenergic Receptors

α_2-ARs play an important role in multiple physiological functions, especially in the cardiovascular and central nervous systems. α_2-ARs are highly expressed in the rostral ventrolateral medulla *(48)*, on vascular smooth muscle cells *(49)*, and in nerve terminals *(50)*. Within all AR subtypes, α_2-receptors are the only presynaptic inhibitory ARs described.

Centrally, α_2-AR agonists decrease sympathetic outflow and reduce arterial blood pressure and heart rate by acting at the presynaptic level and inhibiting norepinephrine release *(51)*. In the periphery, stimulation of α_2-ARs on vascular smooth muscle cells induces a transient hypertensive response by causing vasoconstriction *(52)*. By coupling to G_i, α_2-ARs inhibit AC activity *(53)* and activate

G protein-gated K^+ channels *(54)*, resulting in membrane hyperpolarization. α_2-ARs can also inhibit voltage-sensitive Ca^{2+} channels by coupling to G_o *(55)*. Three different subtypes of α_2-AR have been identified on the basis of pharmacology *(56)* and molecular cloning *(57)*: α_{2A}, α_{2B}, and α_{2C}. Genetic approaches using deletions, mutations, or overexpression of specific α_2-AR subtypes have elucidated subtype-specific functions. Mice with deletions of α_{2A}-, α_{2B}-, and α_{2C}-subtypes have been generated *(58–60)*, as have double-knockout mice, in which both α_{2A} and α_{2C} *(61)* have been deleted. Mice overexpressing a mutated form of the α_{2A}-AR gene (α_{2A}-D79N) were also developed *(51)*, and they served as another functional knockout.

3.1. α_2-ARs and Cardiovascular Function

Studies in both α_{2A}-knockout and α_{2A}-D79N-overexpressing mice indicated that the α_{2A}-subtype is the principal mediator of the classical effects of α_2-ARs agonists. In fact, in both α_{2A}-knockout and α_{2A}-D79N-overexpressing mice, the hypotensive response after administration of α_2-AR agonists was abolished, and the bradycardic response was significantly reduced (Fig. 4) *(51,58)*. In contrast to the α_{2A}-D79N-overexpressing mice, which retained some α_{2A}-AR function, α_{2A}-knockout mice displayed basal tachycardia, and treatment with propanolol abolished the difference in heart rate compared to their WT littermates. These data suggest that the tachycardia was caused by increased sympathetic tone, most likely because of reduced presynaptic inhibition of norepinephrine release *(51,58)*.

Compared to other subtypes, considerably less is known about α_{2B}-ARs. The α_{2B}-ARs appear to have an important role in eliciting the hypertensive response to α_2-adrenergic agonists because in α_{2B}-knockout mice this response was abolished, and the hypotensive effect was immediate and accentuated *(60)*. Moreover, α_{2B}-ARs have been implicated in salt-induced hypertension because α_{2B}-knockout mice showed little hypertensive response after subtotal nephrectomy and dietary salt loading compared to WT mice *(62)*.

3.2. α_2-ARs and Neurological Function

Several lines of evidence support a role for α_{2A}-ARs in sedation, nociception, and development of seizures *(63–65)*. For example, α_{2A}-D79N-overexpressing mice treated with α_2-ARs agonists were unable to induce sedation and analgesia *(66,67)*, and in a kindling model of epileptogenesis, α_{2A}-D79N mice achieved kindling more rapidly and showed a twofold increase in the duration of their seizures *(65)*.

α_{2C}-ARs seem to be exclusively expressed in the central nervous system and do not appear to play a major direct role in the cardiovascular system. The effect of altered α_{2C}-AR overexpression has been tested in several behavioral systems.

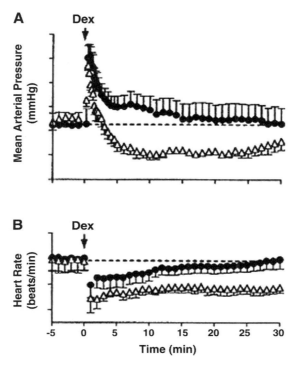

Fig. 4. Hemodynamic effects of nonselective α_2-agonist infusion in WT and α_{2A}-D79N mice. (**A**) Infusion of nonselective α_2-agonist dexmedetomidine (Dex) in unrestrained, conscious, WT (open triangle) mice produced a biphasic blood pressure response. (**B**) Dexmedetomidine failed to reduce blood pressure in α_{2A}-D79N overexpressing mice (closed circle) and administration of α_2-agonist caused a marked decrease in heart rate in both groups of mice, but the maximal bradycardic response to dexmedetomidine was significantly reduced in mice overexpressing α_{2A}-D79N compared to WT. (Reprinted with permission from ref. *51*. © 1996 AAAS.)

The α_{2C}-knockout and -overexpressing mice showed opposite effects on dopamine and homovanillic acid levels, suggesting that α_{2C}-ARs may regulate the dopamine system in the brain *(68)*. Also, α_{2C}-knockout mice showed increased locomotor activity in response to amphetamine challenge compared to WT mice, whereas mice overexpressing α_{2C}-ARs displayed an opposite phenotype *(69)*. In a forced swimming test used to test behavioral despair, opposite effects were also observed in mice that were either knockout or overexpressing α_{2C}-ARs, suggesting a role for these receptors and stress-dependent depression *(70)*. α_{2C}-ARs were impaired in spatial and nonspatial water maze tests, and α_2-antagonist treatment fully reversed this abnormality *(71)*, supporting the concept that these receptors are involved in modulating motor behavior *(71,72)*. Unfortunately, in all the behavioral systems tested, it is unclear whether the α_{2C}-ARs exerted a direct effect or rather influenced metabolism or the regulation of other neurotransmitter systems.

4. β-Adrenergic Receptors

All three subtypes of β-ARs are expressed in the heart *(73)*. Despite the existence of species-related differences (reviewed in ref. *74*), β_1-ARs are the predominant form of ARs. The positive chronotropic and inotropic response of the heart to catecholamine stimulation is mediated almost exclusively by β_1-ARs *(75–77)*. Coupling of β_2-ARs to cardiac contractility is less defined and species related, showing a positive effect in human hearts *(77)* but not affecting contractility in the mouse *(75)*. Better defined is the role of β_2-ARs in the regulation of vascular tone and blood pressure *(78)*. β_3-ARs, "atypical β-ARs," are expressed in the adipose tissue, where they mediate lipolysis and thermogenesis *(79,80)*, and in smooth muscle cells, where they mediate vasorelaxation *(81)*.

All known β-AR subtypes couple to G_s and activate AC, resulting in elevated cyclic adenosine 5′-monophosphate (cAMP) levels and subsequent activation of PKA (reviewed in ref. *82*). PKA activation is a critical step in the mediation of contractility through phosphorylation of L-type calcium channels and regulation of calcium influx and reuptake (reviewed in ref. *74*). Despite the dominant role of the G_s/AC/cAMP pathway in β-AR signaling (particularly that of β_1-ARs), different subtypes of β-ARs are capable of coupling to other G proteins, thereby activating more than one intracellular signaling pathway. In addition to G_s, β_2-ARs were shown to couple to G_i both in vitro *(83)* and in the heart *(74,84–86)*. A large body of data indicates that β_2-ARs have the capacity to utilize alternative compensatory mechanisms under conditions of altered/defective β-AR/G_s/AC coupling *(87–89)*.

4.1. β_1 and β_2 Adrenergic Receptors

β-AR abnormalities have been recognized in a number of human diseases. Undoubtedly, the alterations that take place during the progression of heart failure are the best studied and characterized *(90)*. Bristow et al. first observed in the failing human heart a reduction of cardiac β_1-AR density and desensitization of the remaining receptors *(91)*. Chronic exposure to high levels of circulating catecholamines during heart failure results in marked impairment in the ability of both β_1- and β_2-ARs to couple to their respective G proteins *(92)*. Studies in transgenic animals overexpressing G_s confirmed that increased signaling in the β-AR/G_s/AC pathway initially leads to increased cardiac function but is detrimental to the heart in the long run *(93)*. Overexpression of β_1-ARs in a transgenic mouse model was also shown to cause hypertrophy and interstitial fibrosis in

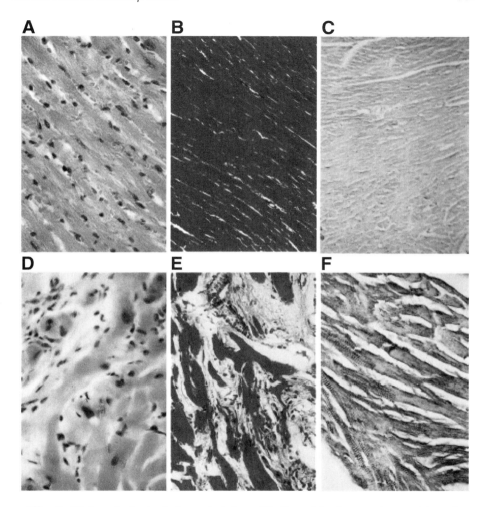

Fig. 5. Histopathological characteristics of left ventricular specimens taken from mice overexpressing the human β_1-AR. The upper panels show (**A**) H&E stain, (**B**) Masson's Trichrome stain, and (**C**) signal for epitope-tagged human β_1-AR protein in control hearts. The lower panels (**D–F**) show representative sections from transgenic mice overexpressing the human β_1-AR. (*See* Color Plate 4 following p. 148; from ref. *95*, © 2000, with permission from Elsevier.)

young animals (Fig. 5; *see* Color Plate 4 following p. 148.), which proceeded to cardiac dysfunction (~50% reduction in contractility) as the animals aged *(94,95)*. Hemodynamic studies in these mice showed that, although maximal contractility and rate of isovolumic relaxation were initially increased in young animals, systolic and diastolic functions were already impaired and progressed to a steady decline of left ventricular contractility and relaxation *(96)*. Although overexpression of WT β_1-AR in the healthy myocardium clearly is deleterious, it remains to be determined whether it is advantageous under conditions of chronic downregulation.

As opposed to a specific marked downregulation of β_1-ARs, there is no significant change in the levels of β_2-ARs in the failing heart *(92)*. The result is a change in the ratio of β_1- to β_2-ARs and suggests a prominent role for β_2-ARs when β_1-AR signaling is suppressed. Importantly, failing hearts also display a significant elevation in the levels of G_i *(97)*. Because β_1-:β_2-AR ratios are significantly altered in heart failure, coupling of β_2-ARs to G_i is likely to play an important role in heart failure pathophysiology.

Several studies addressed the issue of whether β_2-ARs are advantageous or deleterious during cardiac hypertrophy and failure. Mice with extremely high levels of β_2-ARs in the myocardium (200- to 350-fold over endogenous levels) *(98)* displayed a phenotype of maximal activation of β-AR signaling in basal conditions, with no additional response to ISO stimulation (Fig. 6) *(98)*. It is possible that the activation of the receptors in the absence of agonist was caused by the extremely high expression levels, causing an increase in spontaneously isomerized receptors in the active conformation. However, lower levels of β_2-ARs (60 times higher) also resulted in enhanced AC activation and cardiac function *(99)*. Enhanced baseline function in these mice occurred in the absence of any pathological signs over a 1-yr period *(99)*. Conversely, mice with 350 times higher expression levels of β_2-ARs showed rapidly progressive fibrosis, heart failure, and premature death *(99)*.

Interestingly, intrinsic receptor activity was observed only in the highest expression levels line *(99)*, suggesting that expression of β_2-ARs at a level that improves cardiac performance but is not associated with ligand-independent signaling may be beneficial without exerting long-term deleterious effects. Importantly, in all β_2-AR-overexpressing lines, cyclase activity was reduced on forskolin/NaF stimulation, suggesting that significant coupling to G_i takes place in these animals *(37,98,99)*. Indeed, disruption of G_i signaling by PTX was found to totally rescue the contractile response to β_2-agonists in ventricular myocytes from β_2-AR-overexpressing mice *(74)*, suggesting that β_2-AR/G_i coupling contributes to adequate regulation of contractility. It is important that failing hearts also display a significant elevation in the levels of G_i *(97)*. Because β_1-:β_2-AR ratios are significantly altered in heart failure, coupling of β_2-AR to G_i is likely to play an important role in heart failure pathophysiology. For example, it has been demonstrated that although activation of β_1-AR in mouse cardiac myocytes leads to cellular apoptosis, β_2-AR stimulation results in activation of a G_i-$G_{\beta\gamma}$-PI3K-mediated survival pathway *(100,101)* (reviewed in ref. *102*). Therefore, it has been suggested that β_2-AR/G_i coupling may act to activate a protective

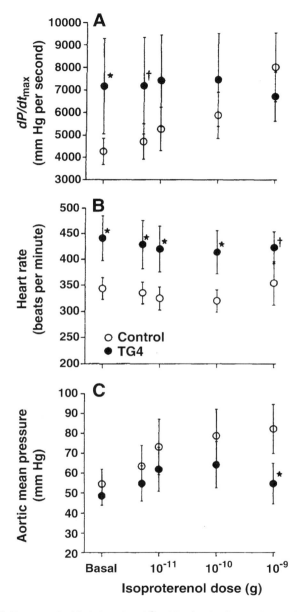

Fig. 6. Extremely high levels of β_2-ARs in the heart determine maximal activation of β-AR signaling in basal conditions. Mice overexpressing at very high levels of β_2-ARs (TG4, open circle; $\bigcirc$) and corresponding WT controls (control, closed circle; $\bullet$) were anesthetized, and their hemodynamic parameters were invasively studied: **(A)** dp/dt max; **(B)** heart rate; **(C)** aortic mean pressure. (Reprinted with permission from ref. *98;* © 1994 AAAS.)

antiapoptotic pathway during hyperactivation of β_1-ARs by excess catecholamines *(103)*.

In this regard, adenoviral-mediated transfer of the human β_2-ARs to ventricular myocytes from chronically paced rabbits led to restoration of β-AR signaling in vitro *(37)*. Hence, expression of β_2-ARs may be advantageous in some conditions and deleterious in others, depending on the expression levels and on the types of signals that are initiated.

Besides downregulation of β_1-ARs, human failing hearts are characterized by profound desensitization of remaining receptors *(92,104)*. Desensitization of ARs in patients with heart failure is attributed in part to a significant increase in the levels of β-adrenergic receptor kinase (ARK) 1 *(105)*. The role of β-ARK1 in myocardial contractility and its potential therapeutic role have been studied extensively (for reviews, *see* refs. *13,106,107*) and is not discussed here. Because recent data have shown that β-ARK1 and PI3K form a cytosolic complex that is recruited to the membrane on agonist binding *(12)*, long-term pressure overload in transgenic mice has been used as a model to study the role of PI3K in the transition from hypertrophy to heart failure. These experiments showed that short-term transverse aortic constriction (TAC) results in specific activation of p110γ (PI3Kγ) *(108)*. Activation of PI3Kγ on pressure overload was completely absent in mice overexpressing the C-terminus of β-ARK (β-ARKct), which binds and sequesters $G_{\beta\gamma}$-subunits *(6)*, suggesting that PI3K activation in pressure overload is $G_{\beta\gamma}$ dependent *(108)*.

The evidence that PI3Kγ is activated during the hypertrophic process and that it may play a role in the transition to heart failure led to the investigation of the hypothesis that downregulation of β-ARs under conditions of chronic catecholamine stimulation can be prevented through interference with PI3K interaction with the receptor complex *(109)*. By displacing endogenous PI3K from β-ARK, transgenic overexpression of the catalytically inactive mutant of PI3Kγ prevented the development of heart failure after pressure overload (Fig. 7) *(109)*. These data establish a novel role for receptor-localized PI3K in regulation of β-AR turnover in vivo and show that a strategy that blocks membrane association of PI3K may provide a novel therapeutic approach to restore normal β-AR signaling and preserve cardiac function.

Besides the effects of receptor levels, it is becoming evident that genetic heterogeneity in the structure of both β_1- and β_2-ARs has a remarkable effect on heart failure predisposition. Human β_1-ARs were found to be polymorphic at amino acid residue 389 (substitute of Arg to Gly). Overexpression of the Arg389 in mice was found to induce an initial increase in receptor function and contractility, followed by marked deterioration in both parameters, suggesting predisposition of Arg389 to heart failure *(110)*. Together with the findings in β_1-AR-overexpressing mice *(94,95)*, these results suggest that initial hyper-

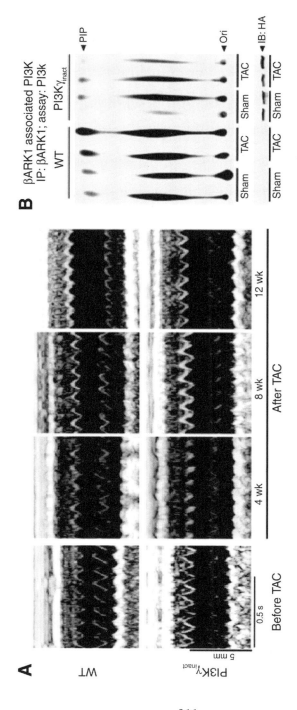

Fig. 7. Displacement of endogenous PI3K from β-ARK prevents the development of heart failure after pressure overload. (**A**) Representative echocardiograms in conscious wild-type (WT) and transgenic mice overexpressing a catalytically inactive mutant of PI3Kγ after 4, 8, and 12 wk of pressure overload. (**B**) β-ARK-associated PI3K activity in membrane fractions from hearts of WT and transgenic mice overexpressing a catalytically inactive mutant of PI3Kγ. (From ref. *109*, with permission.)

stimulation of the β_1-AR system may culminate in depressed receptor function and ventricular dysfunction.

4.2. β_3-Adrenergic Receptors

β_3-ARs, "atypical β-ARs," are highly expressed in the white and brown adipose tissue *(111)* to induce lipolysis or thermogenesis by coupling mainly to G_s. In cultured adipocytes, they have also been shown to couple to G_i and activate the MAPK pathway with a cAMP-independent mechanism *(112)*. Two distinguishing features of β_3-ARs are (1) much lower affinity for catecholamines compared to other β-ARs and (2) relative resistance to desensitization and downregulation. The β_3-selective agonists potently stimulate energy expenditure, and a missense mutation in the human β_3-AR gene has been associated with obesity, reduced insulin sensitivity, and earlier onset of non-insulin-dependent diabetes *(113–115)*. Mice with targeted disruption of β_3-ARs completely lacked AC activation on selective β_3-agonist stimulation and showed an increase in fat stores *(79)*. Interestingly, β_3 knockout mice also showed a selective upregulation of β_1-AR mRNA, indicating that cross talk between β_1- and β_3-gene expression exists *(79)*.

Although β_3-ARs have been detected in both murine and human hearts, their physiological role in the regulation of cardiac function is still not well understood. Stimulation of human ventricular biopsies with β_3-agonists induced a PTX-sensitive negative inotropic effect *(116)*, initially suggesting that, in the heart, β_3-ARs are preferentially coupled to G_i. Similarly, ISO infusion induced an augmented contractile response in β_3-knockout mice compared with WT littermates *(117)*, indicating that β_3-adrenergic stimulation can lead to a negative inotropic effect. However, in transgenic mice with cardiac-specific overexpression of the human β_3-AR, stimulation with selective β_3-agonist induced a significant increase in AC activity and cardiac *(118)* and basal contractility, investigated with a load-independent pressure–volume loop analysis, showed similar cardiac function in β_3-overexpressing mice and their WT littermates *(118)*. β_3-AR-overexpressing mice were also characterized by 50% downregulation of endogenous β_1-ARs *(118)*, confirming a previously described compensatory regulation between β_1- and β_3-gene expression *(79)*. Moreover, PTX had no effect on the enhancement of cardiac contractility to β_3-agonists, indicating little coupling to G_i. The reason for the discrepancy between these studies is not clear but may be caused by the use of different selective β_3-agonists or species differences.

Interestingly, unlike β_1-ARs, β_3-ARs are upregulated in human heart failure *(119)*. Taken together, these studies highlight a potential therapeutic role for β_3-ARs in heart failure by providing receptors that are functionally inactive in basal conditions and become activated on selective agonist administration.

References

1. Rockman HA, Koch WJ, Lefkowitz RJ. Seven-transmembrane-spanning receptors and heart function. Nature 2002;415:206–212.
2. Pitcher JA, Freedman NJ, Lefkowitz RJ. G protein-coupled receptor kinases. Annu Rev Biochem 1998;67:653–692.
3. Lefkowitz RJ. G protein-coupled receptors. III. New roles for receptor kinases and β-arrestins in receptor signaling and desensitization. J Biol Chem 1998;273: 18,677–18,680.
4. Prasad SV, Perrino C, Rockman HA. Role of phosphoinositide 3-kinase in cardiac function and heart failure. Trends Cardiovasc Med 2003;13:206–212.
5. Inglese J, Freedman NJ, Koch WJ, Lefkowitz RJ. Structure and mechanism of the G protein-coupled receptor kinases. J Biol Chem 1993;268:23,735–23,738.
6. Iaccarino G, Rockman HA, Shotwell KF, Tomhave ED, Koch WJ. Myocardial overexpression of GRK3 in transgenic mice: evidence for in vivo selectivity of GRKs. Am J Physiol 1998;275:H1298–H1306.
7. Perry SJ, Lefkowitz RJ. Arresting developments in heptahelical receptor signaling and regulation. Trends Cell Biol 2002;12:130–138.
8. Laporte SA, Oakley RH, Holt JA, Barak LS, Caron MG. The interaction of β-arrestin with the AP-2 adaptor is required for the clustering of β$_2$-adrenergic receptor into clathrin-coated pits. J Biol Chem 2000;275:23,120–23,126.
9. Luttrell LM, Ferguson SS, Daaka Y, et al. β-arrestin-dependent formation of β$_2$ adrenergic receptor-Src protein kinase complexes. Science 1999;283:655–661.
10. DeFea KA, Zalevsky J, Thoma MS, Dery O, Mullins RD, Bunnett NW. β-Arrestin-dependent endocytosis of proteinase-activated receptor 2 is required for intracellular targeting of activated ERK1/2. J Cell Biol 2000;148:1267–1281.
11. Claing A, Laporte SA, Caron MG, Lefkowitz RJ. Endocytosis of G protein-coupled receptors: roles of G protein-coupled receptor kinases and β-arrestin proteins. Prog Neurobiol 2002;66:61–79.
12. Naga Prasad SV, Barak LS, Rapacciuolo A, Caron MG, Rockman HA. Agonist-dependent recruitment of phosphoinositide 3-kinase to the membrane by β-adrenergic receptor kinase 1. A role in receptor sequestration. J Biol Chem 2001;276: 18,953–18,959.
13. Naga Prasad SV, Laporte SA, Chamberlain D, Caron MG, Barak L, Rockman HA. Phosphoinositide 3-kinase regulates β$_2$-adrenergic receptor endocytosis by AP-2 recruitment to the receptor/beta-arrestin complex. J Cell Biol 2002;158: 563–575.
14. Forray C, Bard JA, Wetzel JM, et al. The α$_1$-adrenergic receptor that mediates smooth muscle contraction in human prostate has the pharmacological properties of the cloned human alpha 1c subtype. Mol Pharmacol 1994;45:703–708.
15. Faure C, Pimoule C, Vallancien G, Langer SZ, Graham D. Identification of α$_1$-adrenoceptor subtypes present in the human prostate. Life Sci 1994;54:1595–1605.
16. Garcia-Sainz JA, Romero-Avila MT, Torres-Marquez ME. Characterization of the human liver α$_1$-adrenoceptors: predominance of the α$_{1A}$ subtype. Eur J Pharmacol 1995;289:81–86.

17. Price DT, Lefkowitz RJ, Caron MG, Berkowitz D, Schwinn DA. Localization of mRNA for three distinct α_1-adrenergic receptor subtypes in human tissues: implications for human a adrenergic physiology. Mol Pharmacol 1994;45:171–175.

18. Wu D, Katz A, Lee CH, Simon MI. Activation of phospholipase C by α_1- adrenergic receptors is mediated by the α subunits of G_q family. J Biol Chem 1992;267: 25,798–25,802.

19. Minneman KP. α_1-Adrenergic receptor subtypes, inositol phosphates, and sources of cell Ca^{2+}. Pharmacol Rev 1988;40:87–119.

20. Stull JT, Bowman BF, Gallagher PJ, et al. Myosin phosphorylation in smooth and skeletal muscles: regulation and function. Prog Clin Biol Res 1990;327:107–126.

21. Llahi S, Fain JN. α_1-Adrenergic receptor-mediated activation of phospholipase D in rat cerebral cortex. J Biol Chem 1992;267:3679–3685.

22. Perez DM, DeYoung MB, Graham RM. Coupling of expressed α_{1B}- and α_{1D}-adrenergic receptor to multiple signaling pathways is both G protein and cell type specific. Mol Pharmacol 1993;44:784–795.

23. Simpson P. Norepinephrine-stimulated hypertrophy of cultured rat myocardial cells is an α_1 adrenergic response. J Clin Invest 1983;72:732–738.

24. Starksen NF, Simpson PC, Bishopric N, et al. Cardiac myocyte hypertrophy is associated with c-myc protooncogene expression. Proc Natl Acad Sci USA 1986; 83:8348–8350.

25. Zhong H, Minneman KP. Differential activation of mitogen-activated protein kinase pathways in PC12 cells by closely related α_1-adrenergic receptor subtypes. J Neurochem 1999;72:2388–2396.

26. Graham RM, Perez DM, Hwa J, Piascik MT. α_1-Adrenergic receptor subtypes. Molecular structure, function, and signaling. Circ Res 1996;78:737–749.

27. Knowlton KU, Michel MC, Itani M, et al. The α_{1A}-adrenergic receptor subtype mediates biochemical, molecular, and morphologic features of cultured myocardial cell hypertrophy. J Biol Chem 1993;268:15,374–15,380.

28. Autelitano DJ, Woodcock EA. Selective activation of α_{1A}-adrenergic receptors in neonatal cardiac myocytes is sufficient to cause hypertrophy and differential regulation of α_1-adrenergic receptor subtype mRNAs. J Mol Cell Cardiol 1998;30: 1515–1523.

29. Lin F, Owens WA, Chen S, et al. Targeted α_{1A} adrenergic receptor overexpression induces enhanced cardiac contractility but not hypertrophy. Circ Res 2001;89:343–350.

30. D'Angelo DD, Sakata Y, Lorenz JN, et al. Transgenic $G_{\alpha q}$ overexpression induces cardiac contractile failure in mice. Proc Natl Acad Sci USA 1997;94:8121–8126.

31. Paradis P, Dali-Youcef N, Paradis FW, Thibault G, Nemer M. Overexpression of angiotensin II type I receptor in cardiomyocytes induces cardiac hypertrophy and remodeling. Proc Natl Acad Sci USA 2000;97:931–936.

32. Akhter SA, Luttrell LM, Rockman HA, Iaccarino G, Lefkowitz RJ, Koch WJ. Targeting the receptor–G_q interface to inhibit in vivo pressure overload myocardial hypertrophy. Science 1998;280:574–577.

33. O'Connell TD, Ishizaka S, Nakamura A, et al. The $\alpha_{1A/C}$- and α_{1B}-adrenergic receptors are required for physiological cardiac hypertrophy in the double-knockout mouse. J Clin Invest 2003;111:1783–1791.

34. Cavalli A, Lattion AL, Hummler E, et al. Decreased blood pressure response in mice deficient of the α_{1B}-adrenergic receptor. Proc Natl Acad Sci USA 1997;94: 11,589–11,594.
35. Milano CA, Dolber PC, Rockman HA, et al. Myocardial expression of a constitutively active α_{1B}-adrenergic receptor in transgenic mice induces cardiac hypertrophy. Proc Natl Acad Sci USA 1994;91:10,109–10,113.
36. Wang BH, Du XJ, Autelitano DJ, Milano CA, Woodcock EA. Adverse effects of constitutively active α_{1B} adrenergic receptors after pressure overload in mouse hearts. Am J Physiol Heart Circ Physiol 2000;279:H1079–H1086.
37. Akhter SA, Milano CA, Shotwell KF, et al. Transgenic mice with cardiac overexpression of α_{1B}-adrenergic receptors. In vivo α_1-adrenergic receptor-mediated regulation of β-adrenergic signaling. J Biol Chem 1997;272:21,253–21,259.
38. Grupp IL, Lorenz JN, Walsh RA, Boivin GP, Rindt H. Overexpression of α_{1B}-adrenergic receptor induces left ventricular dysfunction in the absence of hypertrophy. Am J Physiol 1998;275:H1338–H1350.
39. Zuscik MJ, Chalothorn D, Hellard D, et al. Hypotension, autonomic failure, and cardiac hypertrophy in transgenic mice overexpressing the α_{1B}-adrenergic receptor. J Biol Chem 2001;276:13,738–13,743.
40. Rudner XL, Berkowitz DE, Booth JV, et al. Subtype specific regulation of human vascular α_1 adrenergic receptors by vessel bed and age. Circulation 1999;100: 2336–2343.
41. Piascik MT, Hrometz SL, Edelmann SE, Guarino RD, Hadley RW, Brown RD. Immunocytochemical localization of the α_{1B} adrenergic receptor and the contribution of this and the other subtypes to vascular smooth muscle contraction: analysis with selective ligands and antisense oligonucleotides. J Pharmacol Exp Ther 1997; 283:854–868.
42. Hrometz SL, Edelmann SE, McCune DF, et al. Expression of multiple α_1-adrenoceptors on vascular smooth muscle: correlation with the regulation of contraction. J Pharmacol Exp Ther 1999;290:452–463.
43. Rokosh DG, Simpson PC. Knockout of the $\alpha_{1A/C}$-adrenergic receptor subtype: the $\alpha_{1A/C}$ is expressed in resistance arteries and is required to maintain arterial blood pressure. Proc Natl Acad Sci USA 2002;99:9474–9479.
44. Tanoue A, Nasa Y, Koshimizu T, et al. The α_{1D} adrenergic receptor directly regulates arterial blood pressure via vasoconstriction. J Clin Invest 2002;109:765–775.
45. Stone EA, Zhang Y, Rosengarten H, Yeretsian J, Quartermain D. Brain α_1-adrenergic neurotransmission is necessary for behavioral activation to environmental change in mice. Neuroscience 1999;94:1245–1252.
46. Sirvio J, Lahtinen H, Riekkinen P Jr, Riekkinen PJ. Spatial learning and noradrenaline content in the brain and periphery of young and aged rats. Exp Neurol 1994;125:312–315.
47. Zuscik MJ, Sands S, Ross SA, et al. Overexpression of the α_{1B}-adrenergic receptor causes apoptotic neurodegeneration: multiple system atrophy. Nat Med 2000;6: 1388–1394.
48. Guyenet PG, Stornetta RL, Riley T, Norton FR, Rosin DL, Lynch KR. α_{2A}-Adrenergic receptors are present in lower brainstem catecholaminergic and serotonergic neurons innervating spinal cord. Brain Res 1994;638:285–294.

49. Chen DG, Dai XZ, Bache RJ. Postsynaptic adrenoceptor-mediated vasoconstriction in coronary and femoral vascular beds. Am J Physiol 1988;254:H984–H992.

50. Langer SZ. Presynaptic regulation of the release of catecholamines. Pharmacol Rev 1980;32:337–362.

51. MacMillan LB, Hein L, Smith MS, Piascik MT, Limbird LE. Central hypotensive effects of the α_{2A}-adrenergic receptor subtype. Science 1996;273:801–803.

52. Chotani MA, Mitra S, Su BY, et al. Regulation of α_2-adrenoceptors in human vascular smooth muscle cells. Am J Physiol Heart Circ Physiol 2004;286:H59–H67.

53. Bylund DB. Subtypes of α_1- and α_2-adrenergic receptors. FASEB J 1992;6:832–839.

54. Arima J, Kubo C, Ishibashi H, Akaike N. α_2-Adrenoceptor-mediated potassium currents in acutely dissociated rat locus coeruleus neurones. J Physiol 1998;508 (Pt 1):57–66.

55. Caulfield MP, Jones S, Vallis Y, et al. Muscarinic M-current inhibition via $G_{\alpha q}/11$ and α-adrenoceptor inhibition of Ca^{2+} current via G α o in rat sympathetic neurones. J Physiol 1994;477(Pt 3):415–422.

56. Bylund DB. Subtypes of α_2-adrenoceptors: pharmacological and molecular biological evidence converge. Trends Pharmacol Sci 1988;9:356–361.

57. Lomasney JW, Cotecchia S, Lefkowitz RJ, Caron MG. Molecular biology of α-adrenergic receptors: implications for receptor classification and for structure-function relationships. Biochim Biophys Acta 1991;1095:127–139.

58. Altman JD, Trendelenburg AU, MacMillan L, et al. Abnormal regulation of the sympathetic nervous system in α_{2A}-adrenergic receptor knockout mice. Mol Pharmacol 1999;56:154–161.

59. Link RE, Stevens MS, Kulatunga M, Scheinin M, Barsh GS, Kobilka BK. Targeted inactivation of the gene encoding the mouse α_{2C}-adrenoceptor homolog. Mol Pharmacol 1995;48:48–55.

60. Link RE, Desai K, Hein L, et al. Cardiovascular regulation in mice lacking α_2-adrenergic receptor subtypes b and c. Science 1996;273:803–805.

61. Hein L, Altman JD, Kobilka BK. Two functionally distinct α_2-adrenergic receptors regulate sympathetic neurotransmission. Nature 1999;402:181–184.

62. Makaritsis KP, Handy DE, Johns C, Kobilka B, Gavras I, Gavras H. Role of the α_{2B}-adrenergic receptor in the development of salt-induced hypertension. Hypertension 1999;33:14–17.

63. Nicholas AP, Hokfelt T, Pieribone VA. The distribution and significance of CNS adrenoceptors examined with *in situ* hybridization. Trends Pharmacol Sci 1996;17:245–255.

64. Eisenach JC, De Kock M, Klimscha W. α_2 Adrenergic agonists for regional anesthesia. A clinical review of clonidine (1984–1995). Anesthesiology 1996;85:655–674.

65. Janumpalli S, Butler LS, MacMillan LB, Limbird LE, McNamara JO. A point mutation (D79N) of the α_{2A} adrenergic receptor abolishes the antiepileptogenic action of endogenous norepinephrine. J Neurosci 1998;18:2004–2008.

66. Lakhlani PP, MacMillan LB, Guo TZ, et al. Substitution of a mutant α_{2A}-adrenergic receptor via "hit and run" gene targeting reveals the role of this subtype in

sedative, analgesic, and anesthetic-sparing responses in vivo. Proc Natl Acad Sci USA 1997;94:9950–9955.

67. Hunter JC, Fontana DJ, Hedley LR, et al. Assessment of the role of α_2-adrenoceptor subtypes in the antinociceptive, sedative and hypothermic action of dexmedetomidine in transgenic mice. Br J Pharmacol 1997;122:1339–1344.

68. Sallinen J, Link RE, Haapalinna A, et al. Genetic alteration of α_{2C}-adrenoceptor expression in mice: influence on locomotor, hypothermic, and neurochemical effects of dexmedetomidine, a subtype-nonselective α_2-adrenoceptor agonist. Mol Pharmacol 1997;51:36–46.

69. Sallinen J, Haapalinna A, Viitamaa T, Kobilka BK, Scheinin M. d-Amphetamine and L-5-hydroxytryptophan-induced behaviours in mice with genetically-altered expression of the α_{2C}-adrenergic receptor subtype. Neuroscience 1998;86: 959–965.

70. Sallinen J, Haapalinna A, MacDonald E, et al. Genetic alteration of the α_2-adrenoceptor subtype c in mice affects the development of behavioral despair and stress-induced increases in plasma corticosterone levels. Mol Psychiatry 1999;4: 443–452.

71. Bjorklund M, Sirvio J, Riekkinen M, Sallinen J, Scheinin M, Riekkinen P Jr. Overexpression of α_{2C}-adrenoceptors impairs water maze navigation. Neuroscience 2000;95:481–487.

72. Bjorklund M, Sirvio J, Puolivali J, et al. α_{2C}-Adrenoceptor-overexpressing mice are impaired in executing nonspatial and spatial escape strategies. Mol Pharmacol 1998;54:569–576.

73. Brodde OE, Michel MC. Adrenergic and muscarinic receptors in the human heart. Pharmacol Rev 1999;51:651–690.

74. Xiao RP, Avdonin P, Zhou YY, et al. Coupling of β_2-adrenoceptor to G_i proteins and its physiological relevance in murine cardiac myocytes. Circ Res 1999;84: 43–52.

75. Rohrer DK, Desai KH, Jasper JR, et al. Targeted disruption of the mouse β_1-adrenergic receptor gene: developmental and cardiovascular effects. Proc Natl Acad Sci USA 1996;93:7375–7380.

76. Rohrer DK, Schauble EH, Desai KH, Kobilka BK, Bernstein D. Alterations in dynamic heart rate control in the β_1-adrenergic receptor knockout mouse. Am J Physiol 1998;274:H1184–H1193.

77. Brodde OE. β_1- and β_2-adrenoceptors in the human heart: properties, function, and alterations in chronic heart failure. Pharmacol Rev 1991;43:203–242.

78. Chruscinski AJ, Rohrer DK, Schauble E, Desai KH, Bernstein D, Kobilka BK. Targeted disruption of the β_2 adrenergic receptor gene. J Biol Chem 1999;274: 16,694–16,700.

79. Susulic VS, Frederich RC, Lawitts J, et al. Targeted disruption of the β_3-adrenergic receptor gene. J Biol Chem 1995;270:29,483–29,492.

80. Revelli JP, Preitner F, Samec S, et al. Targeted gene disruption reveals a leptin-independent role for the mouse β_3-adrenoceptor in the regulation of body composition. J Clin Invest 1997;100:1098–1106.

81. Guimaraes S, Moura D. Vascular adrenoceptors: an update. Pharmacol Rev 2001;53:319–356.

82. Brodde OE, Michel MC, Zerkowski HR. Signal transduction mechanisms controlling cardiac contractility and their alterations in chronic heart failure. Cardiovasc Res 1995;30:570–584.

83. Abramson SN, Martin MW, Hughes AR, et al. Interaction of β-adrenergic receptors with the inhibitory guanine nucleotide-binding protein of adenylate cyclase in membranes prepared from cyc- S49 lymphoma cells. Biochem Pharmacol 1988;37:4289–4297.

84. Xiao RP, Ji X, Lakatta EG. Functional coupling of the β_2-adrenoceptor to a pertussis toxin-sensitive G protein in cardiac myocytes. Mol Pharmacol 1995;47:322–329.

85. Communal C, Singh K, Sawyer DB, Colucci WS. Opposing effects of β_1 and β_2-adrenergic receptors on cardiac myocyte apoptosis: role of a pertussis toxin-sensitive G protein. Circulation 1999;100:2210–2212.

86. Kilts JD, Gerhardt MA, Richardson MD, et al. β_2 Adrenergic and several other G protein-coupled receptors in human atrial membranes activate both G(s) and G(i). Circ Res 2000;87:705–709.

87. Daaka Y, Luttrell LM, Lefkowitz RJ. Switching of the coupling of the β_2-adrenergic receptor to different G proteins by protein kinase A. Nature 1997;390:88–91.

88. Pavoine C, Magne S, Sauvadet A, Pecker F. Evidence for a β_2-adrenergic/arachidonic acid pathway in ventricular cardiomyocytes. Regulation by the β_1-adrenergic/camp pathway. J Biol Chem 1999;274:628–637.

89. Pavoine C, Behforouz N, Gauthier C, et al. β_2-Adrenergic signaling in human heart: shift from the cyclic AMP to the arachidonic acid pathway. Mol Pharmacol 2003;64:1117–1125.

90. Brodde OE. β-Adrenoceptors in cardiac disease. Pharmacol Ther 1993;60:405–430.

91. Bristow MR, Minobe WA, Raynolds MV, et al. Reduced beta 1 receptor messenger RNA abundance in the failing human heart. J Clin Invest 1993;92:2737–2745.

92. Bristow MR. Why does the myocardium fail? Insights from basic science. Lancet 1998;352(Suppl 1):SI8–SI14.

93. Iwase M, Bishop SP, Uechi M, et al. Adverse effects of chronic endogenous sympathetic drive induced by cardiac $G_{s\alpha}$ overexpression. Circ Res 1996;78:517–524.

94. Engelhardt S, Hein L, Wiesmann F, Lohse MJ. Progressive hypertrophy and heart failure in β_1-adrenergic receptor transgenic mice. Proc Natl Acad Sci USA 1999;96:7059–7064.

95. Bisognano JD, Weinberger HD, Bohlmeyer TJ, et al. Myocardial-directed overexpression of the human β_1 adrenergic receptor in transgenic mice. J Mol Cell Cardiol 2000;32:817–830.

96. Engelhardt S, Boknik P, Keller U, Neumann J, Lohse MJ, Hein L. Early impairment of calcium handling and altered expression of junction in hearts of mice overexpressing the β_1-adrenergic receptor. FASEB J 2001;15:2718–2720.

97. Feldman AM, Cates AE, Veazey WB, et al. Increase of the 40,000-mol wt pertussis toxin substrate (G protein) in the failing human heart. J Clin Invest 1988;82:189–197.

98. Milano CA, Allen LF, Rockman HA, et al. Enhanced myocardial function in transgenic mice overexpressing the β_2-adrenergic receptor. Science 1994;264: 582–586.
99. Liggett SB, Tepe NM, Lorenz JN, et al. Early and delayed consequences of β_2 adrenergic receptor overexpression in mouse hearts: critical role for expression level. Circulation 2000;101:1707–1714.
100. Zhu WZ, Zheng M, Koch WJ, Lefkowitz RJ, Kobilka BK, Xiao RP. Dual modulation of cell survival and cell death by β_2 adrenergic signaling in adult mouse cardiac myocytes. Proc Natl Acad Sci USA 2001;98:1607–1612.
101. Condorelli G, Drusco A, Stassi G, et al. Akt induces enhanced myocardial contractility and cell size in vivo in transgenic mice. Proc Natl Acad Sci USA 2002;99: 12,333–12,338.
102. Singh K, Xiao L, Remondino A, Sawyer DB, Colucci WS. Adrenergic regulation of cardiac myocyte apoptosis. J Cell Physiol 2001;189:257–265.
103. Xiang Y, Devic E, Kobilka B. The PDZ binding motif of the β_1 adrenergic receptor modulates receptor trafficking and signaling in cardiac myocytes. J Biol Chem 2002;277:33,783–33,790.
104. Bristow MR, Minobe WA, Raynolds MV, et al. Reduced β_1 receptor messenger RNA abundance in the failing human heart. J Clin Invest 1993;92:2737–2745.
105. Ungerer M, Bohm M, Elce JS, Erdmann E, Lohse MJ. Altered expression of β-adrenergic receptor kinase and β_1-adrenergic receptors in the failing human heart. Circulation 1993;87:454–463.
106. Iaccarino G, Lefkowitz RJ, Koch WJ. Myocardial G protein-coupled receptor kinases: implications for heart failure therapy. Proc Assoc Am Physicians 1999; 111:399–405.
107. Petrofski JA, Koch WJ. The β-adrenergic receptor kinase in heart failure. J Mol Cell Cardiol 2003;35:1167–1174.
108. Naga Prasad SV, Esposito G, Mao L, Koch WJ, Rockman HA. $G_{\beta\gamma}$-dependent phosphoinositide 3-kinase activation in hearts with in vivo pressure overload hypertrophy. J Biol Chem 2000;275:4693–4698.
109. Nienaber JJ, Tachibana H, Naga Prasad SV, et al. Inhibition of receptor-localized PI3K preserves cardiac β-adrenergic receptor function and ameliorates pressure overload heart failure. J Clin Invest 2003;112:1067–1079.
110. Mialet Perez J, Rathz DA, Petrashevskaya NN, et al. β_1-Adrenergic receptor polymorphisms confer differential function and predisposition to heart failure. Nat Med 2003;9:1300–1305.
111. Strosberg AD. Structure and function of the β_3-adrenergic receptor. Annu Rev Pharmacol Toxicol 1997;37:421–450.
112. Soeder KJ, Snedden SK, Cao W, et al. The β_3-adrenergic receptor activates mitogen-activated protein kinase in adipocytes through a G_i-dependent mechanism. J Biol Chem 1999;274:12,017–12,022.
113. Walston J, Silver K, Bogardus C, et al. Time of onset of non-insulin-dependent diabetes mellitus and genetic variation in the β_3-adrenergic-receptor gene. N Engl J Med 1995;333:343–347.
114. Widen E, Lehto M, Kanninen T, Walston J, Shuldiner AR, Groop LC. Association of a polymorphism in the β_3-adrenergic-receptor gene with features of the insulin resistance syndrome in Finns. N Engl J Med 1995;333:348–351.

115. Clement K, Vaisse C, Manning BS, et al. Genetic variation in the β_3-adrenergic receptor and an increased capacity to gain weight in patients with morbid obesity. N Engl J Med 1995;333:352–354.

116. Gauthier C, Tavernier G, Charpentier F, Langin D, Le Marec H. Functional β_3-adrenoceptor in the human heart. J Clin Invest 1996;98:556–562.

117. Varghese P, Harrison RW, Lofthouse RA, Georgakopoulos D, Berkowitz DE, Hare JM. β_3 Adrenoceptor deficiency blocks nitric oxide-dependent inhibition of myocardial contractility. J Clin Invest 2000;106:697–703.

118. Kohout TA, Takaoka H, McDonald PH, et al. Augmentation of cardiac contractility mediated by the human β_3 adrenergic receptor overexpressed in the hearts of transgenic mice. Circulation 2001;104:2485–2491.

119. Moniotte S, Kobzik L, Feron O, Trochu JN, Gauthier C, Balligand JL. Upregulation of β_3 adrenoceptors and altered contractile response to inotropic amines in human failing myocardium. Circulation 2001;103:1649–1655.

120. Knauber J, Muller WE. Decreased exploratory activity and impaired passive avoidance behaviour in mice deficient for the α_{1B}. Eur Neuropsychopharmacol 2000; 10:423–427.

121. Tanoue A, Koba M, Miyawaki S, et al. Role of the α_{1D}-adrenergic receptor in the development of salt-induced hypertension. Hypertension 2002;40:101–106.

122. Harasawa I, Honda K, Tanoue A, et al. Responses to noxious stimuli in mice lacking α_{1D} adrenergic receptors. Neuroreport 2003;14:1857–1860.

123. Rohrer DK, Chruscinski A, Schauble EH, Bernstein D, Kobilka BK. Cardiovascular and metabolic alterations in mice lacking both β_1- and β_2-adrenergic receptors. J Biol Chem 1999;274:16,701–16,708.

12

Adrenergic Receptor Signaling Components in Gene Therapy

Andrea D. Eckhart and Walter J. Koch

Summary

Adrenergic receptor (AR) signaling is a key regulator of normal cardiopulmonary homeostasis. Under pathophysiological conditions, such as heart failure, asthma, and hypertension, there are alterations in the signaling cascades. Advances in the ability to manipulate the adenoviral genome have allowed the development of gene therapy in which transgenes of interest are inserted into the adenovirus and transferred to mammals in an organ-specific manner based on delivery methods. These transgenes have included components of the AR signaling pathway that have gone awry at the level of the AR itself or the G protein it activates, the G protein-coupled receptor kinases (GRKs), and regulators of G protein signaling (RGS) proteins that regulate AR desensitization, or the adenylyl cyclase that subsequently activates protein kinase A activity. The use of these vectors in both the heart and the lung has offered promising novel benefits for animal models of disease, including heart failure and lung disorders, and it remains to be determined whether these will be successful future therapeutic strategies in human disease.

Key Words: Adenovirus; adenylyl cyclase; β-adrenergic receptor signaling; G protein; G protein-coupled receptor kinase; heart failure; regulator of G protein signaling (RGS) protein.

1. Introduction

Adrenergic receptor (AR) signaling components are essential for the establishment and maintenance of overall homeostasis. Pathophysiologies and dis-

From: *The Receptors: The Adrenergic Receptors: In the 21st Century*
Edited by: D. Perez © Humana Press Inc., Totowa, NJ

ease states can arise when there are aberrations in the AR signaling cascades, and dysfunctional AR signaling can be associated with different disorders. This phenomenon has been best characterized in the cardiovascular and respiratory systems. A goal in the generation of novel therapeutics to treat heart failure, hypertension, and lung disorders has been either to augment or to attenuate abnormal adrenergic signaling cascades using gene therapy. Although not yet at the clinical stage, these methods have been extensively studied in animal models of human disease.

At present, gene therapy is primarily accomplished using adenoviral vectors *(1)*. The adenovirus used has been engineered such that it lacks an envelope and has a 36-kb double-stranded deoxyribonucleic acid (DNA) genome, and it is no longer capable of viral replication *(1)*. The virus is not integrated into host DNA, but rather it persists in the cell as episomal DNA. Adenovirus has produced robust transgene expression in cardiomyocytes, and it can easily be produced in quantities sufficient for experimentation. The advent of adenoviral-mediated gene transfer has provided researchers with a powerful tool to examine signaling pathways in animal models of disease, and it has the potential to provide clinicians with an effective new therapeutic tool.

2. Potential Gene Therapy Targets

2.1. Adrenergic Receptors

The signaling cascade activated with AR stimulation is similar between the three major subclasses of ARs: α_1, α_2, and β (Fig. 1). Agonist binding to the AR causes a conformational change that stimulates a heterotrimeric protein, which acts as a molecular transducer. The heterotrimeric G proteins coupled to ARs (G_s, G_q, or G_i) differ depending on the specific AR activated and can even vary depending on the modification status of a single AR (Fig. 1). The activated heterotrimeric protein dissociates into α– and $\beta\gamma$-components *(2)*, each of which can transduce signals and modulate different second messengers, including activation of adenylyl cyclase (G_s), phospholipase C (G_q), and inhibition of adenylyl cyclase (G_i).

Also integral to the AR signaling cascade is the densensitization and downregulation of AR signaling. This is accomplished primarily by the G protein-coupled receptor kinases (GRKs), which phosphorylate activated ARs, allowing for the subsequent association of the arrestins. The arrestin association leads to inhibition of classical signaling cascades described above via the endocytic process and activation of newly appreciated signaling cascades, including mitogen-activated protein kinases (MAPKs) *(3)*.

2.1.1. β-AR in Heart Failure

The ARs most predominant in both the cardiac and respiratory setting include β-ARs. The β-AR family consists of three subtypes, β_1, β_2, and β_3. The majority of

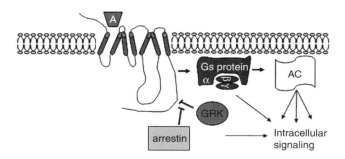

Fig. 1. The β-AR system in cardiomyocytes. On agonist binding to β-ARs, the G_s heterotrimeric protein dissociates into α- and βγ-components. The α-component activates adenylyl cyclase (AC), which results in cAMP accumulation. cAMP activates protein kinase A, which leads to downstream signaling effects, including phosphorylation of L-type calcium channels, phospholamban, troponin I, ryanodine receptors, myosin-binding protein C, and protein phosphatase inhibitor-1 *(4)*. β-ARK1 (or GRK2) is brought to the membrane via association with the G protein βγ-subunits, whereas GRK5 is already associated with the membrane. Either of these GRKs is capable of phosphorylating the agonist-activated β-AR and subsequently desensitizing the receptor. On GRK phosphorylation, a member of the arrestin protein family binds and stimulates an entirely new signaling cascade unique from the adenylyl cyclase. This signaling cascade activates the family of MAPKs.

research to date has primarily focused on the $β_1$- and $β_2$-AR subtypes, and the role of the $β_3$-AR remains controversial *(4)*. The β-AR system is compromised in both the failing heart *(4)* and asthmatic lungs *(5)*. The alterations that take place in the β-AR system during the progression of heart failure are best characterized *(6)*. As the heart begins to fail, compensatory mechanisms are initiated to maintain cardiac output and systemic blood pressure. One of these mechanisms involves the sympathetic nervous system, which increases its myocardial outflow of norepinephrine in an attempt to stimulate contractility *(7)*, leading to β-AR desensitization. There is a reduction of cardiac β-AR density in the failing human heart, and the remaining receptors appear to be desensitized *(8)*. $β_1$-ARs have been shown to be selectively reduced, and $β_2$-ARs are not altered *(9,10)*.

Interestingly, the levels of β-adrenergic receptor kinase 1 (β-ARK1, otherwise known as GRK2) are significantly elevated in human heart failure, representing a potential mechanism for loss of β-AR responsiveness seen in this disease *(9)*. The loss of cardiac $β_1$-ARs is critical because this translates to a larger percentage of $β_2$-ARs and $α_1$-ARs. Thus, signaling from these ARs becomes more important in heart failure. Another potential contributing factor to overall decreased β-AR signaling in heart failure is increased levels of $G_{αi}$ *(11)*. These collective β-AR changes are thought to be adaptive to protect the heart against chronic activation *(6,12)*.

2.1.1.1. COMPARTMENTALIZATION OF β-ARs

Although at the macroscopic level β_1- and β_2-AR signaling appears similar, evidence suggests that their signaling consequences are not only distinct, but also they are uniquely regulated. There appears to be compartmentalization *(13)*. The β_2-AR subtype is copurified with cardiomyocyte caveolae, whereas the β_1-AR subtype is more evenly distributed *(14)*. In addition, these two subtypes of β-AR possess distinct abilities to activate adenylyl cyclase, resulting in accumulated cyclic adenosine 5′-monophosphate (cAMP) *(4)*. Furthermore, activation of protein kinase A subsequent to cAMP accumulation phosphorylates β_2-AR, which then allows the receptor to switch from coupling with G_s to G_i, whereas β_1-AR does not undergo this same phenomenon *(15)*. The differences between β_1- and β_2-ARs become even more apparent when the studies are conducted in vivo.

2.1.1.2. β₂-ARs IN CARDIAC GENE TRANSFER TO NORMAL HEARTS

Through several key in vitro and in vivo studies, it appears that genetic enhancement of β_2-AR density has therapeutic potential for cardiovascular and pulmonary disorders. The benefits of cardiac-specific β_2-AR overexpression were first studied in transgenic mice. With more than 200-fold *(16)* cardiac-specific overexpression of β_2-AR using the α-myosin heavy chain promoter, mice demonstrated significantly greater indices of cardiac performance, including enhanced systolic function and myocardial relaxation *(16,17)*. These mice, when compared with their nontransgenic littermate controls, have the phenotype of maximal β-AR myocardial signaling, both biochemically and physiologically *(16)*. Baseline, nonstimulated cardiac function in mice with cardiac-specific overexpression of β_2-AR is equal to or greater than function in control mice with maximum doses of the β-AR agonist isoproterenol. In addition, there is minimal pathology associated with cardiac β_2-AR overexpression up to 1 yr of age, including negligible fibrosis and collagen replacement *(18)*. A similar phenotype was seen in mouse models with more modest (30- to 50-fold) cardiac β_2-AR overexpression *(19,20,21)*. However, too much β_2-AR overexpression (>200-fold) can lead to cardiac toxicity *(21)*. Importantly, moderate overexpression of the β_2-AR in the heart, using hybrid breeding strategies in a mouse model of heart failure, restores ventricular function and reverses cardiac hypertrophy *(20)*. Therefore, this suggests that β_2-AR supplementation is a potential for gene therapy as a means of enhancing ventricular function.

Gene therapy using an adenovirus that expresses the β_2-AR (adeno-β_2-AR) has been used both in vitro in cultured cardiac myocytes and in vivo. In cultured myocytes, adeno-β_2-AR enhanced adrenergic signaling in cells isolated from hearts of adult control rabbits and those with heart failure *(22,23)*. In vivo delivery of the adeno-β_2-AR using open chest intracoronary injection (aortic cross-clamp) to normal rabbit hearts produced diffuse multichamber myocardial expression with a reproducible 5- to 10-fold β-AR overexpression in the heart, which at 7 and 21 d after delivery resulted in increased in vivo hemodynamic function compared with control rabbits that received an empty adenovirus *(24)*. Several physiological parameters, including contractility, were significantly enhanced basally and showed increased responsiveness to the β-AR agonist isoproterenol *(24)*. Percutaneous left circumflex artery-mediated gene transfer of adeno-β_2-AR to normal rabbit hearts produced expression in a chamber-specific manner, with approx 10-fold overexpression of the β_2-AR *(25)*. Delivery of a control virus that expresses the β-galactosidase gene did not alter in vivo left ventricular systolic function, whereas overexpression of β_2-ARs in the left ventricle improved global left ventricular contractility at baseline and in response to isoproterenol *(25)*. In addition, in a rat model of heterotopic cardiac transplantation, ex vivo delivery of adeno-β_2-AR prior to heterotopic transplantation resulted in enhanced function 1 wk later *(26)*. Therefore, similar to what was seen in transgenic mice, cardiac-specific overexpression of β_2-ARs using adenovirus in either a global or chamber-specific manner or ex vivo in a transplant situation is sufficient to improve baseline and agonist-stimulated cardiac function.

2.1.1.3. β_2-ARs IN CARDIAC GENE TRANSFER TO FAILING HEARTS

Adenoviral transfer of the β_2-AR is also capable of improving failing hearts. Pressure overload is a method used in animals to induce cardiac hypertrophy and failure. Concomitant with the failure, there is a decrease in β-AR responsiveness and receptor number *(1)*. In vivo transfection of β_2-AR enhances the cardiac response to isoproterenol in the pressure-overloaded rat heart, thus preserving myocardial function *(27)*. In addition, as a model of cardiac unloading, such as that which occurs with the use of left ventricular assist devices, rabbits undergoing heterotopic transplantation of failing hearts with prior treatment with intracoronary delivery of adeno-β_2-AR functionally recovered rapidly, and this improvement in function was comparable to nonfailing hearts *(28)*. These data suggest that β_2-AR may be a useful molecular adjunct to existing therapies in select patients with heart failure.

Interestingly, because of the dual coupling of β_2-AR, and not β_1-AR, to both G_s and G_i, it appears that β_2-AR–G_i coupling conveys a significant cell survival signal that counteracts apoptosis induced by concurrent $\beta_{1/2}$-AR–G_s-mediated and other signaling pathways *(29)*. This survival pathway sequentially involves G_i, $G_{\beta\gamma}$, phosphoinositide-3 kinase, and Akt *(29)*. This suggests that selective activation of cardiac β_2-ARs may provide beneficial effects to the failing heart via catecholamine-dependent inotropic support without cardiotoxic consequences *(29)*. Further, it suggests that β_2-ARs are excellent targets for gene transfer-based gene therapy in the failing heart.

2.1.1.4. β₂-AR Gene Transfer
for Arrhythmias and Heart Rate Control

Arrhythmias and heart rate control are complicating factors associated with heart failure. β-ARs can affect the automaticity of myocardium; accordingly, the use of β₂-AR gene transfer has been explained for this purpose. Studies were done that injected β₂-AR plasmid constructs into the right atrium of native murine hearts *(30)*. Mouse hearts that were transfected with β₂-AR and subsequently heterotopically transplanted had a marked increase in cardiac rate as compared with mice transfected with control plasmids *(30)*. Minimal changes were noted in the electrocardiograms of β₂-AR-transfected hearts, suggesting that electrical conduction is unaltered except for the increased basal heart rate. These studies demonstrated that the basal heart rate can be enhanced by local delivery of β₂-ARs, improving cardiac automaticity and suggesting that the β₂-AR may be a successful candidate gene to act as an in vivo alternative to pacemaker implantation.

2.1.1.5. β₂-AR in Pulmonary Disease

Not only has gene transfer of the β₂-AR been successful in the improvement of heart function, β₂-AR gene therapy has also been successful in the treatment of animal models of asthma and pulmonary edema *(31)*. β-AR agonists accelerate the clearance of edema from the alveolar airspace by increasing the function of epithelial transport proteins. Adeno-β₂-AR was used to cause a significant increase in β₂-AR number and function in the alveolar epithelium of normal rats *(31)*. β₂-AR overexpression upregulates alveolar fluid clearance, improves responsiveness to endogenous catecholamines, and prevents receptor desensitization, suggesting a therapeutic role for the β₂-AR in the treatment of pulmonary edema *(31)*. In lung airway smooth muscle, β₂-ARs also act to relax the muscle, resulting in bronchodilation, and contribute to bronchomotor tone *(32)*. In asthma, there is excessive bronchial smooth muscle contraction, and airway epithelial and smooth muscle β₂-AR function is depressed *(32)*. Although current therapy for the disease includes the regular use of β-agonists for bronchodilation, this therapy also results in β-AR desensitization, thus potentially worsening obstruction and limiting the effectiveness of therapy *(32)*. β₂-AR gene delivery may be a successful strategy to treat asthma because transgenic overexpression of β₂-AR in airway smooth muscle results in mice resistant to an animal model of bronchoconstriction *(33)* and hyperreactivity *(34)*, although it remains to be determined whether this is the case.

2.1.2. β₁-ARs in Heart Disease

Interestingly, although β₂-ARs appear to be beneficial during disease states, it appears that β₁-ARs, the most abundant β-AR subtype in the human heart, are pathological *(1)*. Even at modest levels of cardiac-specific β_1-AR overexpression in the range of 3- to 15-fold, transgenic mice present with myocardial hypertrophy with rapid progression to failure *(35,36)*. In vitro studies of cardiac myocytes demonstrated that prolonged stimulation of β_1-AR induces cAMP-independent calcium-calmodulin kinase II-dependent apoptosis *(37)*, whereas β_2-AR stimulation may actually prevent apoptosis *(29)*. In addition, it appears that β_1-AR stimulation also leads to cardiac fibrosis and accumulation of extracellular matrix *(38)*. Therefore, at least with respect to cardiac failure, it does not appear that overexpression of the β_1-AR would be a successful approach to improve cardiac function. However, data suggest that the use of antisense therapy against the β_1-AR could be a useful strategy to combat high blood pressure *(39)*, and perhaps this strategy could also be used in the heart to minimize the detrimental β_1-AR effects caused by prolonged stimulation.

2.2. G Proteins in Heart Failure

2.2.1. G_i

In addition to enhancing β_2-ARs or inhibiting β_1-ARs, potential gene therapy can also be administered downstream of the AR in the signaling cascade. As determined using mice with G_{i2} gene ablation, G_{i2} is critical for the prevention of hypertrophy and survival of mice with chronic β_2-AR signaling *(40)*. Although it remains unclear whether $G_{\alpha i2}$ upregulation is part of the diminished positive inotropic effect after β-AR stimulation or whether it represents a protective mechanism to attenuate the effect of adrenergic overstimulation, gene transfer of $G_{\alpha i2}$ severely attenuated the β_1-adrenergic contractile response in cardiac myocytes isolated from normal adult female rabbits *(41)*. Therefore, this would suggest that it may be advantageous to increase $G_{\alpha i2}$ levels such that beneficial antiapoptotic G_i-mediated β_2-AR signaling *(29)* is enhanced and detrimental β_1-AR signaling, in the setting of heart failure, is diminished. Another possibility is the use of gene therapy of the $G_{\alpha i2}$ as an antiarrhythmic strategy. $G_{\alpha i2}$ overexpression in the atrioventricular node using adenoviral gene transfer suppressed baseline atrioventricular conduction and slowed the heart rate during atrial fibrillation without producing complete heart block *(42)*. In essence, the $G_{\alpha i2}$ was acting as a directed β-AR antagonist again, inhibiting detrimental β-AR signaling. Therefore, gene therapy for cardiac-specific overexpression of the $G_{\alpha i2}$ warrants further investigation to determine whether it is a successful strategy to augment beneficial and attenuate detrimental β-AR signaling with respect to cardiac contractility and pacing.

2.2.2. G_s

In contrast to $G_{\alpha i}$ signaling, which is enhanced in heart failure, $G_{\alpha s}$ protein levels are unchanged *(43)*. However, studies have been done using transgenic cardiac overexpression of $G_{\alpha s}$, and it was found that the efficacy of the β-AR–G_s–adenylyl cyclase signaling pathway is enhanced (44). This increased G_s activity leads to amplified inotropic and chronotropic responses to endogenous sympathetic stimulation, which over the life of the animal results in myocardial damage characterized by cellular degeneration, necrosis, fibrosis, and compensatory hypertrophy (44). Therefore, similar to $β_1$-AR, a gene therapy approach targeting this molecule would not be to enhance but rather to inhibit signaling. This could be accomplished through the use of a peptide inhibitor of G_s signaling (45) engineered in a similar manner to that described for G_q signaling in the heart (46), although this remains to be determined.

2.2.3. G_q

Activation of $G_{\alpha q}$ signaling in the heart through either cardiac overexpression of $G_{\alpha q}$ (20) or excessive activation of receptors that couple to G_q, including $α_1$-ARs, can induce cardiomyocyte hypertrophy (47). Thus, inhibition of G_q and its signals was envisioned by us as a potential therapeutic intervention to limit cardiac hypertrophy, which often leads to heart failure in humans. To achieve class-specific G protein inhibition and inhibit the signaling of all receptors that employ G_q, we targeted the receptor–G_q interface (46). This therapeutic strategy eliminates the need for multiple receptor antagonists in a variety of diseases, including pressure overload cardiac hypertrophy. We designed an inhibitor carboxyl-terminal peptide of $Gα_q$ that contains the region of the $G_{\alpha q}$ subunit that interacts with the intracellular domains of agonist-occupied receptors (GqI) and created transgenic mice with cardiac-specific overexpression of this GqI peptide (46). When pressure overload was surgically induced, the GqI transgenic mice developed significantly less ventricular hypertrophy than control animals; therefore, inhibition of myocardial G_q may be a possible strategy for preventing pathophysiological signaling by simultaneously blocking multiple receptors coupled to G_q (46). This peptide inhibitor strategy is particularly amenable to targeted gene therapy strategies because it would permit organ-specific inhibition of an entire class of receptors and minimize side effects. In addition to cardiac hypertrophy, this strategy of targeting G_q signaling may be amenable for hypertension because G_q signaling can cause vasoconstriction, which plays a role in this vascular disorder. Further studies will be directed in this area.

2.3. GRKs in Cardiovascular Disease

2.3.1. β-ARK1 (GRK2)

Much work on cardiovascular gene therapy has been done in our lab targeting the manipulation of β-ARK1 (GRK2) activity. Signaling via ARs is regulated by GRKs, and β-ARK1 is upregulated in heart failure (9). Evidence from transgenic mouse models suggests that inhibiting β-ARK1 may be beneficial in the setting of heart failure. On agonist binding, β-ARK1 is translocated to the membrane via the βγ-subunits of the heterotrimeric G protein *(18)*. Overexpression of the carboxyl terminal portion of β-ARK1 (β-ARKct) competes with endogenous β-ARK1 and prevents the translocation of β-ARK1 and its subsequent phosphorylation and desensitization of its target G protein-coupled receptor *(48)*. There are numerous different G protein-coupled receptors in the heart that β-ARK1 desensitizes *(18)*. In addition, β-ARKct also interferes with βγ-signaling, including activation of the family of MAPKs *(48)*. However, in the heart, the β-ARs are the predominant receptor; therefore, it is believed that the majority of β-ARKct actions are caused by inhibition of β-ARK1 activity rather than effects on other signaling systems, although this remains to be determined *(2)*.

Importantly, mice with transgenic cardiac-specific expression of the β-ARK1 demonstrated attenuation of agonist-stimulated left ventricular contractility in vivo, dampening of myocardial adenylyl cyclase activity, and reduced functional coupling of β-ARs *(48)*, similar to what is observed in heart failure. In contrast, mice expressing the β-ARKct displayed enhanced cardiac contractility in vivo both basally and with agonist stimulation *(48)*, indicating an important role for β-ARK1 in normal cardiac regulation and function *(1)*. In fact, the β-ARKct has been able to restore normal β-AR function and improve left ventricular function and remodeling, cardiac hypertrophy, and survival rates in several different mouse models of heart failure *(1)*. Therefore, these studies were applied to larger animal models of heart failure to determine whether gene therapy using an adeno-β-ARKct would be a successful therapeutic strategy.

Adeno-β-ARKct infection transmitted globally to the entire heart was able to prevent the development of heart failure in a rabbit following left circumflex artery ligation if given at the time of ligation *(49)* or reverse the heart failure phenotype if given 3 wk following myocardial infarction via percutaneous subselective coronary artery catheterization *(50)*. In addition, inhibition of β-ARK1 activation using adeno-β-ARKct was able to restore β-AR signaling and contractile function in donor hearts that had undergone cardioplegic arrest and cold ischemia for up to 4 h prior to transplant. Thus, β-ARK1 inhibition may represent a novel target in limiting depressed ventricular function after cardiopulmonary bypass *(51)*. Interestingly, β-ARK1 levels are also increased in human hypertensive patients *(52)*. Therefore, it would be interesting to determine whether adeno-β-ARKct would be a successful antihypertensive therapeutic strategy. Importantly, we have data supporting this idea as we overexpressed β-ARK1 in the vascular smooth muscle of transgenic mice, and this was sufficient to cause hypertension *(53)*.

2.3.2. GRK5

Unlike human heart failure, for which there has been no change in GRK5 documented, in some animal models of heart failure such as the pacing-induced pig model *(54)*, cardiomyopathic hamsters *(55)*, and rats with surgically induced myocardial infarction *(56)* and hypertension *(57)*, GRK5 levels are increased. GRK5 also phosphorylates and desensitizes β-ARs as well as other ARs. Therefore, it might be of potential therapeutic benefit to inhibit GRK5 using an adenoviral approach to express small molecule interfering RNA (RNAi) inhibitors that could prevent RNA transcription of the GRK5 gene. Alternatively, some sort of peptide inhibitors of GRK5 could be derived that would inhibit GRK5 function and thus potentially restore heart function.

2.4. Regulators of G Protein Signaling Proteins

In addition to the GRKs, a new class of proteins has been appreciated; the regulators of G protein signaling (RGS) proteins also exhibit specific regulation of G protein-coupled receptor-induced signaling within cells *(58)*. RGS proteins negatively regulate the activity of heterotrimeric G proteins by accelerating guanosine 5′-triphosphate hydrolysis and termination of signaling *(58)*. To date, it has been described that the RGS proteins have a relatively nonspecific negative regulation of G protein-coupled receptor signaling mediated by $G_{i/o}$ and $G_{q/11}$, and an interaction with G_s and G_{12} has not been detected *(58)*. The majority of cardiovascular studies to date have focused on RGS4, although there are 13 different RGS proteins expressed in the heart and vasculature *(58)*. Transgenic mice with cardiac-specific overexpression of RGS4 appear normal basally with no apparent morphological abnormalities *(59)*. However, the hearts of RGS4 mice are markedly compromised in their ability to adapt to pressure overload induced by transverse aortic constriction, and they had elevated postoperative mortality compared to nontransgenic littermate control mice *(59)*. In contrast, when RGS4 mice were mated with a heart failure mouse model in which $G_{\alpha q}$ signaling is enhanced, the RGS4 was able to delay the progression of heart failure *(60)*. Therefore, the antihypertrophic effects that RGS4 can exert on $G_{\alpha q}$ signaling in the heart can be either beneficial or detrimental depending on the physiology or pathophysiological context, suggesting that further studies are needed to explore whether the RGS family of proteins may be a potentially important therapeutic target to either enhance or inhibit, depending on circumstances.

2.5. Adenylyl Cyclase Gene Transfer in Heart Disease

β-AR signaling is coupled to adenylyl cyclase. When β-ARs are coupled with G_s, as is primarily the case, β-AR stimulation activates adenylyl cyclase, resulting in an accumulation of cAMP and activation of protein kinase A, which in the heart lead to increased chronotropy and inotropy. Protein kinase A activity phosphorylates a number of important and interesting substrates, including β_2-AR, such that the β_2-AR is now capable of coupling to G_i, inhibiting adenylyl cyclase activity and preventing apoptosis *(29)*. Adenylyl cyclase 5 and 6 are the most abundantly expressed cyclases in the heart *(61)*. Interestingly, cardiac-specific overexpression of adenylyl cyclase 6 alone had normal cardiac function with no change in myocardial β-AR; G protein or cAMP expression and signaling were only altered when transmembrane receptors were activated *(62,63)*. Cardiac-specific adenylyl cyclase 6 mice were mated with a mouse model of heart failure, and the hybrid mice had increased survival, restored cAMP-generating capacity, improved basal heart function, and increased β-AR responsiveness *(64)*. This suggested that adenylyl cyclase 6 may be a powerful therapeutic target. In fact, intracoronary injection of a recombinant adenovirus encoding adenylyl cyclase 6 into normal pigs provided persistent increases in cardiac function, whereas basal heart rate and blood pressure were unchanged *(65)*. Therefore, although further study is needed, these data suggest that long-term exposure to cardiac-selective overexpression is beneficial and that this may also be an important method for increasing function in the setting of heart failure.

3. Conclusions

Gene therapy is a powerful research and therapeutic tool that allows for organ-specific expression of transgenes. As an investigational tool, gene therapy of the AR system is powerful because it allows for acute changes in expression/activity to be studied without developmental issues and chronic expression that is encountered with transgenic mice. As a therapeutic approach, there are many different molecules along the cascade involved in AR signaling pathways that can be considered as targets, which may provide beneficial outcomes in the setting of heart failure, asthma, hypertension, and other diseases of the cardiovascular and pulmonary systems. Further research is needed to determine whether a single target approach would be more successful than a multimolecular approach. In addition, it remains to be determined whether a designer strategy is needed in which transgenes are manipulated and tailored prior to infection such that certain signaling pathways are favored over others *(32)*. What has been established through extensive transgenic mouse models and larger animal models using adenoviral-mediated gene delivery is that the genetic manipulation of several members of the AR signaling cascade has therapeutic potential that may lead to novel strategies to treat diseases for which, overall, current drug treatments are not optimal.

References

1. Williams ML, Koch WJ. Viral-based myocardial gene therapy approaches to alter cardiac function. Annu Rev Physiol 2004;66:1–27.
2. Rockman HA, Koch WJ, Lefkowitz RJ. Seven-transmembrane-spanning receptors and heart function. Nature 2002;415:206–212.
3. Kohout TA, Lefkowitz RJ. Regulation of G protein-coupled receptor kinases and arrestins during receptor desensitization. Mol Pharmacol 2003;63:9–18.
4. Lohse MJ, Engelhardt S, Eschenhagen T. What is the role of β-adrenergic signaling in heart failure? Circ Res 2003;93:896–906.
5. Shore SA, Moore PE. Regulation of β-adrenergic responses in airway smooth muscle. Respir Physiol Neurobiol 2003;137:179–195.
6. Brodde OE. β-Adreneroceptors in cardiac disease. Pharmacol Ther 1993;60: 405–430.
7. Leimbach WN, Wallin G, Victor RG, Aylward PE, Sundlof G, Mark AL. Direct evidence from intraneural recordings for increased central sympathetic outflow in patients with failure. Circulation 1986;73:913–919.
8. Bristow MR, Ginsburg R, Minobe W, et al. Decreased catecholamine sensitivity and β-adrenergic receptor density in failing human hearts. N Engl J Med 1982;307: 205–211.
9. Ungerer M, Bohm M, Elce JS, Erdmann E, Lohse ML. Altered expression of β-adrenergic receptor kinase and β_1-adrenergic receptors in the failing heart. Circulation 1993;87:454–463.
10. Bristow MR, Minobe W, Raynolds MV, et al. Reduced β_1 receptor messenger RNA abundance in the failing human heart. J Clin Invest 1993;92:2737–2745.
11. Feldman AM, Cates AE, Veazey WB, et al. Increase of the 40,000-mol wt pertussis toxin substrate (G protein) in the failing human heart. J Clin Invest 1988;82: 189–197.
12. Bristow MR, Lowes BD. Low-dose inotropic therapy for ambulatory heart failure. Coronary Artery Dis 1994;5:112–118.
13. Steinberg SF, Brunton LL. Compartmentation of G protein-coupled signaling pathways in cardiac myocytes. Annu Rev Pharmacol Toxicol 2001;41:751–773.
14. Rybin VO, Xu X, Lisanti MP, Steinberg SF. Differential targeting of β-adrenergic receptor subtypes and adenylyl cyclase to cardiomyocyte caveolae. A mechanism to functionally regulate the cAMP signaling pathway. J Biol Chem 2000;275: 41,447–41,457.
15. Kuschel M, Zhou YY, Cheng H, et al. G_i protein-mediated functional compartmentalization of cardiac β_2-adrenergic signaling. J Biol Chem 1999;274:22,048–22,052.
16. Milano CA, Allen LF, Rockman HA, et al. Enhanced myocardial function in transgenic mice overexpressing the β_2-adrenergic receptor. Science 1994;264: 582–586.
17. Bittner HB, Chen EP, Milano CA, Lefkowitz RJ, Van Trigt P. Functional analysis of myocardial performance in murine hearts overexpressing the human β_2-adrenergic receptor. J Mol Cell Cardiol 1997;29:961–967.
18. Koch WJ, Lefkowitz RJ, Rockman HA. Functional consequences of altering myocardial adrenergic receptor signaling. Annu Rev Physiol 2000;62:237–260.

19. Turki J, Lorenz JN, Green SA, Donnelly ET, Jacinto M, Liggett SB. Myocardial signaling defects and impaired cardiac function of a human β_2-adrenergic receptor polymorphism expressed in transgenic mice. Proc Natl Acad Sci USA 1996;93: 10,483–10,488.

20. Dorn GW 2nd, Tepe NM, Lorenz JN, Koch WJ, Liggett SB. Low- and high-level transgenic expression of β_2-adrenergic receptors differentially affect cardiac hypertrophy and function in $G_{\alpha q}$-overexpressing mice. Proc Natl Acad Sci USA 1999; 96:6400–6405.

21. Liggett, SB. β-Adrenergic receptors in the failing heart: the good, the bad, and the unknown. J Clin Invest 2001;107:947–948.

22. Drazner MH, Peppel KC, Dyer S, Grant AO, Koch WJ, Lefkowitz RJ. Potentiation of β adrenergic signaling by adenoviral-mediated gene transfer in adult rabbit ventricular myocytes. J Clin Invest 1997;99:288–296.

23. Akhter SA, Skaer CA, Kypson AP, et al. Restoration of β-adrenergic signaling in failing cardiac ventricular myocytes via adenoviral-mediated gene transfer. Proc Natl Acad Sci USA 1997;94:12,100–12,105.

24. Maurice JP, Hata JA, Shah AS, et al. Enhancement of cardiac function after adenoviral-mediated in vivo intracoronary β_2-adrenergic receptor gene delivery. J Clin Invest 1999;194:21–29.

25. Shah AS, Lilly RE, Kypson AP, Tai O, Hata JA, Pippen A, Silvestry SC, Lefkowitz RJ, Glower DD, Koch WJ. Intracoronary adenovirus-mediated delivery and overexpression of the β_2-adrenergic receptor in the heart: prospects for molecular ventricular assistance. Circulation. 2000;101:408-414.

26. Kypson AP, Peppel K, Akhter SA, et al. Ex vivo adenovirus-mediated gene transfer to the adult rat heart. J Thorac Cardiovasc Surg 1998;115:623–630.

27. Kawahira Y, Sawa Y, Nishimura M, et al. In vivo transfer of a β_2-adrenergic receptor gene into the pressure-overloaded rat heart enhances cardiac response to β-adrenergic agonist. Circulation 1998;98:II262–II267.

28. Tevaearai HT, Eckhart AD, Walton GB, Keys JR, Wilson K, Koch WJ. Myocardial gene transfer and overexpression of β_2-adrenergic receptors potentiates the functional recovery of unloaded failing hearts. Circulation 2002;106:124–129.

29. Xiao RP. β-Adrenergic signaling in the heart: dual coupling of the β_2-adrenergic receptor to G_s and G_i proteins. Sci STKE 2001;2001:RE15.

30. Edelberg JM, Aird WC, Rosenberg RD. Enhancement of murine cardiac chronotropy by the molecular transfer of the human β_2 adrenergic receptor cDNA. J Clin Invest 1998;101:337–343.

31. Factor P, Adir Y, Mutlu GM, Burhop J, Dumasius V. Effects of β_2-adrenergic receptor overexpression on alveolar epithelial active transport. J Allergy Clin Immunol 2002;110:S242–S246.

32. Small KM, Brown KM, Forbes SL, Liggett SB. Modification of the β_2-adrenergic receptor to engineer a receptor-effector complex for gene therapy. J Biol Chem 2001;276:31,596–31,601.

33. McGraw DW, Forbes SL, Mak JC, et al. Transgenic overexpression of β_2-adrenergic receptors in airway epithelial cells decreases bronchoconstriction. Am J Physiol Lung Cell Mol Physiol 2000;279:L379–L389.

34. McGraw DW, Forbes SL, Kramer LA, et al. Transgenic overexpression of β_2-adrenergic receptors in airway smooth muscle alters myocyte function and ablates bronchial hyperreactivity. J Biol Chem 1999;274:32,241–32,247.

35. Engelhardt S, Grimmer Y, Fan GH, Lohse MJ. Constitutive activity of the human β_1-adrenergic receptor in β_1-receptor transgenic mice. Mol Pharmacol 2001;60: 712–771.

36. Engelhardt S, Hein L, Wiesmann F, Lohse MJ. Progressive hypertrophy and heart failure in β_1-adrenergic receptor transgenic mice. Proc Natl Acad Sci USA 1999;96: 7059–7064.

37. Zhu WZ, Wang SQ, Chakir K, et al. Linkage of β_1-adrenergic stimulation to apoptotic heart cell death through protein kinase A-independent activation of Ca^{2+}/ calmodulin kinase II. J Clin Invest 2003;111:617–625.

38. O'Callaghan CJ, Williams B. The regulation of human vascular smooth muscle extracellular matrix protein production by α- and β-adrenoceptor stimulation. J Hypertens 2002;20:287–294.

39. Zhang YC, Bui JD, Shen L, Phillips MI. Antisense inhibition of β_1-adrenergic receptor mRNA in a single dose produces a profound and prolonged reduction in high blood pressure in spontaneously hypertensive rats. Circulation 2000;101:682–688.

40. Foerster K, Groner F, Matthes J, Koch WJ, Birnbaumer L, Herzig S. Cardioprotection specific for the G protein G_{i2} in chronic adrenergic signaling through β_2-adrenoceptors. Proc Natl Acad Sci USA 2003;100:14,475–14,480.

41. Janssen PM, Schillinger W, Donahue JK, et al. Intracellular β-blockade: overexpression of $G\alpha_{i2}$ depresses the β-adrenergic response in intact myocardium. Cardiovasc Res 2002;55:300–308.

42. Donahue JK, Heldman AW, Fraser H, et al. Focal modification of electrical conduction in the heart by viral gene transfer. Nat Med 2000;6:1395–1398.

43. Feldman AM, Ray PE, Bristow MR. Expression of α-subunits of G proteins in failing human heart: a reappraisal utilizing quantitative polymerase chain reaction. J Mol Cell Cardiol 1991;23:1355–1358.

44. Iwase M, Bishop SP, Uechi M, et al. Adverse effects of chronic endogenous sympathetic drive induced by cardiac G_S α overexpression. Circ Res 1996;78:517–524.

45. Feldman DS, Zamah AM, Pierce KL, et al. Selective inhibition of heterotrimeric G_s signaling. Targeting the receptor-G protein interface using a peptide minigene encoding the $G_{\alpha s}$ carboxyl terminus. J Biol Chem 2002;277:28,631–28,640.

46. Akhter SA, Luttrell LM, Rockman HA, Iaccarino G, Lefkowitz RJ, Koch WJ. Targeting the receptor–G_q interface to inhibit in vivo pressure overload myocardial hypertrophy. Science 1998;280:574–577.

47. Milano CA, Dolber PC, Rockman HA, et al. Myocardial expression of a constitutively active α_{1B}-adrenergic receptor in transgenic mice induces cardiac hypertrophy. Proc Natl Acad Sci USA 1994;91:10,109–10,113.

48. Koch WJ, Rockman HA, Samama P, et al. Cardiac function in mice overexpressing the β-adrenergic receptor kinase or a βARK inhibitor. Science 1995;268: 1350–1353.

49. White DC, Hata JA, Shah AS, Glower DD, Lefkowitz RJ, Koch WJ. Preservation of myocardial β-adrenergic receptor signaling delays the development of heart failure after myocardial infarction. Proc Natl Acad Sci USA 2000;97:5428–5433.

50. Shah AS, White DC, Emani S, et al. In vivo ventricular gene delivery of a β-adrenergic receptor kinase inhibitor to the failing heart reverses cardiac dysfunction. Circulation 2001;103:1311–1316.
51. Tevaearai HT, Eckhart AD, Shotwell KF, Wilson K, Koch WJ. Ventricular dysfunction after cardioplegic arrest is improved after myocardial gene transfer of a β-adrenergic receptor kinase inhibitor. Circulation 2001;104:2069–2074.
52. Gros R, Benovic JL, Tan CM, Feldman RD. G-protein-coupled receptor kinase activity is increased in hypertension. J Clin Invest 1997;99:2087–2093.
53. Eckhart AD, Ozaki T, Tevaearai H, Rockman HA, Koch WJ. Vascular-targeted overexpression of G protein-coupled receptor kinase-2 in transgenic mice attenuates β-adrenergic receptor signaling and increases resting blood pressure. Mol Pharmacol 2002;61:749–758.
54. Ping P, Anzai T, Gao M, Hammond HK. Adenylyl cyclase and G protein receptor kinase expression during development of heart failure. Am J Physiol 1997;273: H707–H717.
55. Takagi C, Urasawa K, Yoshida I, et al. Enhanced GRK5 expression in the hearts of cardiomyopathic hamsters, J2N-k. Biochem Biophys Res Commun 1999;262: 206–210.
56. Vinge LE, Oie E, Andersson Y, Grogaard HK, Andersen G, Attramadal H. Myocardial distribution and regulation of GRK and β-arrestin isoforms in congestive heart failure in rats. Am J Physiol Heart Circ Physiol 2001;281:H2490–H2499.
57. Ishizaka N, Alexander RW, Laursen JB, et al. G protein-coupled receptor kinase 5 in cultured vascular smooth muscle cells and rat aorta. Regulation by angiotensin II and hypertension. J Biol Chem 1997;272:32,482–32,488.
58. Wieland T, Mittmann C. Regulators of G-protein signalling: multifunctional proteins with impact on signalling in the cardiovascular system. Pharmacol Ther 2003;97:95–115.
59. Rogers JH, Tamirisa P, Kovacs A, et al. RGS4 causes increased mortality and reduced cardiac hypertrophy in response to pressure overload. J Clin Invest 1999; 104:567–576.
60. Rogers JH, Tsirka A, Kovacs A, Blumer KJ, Dorn GW 2nd, Muslin AJ. RGS4 reduces contractile dysfunction and hypertrophic gene induction in $G_{\alpha q}$ overexpressing mice. J Mol Cell Cardiol 2001;33:209–218.
61. Feldman AM. Adenylyl cyclase: a new target for heart failure therapeutics. Circulation 2002;105:1876–1878.
62. Gao MH, Lai NC, Roth DM, et al. Adenylyl cyclase increases responsiveness to catecholamine stimulation in transgenic mice. Circulation 1999;99:1618–1622.
63. Gao MH, Bayat H, Roth DM, et al. Controlled expression of cardiac-directed adenylylcyclase type VI provides increased contractile function. Cardiovasc Res 2002;56:197–204.
64. Roth DM, Bayat H, Drumm JD, et al. Adenylyl cyclase increases survival in cardiomyopathy. Circulation 2002;105:1989–1994.
65. Lai NC, Roth DM, Gao MH, et al. Intracoronary delivery of adenovirus encoding adenylyl cyclase VI increases left ventricular function and cAMP-generating capacity. Circulation 2000;102:2396–2401.

PART V

PHARMACOGENOMICS

13

Genetic, Molecular, and Clinical Characterization of Adrenergic Receptor Polymorphisms

Stephen B. Liggett

Summary

Natural variations in the genes that encode adrenergic receptors have been identified. The variations of major interest for common diseases are those that occur with allele frequencies of 1% or more and are termed polymorphisms. Of the nine adrenergic receptors (α_{1A}, α_{1B}, α_{1D}, α_{2A}, α_{2B}, α_{2C}, β_1, β_2, β_3), seven have been found to have nonsynonymous coding polymorphisms. Because of the distribution of adrenergic receptors throughout the body, there is the potential to explore genotype-phenotype associations in many organ systems and diseases. To date, the most extensively studied have been asthma, hypertension, vascular disease, heart failure, and obesity and related metabolic disorders.

Key Words: Associations; allele; asthma; clinical; disease; haplotypes; heart; polymorphism; SNPs; transgenic.

1. Introduction

Natural variation in the genes that encode adrenergic receptors (ARs) have been identified. The variations of major interest for common diseases are those that occur with allele frequencies $\geq 1\%$ and are termed *polymorphisms*. Within the coding region, polymorphic variation can result in either a change in the encoded amino acid (nonsynonymous) or, because of the redundancy of the genetic code, have no effect on the encoded residue (synonymous). The most common variants are single nucleotide polymorphisms (SNPs), but insertions and deletions are also found. AR polymorphisms have been considered as poten-

From: *The Receptors: The Adrenergic Receptors: In the 21st Century*
Edited by: D. Perez © Humana Press Inc., Totowa, NJ

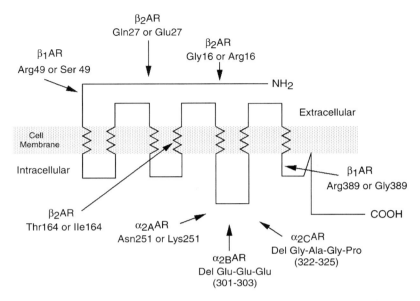

Fig. 1. Localization of nonsynonymous polymorphisms of adrenergic receptors. Schematic representation of a prototypic receptor. Locations are approximate and not to scale. (Reprinted, with permission, from ref. *28;* © 2003 by Annual Reviews, www. annualreviews.org.)

tial risk factors for a disease, as modifiers of a given disease, or as loci that act to alter the response to therapeutic agents targeted to a receptor. In this review, the AR polymorphisms are identified and their molecular properties as determined in cells or genetically altered mice summarized; the physiological/clinical consequences in human disease are discussed.

2. Localization and Population Genomics of Adrenergic Receptor Polymorphisms

Of the nine ARs, seven have been found to have nonsynonymous coding polymorphisms. Although there does not appear to be any pattern regarding the locations of these polymorphisms, certain regions may well be spared (Fig. 1). The nucleotide and amino acid localization, major and minor alleles, and frequencies of these polymorphisms are provided in Table 1. Of particular interest is the difference in allele frequencies for some polymorphisms between those individuals of European vs African descent. For example, the α_{2C}-Del322-325 polymorphism has an allele frequency that is approx 10-fold more common in African Americans *(1)*. On the other hand, the α_{2B}-Del301-303 is threefold more common in Caucasians *(2)*. Combinations of polymorphisms of a gene that are on the same

Table 1
Adrenergic Receptor Polymorphisms

Receptor	Position Nucleotide	Position Amino acid	Alleles Major	Alleles Minor	Minor allele frequency (%) Caucasians	Minor allele frequency (%) African-Americans
α_{1A}-AR	1441	492	Cys[a]	Arg	46	70
α_{2A}-AR	753	251	Asn	Lys	0.4	5
α_{2B}AR	901–909	301–303	No deletion	Delete Glu-Glu-Glu	31	12
α_{2C}-AR	964–975	322–325	No deletion	Delete Gly-Ala-Gly-Pro	4	38
β_1-AR	145	49	Ser	Gly	15	13
	1165	389	Arg	Gly	27	42
β_2-AR	46	16	Gly	Arg	39	50
	79	27	Gln	Glu	43	27
	491	164	Thr	Ile	2–5	2–5
β_3-AR	190	64	Trp	Arg	10	?

[a] In African-Americans, Arg is the major allele.

parental chromosome are termed *haplotypes*. Because of linkage disequilibrium between multiple polymorphisms that are in the same gene, some combinations are uncommon. For the β_2-AR, we have ascertained polymorphic sites within the open reading frame as well as approx 1000 bp 5′ upstream *(3)*. Thirteen SNPs have been identified, and although $2^{13} = 8192$ combinations are possible, only 12 haplotypes were found in a multiethnic population. Using phylogenetic analysis, one can ascertain ancestral alleles and potential recombination events. Such an analysis is shown in Fig. 2 (*see* Color Plate 5 following p. 148.) for the β_2-AR haplotypes.

3. Signaling Consequences of Adrenergic Receptor Polymorphisms

3.1. β_1-AR Polymorphisms

Two nonsynonymous polymorphisms have been identified *(4-6)*, at amino acid 49 within the amino-terminus of the receptor and in the proximal cytoplasmic tail within the proposed eighth α-helix at amino acid 389. There are discrepant reports regarding the effects of the Ser→Gly substitution at position 49 on receptor function. In one report, basal and agonist-stimulated adenylyl cyclase activities were

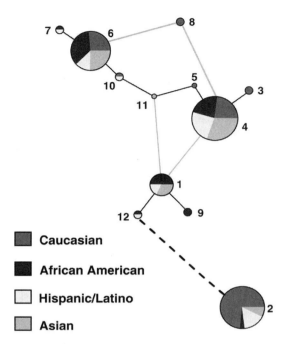

Fig. 2. Phylogenetics of β_2-AR haplotypes. Each circle represents a haplotype with an area that correlates with its frequency in the test population. Sections within each circle show the distribution by race. Connecting lines: solid black, single-site differences; solid blue, two-site differences; dashed, more than two-site differences. Analysis was by the minimum spanning network algorithm. (*See* Color Plate 5 following p. 148; reprinted, with permission, from ref. *3*.)

not different between the two *(6)*; another noted higher activities for β_1-Gly49 *(7)*. There is agreement, though, that agonist-promoted trafficking differs between the two allelic variants. Western blots of transfected HEK-293 cells expressing each receptor revealed different immunoreactive bands (Fig. 3A). For β_1-Ser49, a high molecular weight species (~105 kDa) was identified. This was considered consistent with enhanced glycosylation (N- or O-linked) or dimerization of non-glycosylated receptor (monomer size is ~49 kDa). Although a dimerized form cannot be unequivocally excluded, the high molecular weight form was sensitive to the in vivo glycosylation inhibitor tunicamycin and N-glycosidases in vitro. O-Glycosidases had no effect.

In addition to the lack of this high molecular weight species, β_1-Gly49 has a major immunoreactive species at approx 69 kDa compared to approx 63 kDa for β_1-Ser49. Taken together, it appears that β_1-Gly49 is not expressed in a "mature"

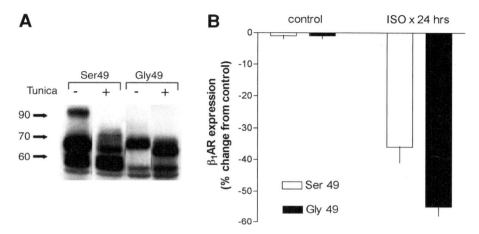

Fig. 3. Phenotype of the position 49 variants of the β₁AR in transfected cells: (**A**) representative autoradiogram of a Western blot from whole cell lysates; (**B**) results from downregulation studies. ISO, isoproterenol. (From ref. 6; with permission from Lippincott Williams & Wilkins.)

form, potentially because of altered glycosylation. It is not clear, however, how a polymorphism at amino acid position 49 can effect N-glycosylation that occurs at Asn15 of the β₁-AR. This altered form of β₁-Gly49 is associated with an increase in agonist-promoted downregulation (net loss of cellular receptor) after 18 h of exposure to the agonist isoproterenol (Fig. 3B). In these experiments, cells were treated with cycloheximide to block new receptor synthesis. Agonist-promoted degradation of receptor was approx 55% for β₁-Gly49 compared to approx 36% for β₁-Ser49. In contrast, degradation in the absence of agonist and agonist-promoted internalization of either receptor were not different. The major phenotype, then, of the β₁-Gly49 receptor is enhanced agonist-promoted down-regulation.

The polymorphism at position 389 has been studied in transfected cells *(4)* and transgenic mice *(8)*. Amino acid 389 is within a proposed α-helix formed by a stretch of intracellular residues from the seventh transmembrane domain (TMD) and the palmitoylated cysteine(s), which forms a membrane anchor. For many receptors, this region is important for coupling to G proteins. Initial agonist-binding studies (Fig. 4A), carried out in the absence of guanine nucleotide, revealed steep and monophasic curves for β₁-Gly389; thus, little high-affinity agonist binding could be detected by this method for this receptor. In contrast, β₁-Arg389 curves could be readily resolved into high- and low-affinity states (Fig. 4B) *(4)*. This suggested that there was greater accumulation of the high-

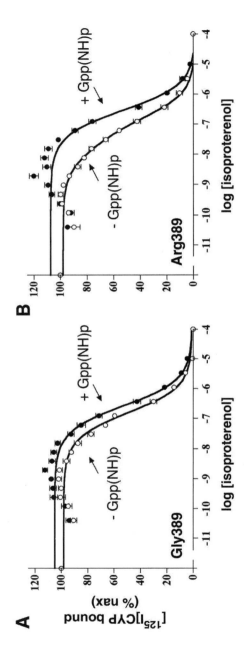

Fig. 4. Phenotype of the β_1-Arg389 and β_1-Gly389 receptors in transfected cells: (**A**) and (**B**) results from agonist competition studies in washed membranes; (**C**) *(Continued on next page)*. *(From ref. 4 with permission.)*

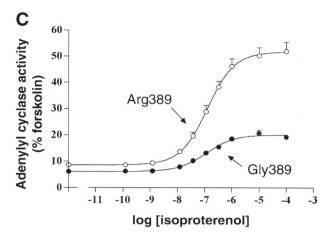

Fig. 4. (C) *(Continued from previous page)* Results from adenylyl cyclase studies. The Arg-389 demonstrated small increases in basal activities and marked increases in agonist-stimulated activities compared with the Gly-389 receptor. (From ref. *4* with permission.)

affinity agonist-receptor-G_s complex for β_1-Arg389 compared to β_1-Gly389, and that the former would display enhanced signal transduction. As shown in Fig. 4C, this turned out to be the case, with basal and isoproterenol-stimulated adenylyl cyclase activities greater for the Arg compared to the Gly allelic variant *(4)*.

Subsequent studies were carried out with transgenic mice, for which in separate lines the two β_1-ARs were expressed on myocytes using the α-myosin heavy chain promoter *(8)*. Lines were selected with equivalent levels of β_1-AR protein expression as assessed by quantitative radioligand binding. The physiological consequences are shown in the work-performing heart studies of Fig. 5A. In 3-mo-old mice, basal and agonist (dobutamine)-stimulated contractility (+dP/dt) is greater for β_1-Arg389 hearts compared to those from β_1-Gly389 mice. In contrast, by 6 mo of age, a contractile response of the β_1-Arg389 hearts to dobutamine was not observed (Fig. 5B). Expression studies revealed a pattern of altered hypertrophy, Ca^{2+}-handling, and signal transduction transcripts or protein in these hearts, which occurred during the 3- to 6-mo window. Some of these changes occurred with both mice; others were specific for β_1-Arg389. These data suggested that the Arg variant evokes a signaling program, which results in adaptation, potentially to protect the heart from persistently enhanced contractility. In the case of these mice, though, this adaptation (which physiologically appears as "autoblockade") is ultimately not successful because β_1-Arg389 mice die of dilated cardiomyopathy by 9 mo of age.

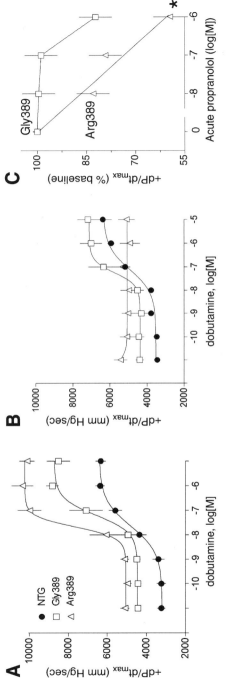

Fig. 5. Physiological consequences of β_1-Arg389 and β_1-Gly389 expression in hearts of transgenic mice: (**A,B**) results from work-performing preparations in hearts from 3- and 6-month-old mice; (**C**) acute response to the β-blocker propranolol. (From ref. 8, with permission from Nature Publishing Group.)

The potential for position 389 of the β_1-AR as a pharmacogenetic locus was assessed in these mice with both acute and chronic dosing of the β-blocker propranolol (Fig. 5C). Acute administration of propranolol in work-performing preparations of 3-mo-old mice revealed increased sensitivity and maximal response to propranolol (decrease in +dP/dt) for the β_1-Arg389 hearts compared to β_1-Gly389 hearts (Fig. 5C). In short-term oral dosing studies, 3-mo-old mice were treated for 5 wk with propranolol, with the decrease in heart rate utilized as the response end point. Only the β_1-Arg389 displayed a decrement. These data suggested that β_1-Arg389 may represent a response locus for β-blockers for the treatment of heart failure.

3.2. β_2-AR Polymorphisms

The most uncommon β_2-AR SNP is at amino acid position 164, where Thr or Ile can be found within the fourth TMD of the receptor *(9)*. The minor allele (Ile) is found in the heterozygous state in approx 2-5% of any population studied to date. Interestingly, a homozygous individual has never been identified, suggesting that it may be developmentally lethal. In transfected cells, β_2-Ile164 displayed two- to threefold lower binding affinity for β_2-agonists and some antagonists. Minimal high-affinity binding was detected, which was consistent with this receptor having substantially decreased basal and agonist-stimulated adenylyl cyclase activities *(9)* (Fig. 6A). This decreased function of the Ile164 variant has also been observed in physiological studies of transgenic mice with targeted overexpression of the β_2-Thr164 and -Ile164 receptors *(10)*. Neither of the transgenic mice exhibited pathological features.

In addition to this uncoupled phenotype, β_2-Ile164 interacts aberrantly with the long-acting β-agonist salmeterol *(11)*. This agonist has a phenylalkyloxyalkyl side chain that "anchors" it to the receptor within the fourth TMD to provide for repetitive binding events and a 12-h duration of bronchodilating action in the treatment of asthma *(12)*. The substitution of Ile for Thr in this region perturbs this anchoring, and functional washout studies in transfected cells *(11)* revealed approx 50% reduction in the duration of action of salmeterol (Fig. 6B).

The prevalent β_2-AR polymorphisms are at amino acid positions 16 and 27 *(13,14)*. Three of the four possible combinations are commonly observed. The phenotypes of the 16/27 polymorphisms appear to be confined to long-term agonist-promoted downregulation. Initial studies revealed no alterations in ligand-binding affinities, coupling to cyclic adenosine 5'-monophosphate (cAMP), the rate of receptor synthesis, or short-term agonist-promoted internalization *(14)*. However, when cells were exposed to isoproterenol for 24 h, a difference in the degree of downregulation was noted (Fig. 7).

The Arg16/Gln27 receptor underwent $26 \pm 3\%$ downregulation. In contrast, the Gly16/Gln27 receptor displayed $41 \pm 3\%$ downregulation. Furthermore, the

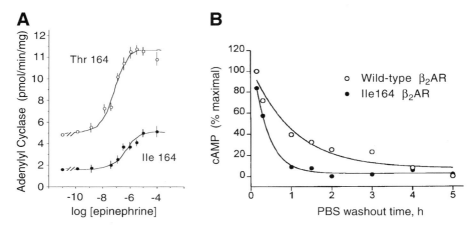

Fig. 6. Signaling characteristics of the β_2-Ile164 polymorphism in transfected cells: **(A)** results from adenylyl cyclase studies reveal decreased coupling of β_2-Ile164; **(B)** washout studies with the agonist salmeterol reveal a shorter duration of action at the β_2-Ile164 receptor compared to the wild-type Thr164. PBS, phosphate-buffered saline. (Reprinted, with permission, from refs. *11* and *28;* © 2003 by Annual Reviews, www.annualreviews.org.)

rare Arg16/Glu27 receptor failed to downregulate. The Gly16/Glu27 receptor displayed a similar level of downregulation ($39 \pm 4\%$) compared to the Gly16/Gln27 receptor. The data suggest that position 16 is the major polymorphic locus that affects agonist-promoted downregulation *(14)*. That is, whenever Gly16 is present, downregulation is enhanced compared to Arg16. The molecular basis of these phenotypes is not clear, but it appears to occur after the internalization process, prior to or during passage through the degradation pathway.

In a study of cultured human airway smooth muscle cells natively expressing several of the β_2-AR genotypic combinations *(15)*, downregulation promoted by 24 h of agonist exposure followed the same pattern as that observed in the transfected cell studies *(14)*. However, another study using human airway smooth muscle cells showed a somewhat different phenotype *(16)*. In this study, changes in receptor expression were not determined, but rather changes in function (cAMP accumulation and cell stiffness) after agonist exposure were examined. The presence of any Glu27 allele was associated with enhanced desensitization of these functions. This finding was observed with both 24-h exposures as well as 1-h exposures to agonist in culture. Because agonist-promoted downregulation of β_2-AR density requires approx 6 h for earliest detection, one must conclude that these protocols serve to study event(s) other than downregulation alone. The

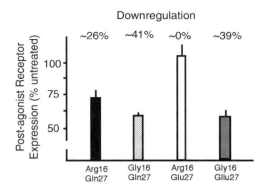

Fig. 7. Downregulation phenotypes of the position 16 and 27 variants of the β_2-AR in transfected cells. These mutations markedly altered the degree of agonist-promoted downregulation of receptor expression after 24-h exposure to 10 μM isoproterenol. (From ref. *28;* © 2003, with permission from Elsevier.)

effect of the position 16 genotype could not be fully assessed because of the distribution of genotypes.

In another study with natively expressing polymorphic β_2-AR, human lung mast cell function (agonist-promoted inhibition of histamine release) was examined *(17)*. Desensitization of this response after 24 h of agonist exposure showed results that were the opposite of that predicted by other studies *(14,15)* in which receptor expression was quantitated by radioligand binding. Although the above studies with endogenous cells from humans utilized different protocols and outcome measures, one must also consider that polymorphisms in other genes with products that are involved in the various pathways investigated may account for some of these apparent discrepancies.

As introduced in Section 1.2., the β_2-AR promoter 5′ untranslated and 5′ leader cistron are highly polymorphic, serving to define at least 12 unique haplotypes *(18,3)*. Although characterization of all the haplotypes has not been carried out, studies of two common Caucasian haplotypes revealed that β_2-AR haplotype 2 *(see* nomenclature from ref. *3)* consistently had higher expression levels in transfected cells compared to haplotype 4. These two differ at eight SNP positions in the gene, including several *cis*-acting elements. As is discussed in Section 4.3., the bronchodilator response to β-agonist is associated with β_2-AR haplotypes in asthmatics, in a direction and magnitude consistent with the in vitro studies *(3)*.

3.3. β_3-AR Polymorphisms

One nonsynonymous polymorphism of the β_3-AR gene has been reported *(19)* that results in a substitution of Arg for Trp (the major human allele) at amino acid position 64. This residue is localized either to the most distal residue within the first transmembrane-spanning domain or the most proximal residue of the first intracellular loop (Fig. 1) of the receptor. It is interesting to note that in virtually all β_3-AR genes cloned from various species, Arg is found at position 64, yet Trp is the major human allele (Table 1). This suggests evolutionary pressure for dominance of the Trp residue in humans. Two studies with discrepant results have been published on the pharmacological effect of the Arg64 substitution in the β_3-AR using recombinant expression. In Chinese hamster ovary (CHO; dhfr-) cells, there were no differences in agonist-binding parameters or agonist stimulation of cellular cAMP accumulation between the Trp64 and Arg64 receptors (20). In contrast, others have reported (21) a decrease in the maximal stimulation of cAMP accumulation in CHO-K1 and HEK-293 cells with the Arg64 β_3-AR compared to its allelic counterpart. It appears, then, that there may be a difference in coupling between Arg64 and Trp64 β_3-ARs, but additional studies are necessary to clarify these pharmacological characteristics.

3.4. α_{2A}-AR Polymorphisms

One nonsynonymous SNP has been reported in the α_{2A}-AR coding region (22), where Asn or Lys can be found at amino acid 251, which is within the third intracellular region (Fig. 1). The SNP is in a region that is highly conserved among species; indeed, Asn is found in the analogous position in genes of all species cloned to date except for human, where the Lys polymorphism has an allele frequency of 0.4% in Caucasians and 5.0% in African Americans (Table 1). The α_{2A}-Lys251 receptor displays enhanced agonist-promoted ^{35}S-GTPγS binding compared to α_{2A}-Asn251, consistent with enhanced coupling to inhibition of adenylyl cyclase and stimulation of mitogen-activated protein kinase p44/42 (Fig. 8) (22).

3.5. α_{2B}-AR Polymorphisms

A nine-nucleotide in-frame deletion resulting in a three-amino acid (Glu-Glu-Glu) deletion representing residues 301-303 of the wild-type α_{2B}-AR has been delineated (22) (Fig. 1). It is common in Caucasians and African Americans. The deletion is within the third intracellular loop of the receptor, within a long string of Glu residues. Studies have shown that this region is important for establishing the acidic environment necessary for G protein-coupled receptor kinase (GRK)-mediated desensitization (23). Expression of wild-type and α_{2B}-Del301-303 receptors in CHO cells revealed a complex phenotype (22). In membrane adenylyl cyclase assays, the polymorphic form displayed a small decrease in maximal inhibition of forskolin-stimulated adenylyl cyclase, and the dose-response curve was right shifted. Thus, one component of the phenotype is decreased coupling to G_i.

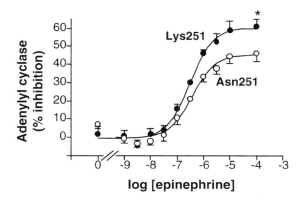

Fig. 8. Enhanced signaling of the α_{2A}Lys251 polymorphic receptor. Adenylyl cyclase activities were determined in the presence of 5.0 μM forskolin and the indicated concentrations of the full agonist epinephrine. Results as shown are the percentage inhibition of forskolin-stimulated activities from clones at matched levels of expression (~2500 fmol/mg). *, $p < 0.05$ for the maximal inhibition compared with wild-type for both agonists. (From ref. *22* with permission.)

Based on the importance of this region for agonist-promoted desensitization, additional studies were carried out to ascertain GRK phosphorylation and desensitization. Cells were cotransfected with GRK2 and the wild-type or α_{2B}-Del301-303 receptor, loaded with ^{32}P-orthophosphate, treated with vehicle or agonist for 10 min, and purified by immunoprecipitation. As shown in Fig. 9A, agonist-promoted phosphorylation of α_{2B}-Del301-303 was reduced by approx 50% compared to wild type. Consistent with these results, agonist-promoted functional desensitization (inhibition of adenylyl cyclase) was absent with the polymorphic receptor compared to 54% for the wild type (Fig. 9B). Thus, the major phenotype of α_{2B}-Del301-303 is a lack of a critical regulatory event: short-term agonist-promoted desensitization by GRK2 phosphorylation.

3.6. α_{2C}-AR Polymorphisms

Like the other two α_2-AR subtypes, the site for polymorphic variation of the α_{2C}-AR is localized to the third intracellular loop *(1)* (Fig. 1). For this subtype, a 12-nucleotide in-frame deletion resulting in a four-amino acid (Gly-Ala-Gly-Pro) loss has been detected, primarily in subjects of African descent (Table 1). In CHO cells, the α_{2C}-Del322-325 displays markedly depressed function as assessed by inhibition of adenylyl cyclase (Fig. 10), stimulation of mitogen-activated protein kinase p44/42, and stimulation of inositol phosphates *(1)*. The basis for this impairment is not clear. Although the third intracellular loop is

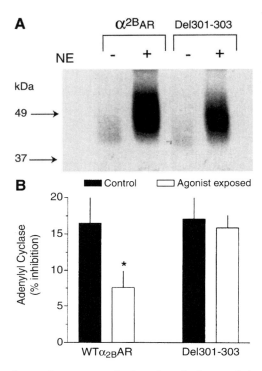

Fig. 9. Decreased agonist-promoted phosphorylation and desensitization of the α_{2B}-Del301-303 polymorphism: **(A)** results of a whole-cell phosphorylation study in cells cotransfected with receptor and GRK2; **(B)** results from adenylyl cyclase studies. The percentage of inhibition of adenylyl cyclase at a submaximal concentration of norepinephrine (NE) in the assay is shown for both conditions, indicating an approx 54% desensitization of wild-type (WT) α_{2B}-AR. The Del301-303 failed to display such desensitization. (From ref. *2* with permission.)

critical for G protein coupling, it is generally felt that the regions near the fifth and sixth TMDs are most important. However, compared to the β_2-AR, the α_2-ARs have large third intracellular loops and minimal cytoplasmic tails. So, there may be complex folding of the third intracellular loop of the α_{2C}-AR that acts to regulate coupling. Other considerations include altered membrane insertion or microdomain localization of the α_{2C}-Del322-325.

3.7. α_1-AR Polymorphisms

To date, only one polymorphism in an α_1-AR subtype gene that alters amino acid sequence has been described (Table 1). This polymorphism is located within the α_{1A}-AR subtype gene, resulting in Arg or Cys at amino acid 492 *(24)*. This

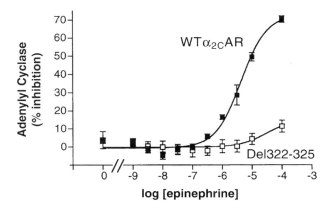

Fig. 10. Depressed function of the α_{2C}-Del322-325 polymorphic receptor. Adenylyl cyclase activities were determined in membranes in response to forskolin (5 μM) and forskolin plus various concentrations of norepinephrine. (From ref. *1* with permission.)

residue is located in the carboxy-terminus of the receptor (Fig. 1). Comparison of the Arg492 and Cys492 α_{1A}-AR functions has been investigated using transfected CHO cells stably expressing each receptor *(24)*. Radioligand-binding studies showed no differences in agonist or antagonist binding. In addition, receptor-mediated calcium signaling and the extent of receptor desensitization following agonist exposure were also similar for both receptors. For the α_{1B}-AR gene, sequence analysis of exonic regions from 51 individuals revealed only two synonymous polymorphisms *(25)*. Studies designed to identify polymorphisms of the α_{1D}-AR have not been described to date.

4. Clinical Relevance of Adrenergic Receptor Polymorphisms

Typically, studies have been carried out to investigate associations between AR polymorphisms and three scenarios: risk factors for disease, modification of disease phenotype, and alteration of the response to therapy *(26)*. These three aspects of genetic variation are interrelated. For example, an apparent direct pharmacogenetic effect of a polymorphism may in fact be caused by its influence on disease severity (i.e., phenotype), thereby associating it with response to therapy. Similarly, the risk for developing a disease if an individual has a given polymorphism may be related to a highly specific clinical subset of the disease, which may be only broadly defined, and thus the risk and disease modification effects can become difficult to distinguish.

Because of the distribution of ARs throughout the body, there is the potential to explore genotype-phenotype associations in many organ systems and dis-

Table 2
Physiologic Phenotypes of Adrenergic Receptor Polymorphisms

Receptor	Disease	Association (−or +)
α_{2A}	Hypertension	(−) Lys251
α_{2B}	Acute coronary events	(+) Del301-303
	Hypertension	(−) and (+) Del301-303
	Reduced metabolic rate	(+) Del301-303
	Body weight	(+) Del301-303
	Fat mass (with β_3-Arg64)	(+) Del301-303
	Vasoconstriction (normals)	(+) Del301-303
α_{2C}	Heart failure	(+) Del322-325
	^{125}I-MIBG uptake (heart failure)	(+) Del322-325
	Hypertension	(−) Del322-325
β_1-AR	Heart failure (with α_{2C}-Del322-325)	(+) Arg389
	Exercise tolerance (heart failure)	(+) Arg389
	Exercise response (normals)	(−) Arg389
	Left ventricular mass	(+) Arg389
	Ex vivo cardiac response (heart failure)	(+) Arg389
	Hypertension	(+) Arg389
	Response to β-blocker (hypertension)	(+) Arg389
	Ventricular tachycardia	(+) Arg389
	Response to β-blocker (heart failure)	(−) Arg389, Gly49
	Response to β-blocker (heart failure)	(+) Arg389
	Survival (heart failure)	(+) Gly49
	Heart rate (normals and hypertension)	(+) Gly49
β_2-AR	Asthma	
	• Nocturnal phenotype	(+) Gly16
	• High immunoglobulin E phenotype	(+) Gln27
	• Bronchial hyperresponsiveness	(−) and (+) 16, 27
	• Altered response to albuterol	(+) Arg16, (+) haplotype (+) 523
	Exercise tolerance (heart failure)	(+) Ile164, (+) Gly16
	Heart rate, QT_C to agonist (normals)	(+) Ile164
	Survival (heart failure)	(+) Ile164, (−) 16/27
	Vascular response to agonist (normals)	(+) 16/27
	Obesity, diabetes, hypertriglyceridemia	Multiple (+) and (−) 16/27
β_3-AR	Obesity, diabetes, hypertriglyceridemia	Multiple (+) and (−) Arg64
α_{1A}-AR	Vascular response to agonist (normals)	(−) 492

(+), An association has been reported; (−), the study revealed no association.

eases. To date, the most extensively studied have been asthma, hypertension, vascular disease, heart failure, and obesity and related metabolic disorders. Physiological studies have also been carried out in normal subjects as well. Table 2 provides results from representative studies. However, it is not comprehensive;

refs. *27* and *28* provide additional discussion of specific diseases. In the follow-ing sections, representative examples of clinical studies that address each of the three aforementioned scenarios are provided and discussed.

4.1. AR Polymorphisms as Risk Factors for Disease

β_2-ARs (and to a lesser extent β_1-ARs) are expressed on vascular smooth muscle, where they serve to vasodilate and, by way of regulating peripheral vascular resistance, have been considered potential genetic loci for hypertension. In addition, β_1-ARs of the kidney regulate renin secretion and subsequent angio-tensin generation. Several studies have addressed whether β_2-AR polymorphisms are associated with essential hypertension. Given the allele frequencies of these SNPs, it was expected that the contribution of an individual SNP or even a haplotype, from one gene, would have a somewhat small contribution to the phenotype. Some of the initial studies may not have been designed in such a way to distinguish small contributions or to take into account population stratification among various ethnic groups *(29,30)*.

A large set of studies by Boerwinkle and colleagues using both pedigrees with sibling pairs discordant for systolic hypertension and two-family studies (total of 2527 individuals) has revealed associations that are the most definitive to date *(31)*. In the sibling pair studies, locus 16 of the β_2-AR was significantly related to blood pressure ($p = 0.009$). In the first family study of 1283 individuals, Arg16 homozygosity was associated with lower diastolic and mean arterial blood pres-sures, accounting for approx 3 mmHg decrease in either parameter. When the second cohort of families was added, the position 27 locus appeared to have a greater effect (they are in strong linkage disequilibrium). Glu27 was associated with increased systolic and mean arterial pressures. The odds ratio for the occur-rence of hypertension for the Glu27 allele was 1.80 (95% confidence interval [CI] 1.08-3.00. Studies with the β_1-AR polymorphisms have been less extensive. Groop and colleagues *(32)* reported associations in a case-control study of unre-lated individuals and in a sibling pair study. In the case-control study, the odds ratio for hypertension for the β_1-Arg389 allele was 1.9 (95% CI 1.3-2.7) when compared to β_1-Gly389 carriers. The sibling study revealed higher diastolic blood pressures for homozygosity at β_1-Arg389, amounting to an approx 3 mmHg increase. A similar observation has also been made in patients with heart failure *(33)*. When stratified by the β_1-AR-389 genotype, those with homozygous β_1-Arg389 had higher systolic blood pressure (by ~12 mmHg) than those who were homozygous for Gly389, with an intermittent value for heterozygotes. This more profound phenotypic effect observed in patients with heart failure compared to those with essential hypertension may be caused by the fact that the former patients have elevated catecholamines, which would be expected to exacerbate the gain-of-function phenotype of β_1-Arg389 *(4)*.

4.2. AR Polymorphisms as Disease Modifiers

In these scenarios, the allele frequency of the variant is not considered to be different between the disease cohort and an appropriate control population. However, the hypothesis being tested is whether the polymorphism is associated with some relevant clinical characteristic, a defined phenotype, or a "clinical subset" of a heterogeneous syndrome. As discussed earlier, it may be difficult to ascertain disease risk when a variant from a single gene is one of several from multiple genes that together ascertain risk. Furthermore, disease modification effects may be part of a pharmacogenetic influence. In many cases, it is not ethical to withdraw or standardize therapy for all patients, so statistical methods need to be utilized to ascertain medication use as a confounder in analysis of a polymorphism's disease modification potential.

Studies of AR polymorphisms in heart failure represent examples of the complexity of the aforementioned issues. Given the highly integrated nature of the sympathetic nervous system, genetic variability of multiple ARs that control cardiac contractility and rate (β_1-β_1-AR), norepinephrine release from cardiac presynaptic nerves (α_{2A}-α_{2C}-AR and β_2-AR), peripheral vascular resistance (α_1-, α_2-, and β-AR subtypes), and other neurohumoral responses to depressed cardiac output, could influence the phenotype. Several studies have concentrated on exercise tolerance as a clinically relevant phenotypic trait, given that it is quantitative (typically, maximal oxygen consumption VO_2 is measured), and it correlates with survival. The β_2-AR expressed on myocytes has a diverse signaling repertoire, which includes coupling to inotropy/chronotropy by stimulation of adenylyl cyclase (via G_s), inhibition of adenylyl cyclase (via G_i), and antiapoptotic signals. The β_2-Ile164 receptor is substantially dysfunctional in transfected cells and transgenic mice (*see* Section 1.2.), so we hypothesized that those carrying this polymorphism who had heart failure (idiopathic dilated or ischemic cardiomyopathies) would have lower VO_2 and increased mortality.

Exercise capacity was measured using a graded treadmill protocol, with VO_2 as the primary outcome measure (34). Those with Ile164 had substantially depressed VO_2 (15.0 ± 0.9 vs 17.9 ± 0.9 mL/kg/min). The odds ratio of having $VO_2 \leq 14$ mL/kg/min was 8.0, $p = 0.009$. Importantly, these patients could not be differentiated by standard clinical tests. Of note, a VO_2 of 14 or below is one of the criteria for placement on the cardiac transplantation list. Cardiac catheterization studies (Fig. 11) in these individuals revealed substantially reduced cardiac output responses as well as decreased vasodilation in response to exercise in the patients with β_2-Ile164 heart failure compared to matched patients homozygous for the wild type (β_2-Thr164). Of note, baseline left ventricular ejection fractions and other clinical characteristics were not different between the two groups. So, even at early stages, a pathophysiological effect of Ile164 is observed.

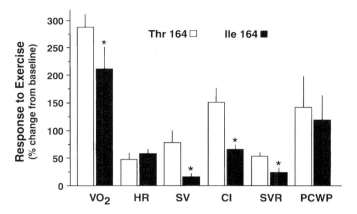

Fig. 11. The hemodynamic response to exercise is influenced by the β_2-Ile164 polymorphism in patients with heart failure. Exercise-induced changes were significantly lower in patients with Ile164 for O_2, stroke volume (SV), cardiac index (CI), and systemic vascular resistance (SVR). All changes represent increases by the indicated percentage, except for SVR, which was a decrease. HR, heart rate. *$p < 0.05$ vs Thr164. VO_2 is maximal oxygen consumption. (Reprinted with permission from ref. *34*.)

A study by Brodde et al. *(35)* with normal volunteers showed mild decreased responsiveness (heart rate and systolic time interval) to infusions of the β_2-AR agonist terbutaline in those with the Ile164 allele compared to Thr164 homozygotes. This indicates that this polymorphism has physiological effects even in the absence of disease, but its effect may be greater in a disease with compromised hemodynamics such as heart failure. Consistent with these findings, a longitudinal study *(36)* with up to 3 yr of follow-up revealed that the adjusted relative risk of death or transplantation for patients with heart failure who carried β_2-Ile164 was 4.81, 95% CI 2-11.5, $p < 0.001$. Because the frequency of this polymorphism is low in the population (Table 1), its relevance to the majority of patients with heart failure is not extensive, but clearly it defines a discreet subset of patients who may require aggressive or alternative therapy. Polymorphisms at positions 16 and 27 of the β_2-AR are not associated with heart failure and do not appear to affect survival *(36)*. However, the position 16 variants do have some effect on exercise tolerance *(34)*.

Similar studies with the two nonsynonymous polymorphisms of the β_1-AR have revealed additional phenotypes. The majority of studies have been with the β_1-AR position 389 variants. Alone, neither allelic variant appears to be associated with heart failure. Of note, the combination of β_1-Arg389 and α_{2C}-Del322-325 appears to impart heart failure risk in African Americans *(37)*. In patients with compensated heart failure, β_1-Arg389 is associated with increased exercise tolerance (VO_2 = 17.7 ± 0.4 mL/kg/min vs 14.5 mL/kg/min, p = 0.006) *(33)*. An additional contribution to VO_2 is provided by the position 49 variants *(33)*. In terms of survival, few studies have addressed this with adequate-size cohorts and control for β-blockers. Nevertheless, β_1-Gly49 has been reported to be associated with improved 5-yr survival (risk = 2.32, 95% CI 1.3–4.20, p = 0.003) *(38)*. This finding appears to be consistent with the Gly49 phenotype in transfected cells, which includes enhanced agonist-promoted downregulation (*see* Fig. 3B), which may provide a protective effect against the high levels of catecholamines in heart failure.

4.3. AR Polymorphisms as Pharmacogenetic Loci

β_2-ARs are expressed on airway smooth muscle and act to relax the constricted airway in asthma. β-Agonists, typically in the inhaled form, are a mainstay of asthma treatment and are used for acute treatment of bronchospasm, prophylaxis prior to a known asthma trigger, or on a regular basis for prevention. "Overuse" of β-agonist, particularly the short-acting forms, has been associated with decreased airway function, increased bronchial hyperreactivity, increased symptoms/exacerbations, and mortality *(49–41)*. Several studies have been carried out to assess whether a β_2-AR SNP or haplotype is predictive of efficacy or unfavorable events during treatment of asthma with the agonist albuterol.

In one study, the various β_2-AR haplotypic combinations (*see* Section 2. for description and ref. *3* for nomenclature) were utilized to assess the acute response to a standard dose (two puffs) of albuterol, with the change in forced expiratory volume in 1 s (FEV_1) as the outcome measure. As shown in Fig. 12, there was a relationship between haplotype pair and FEV_1 response (p = 0.007 by analysis of covariance). The two homozygous haplotype pairs (2 and 4) were further studied in transient transfected cells, with β_2-AR mRNA and protein as measures of expression. Haplotype 4 had approx 50% decreased expression compared to haplotype 2. This was entirely consistent with the physiological data for the asthmatics in that those with the 4/4 haplotype had a lower FEV_1 response to albuterol compared to those with the 2/2 haplotype. Those with the 4/4 haplotype, then, may be the least responsive to acute administration of β-agonist, and either alternative dosing or different agents might be considered for these individuals.

Two studies of the relationship between β_2AR SNPs and the chronic response to albuterol revealed additional findings relevant to those who use the drug on a regularly scheduled basis (i.e., every 6 h regardless of need, which is not an uncommon scenario). Israel and colleagues *(42)* retrospectively genotyped patients with mild asthma from a multicenter trial of albuterol given on an as-needed basis vs regular use. The change in morning and evening peak expiratory flow was the outcome measure. The results stratified by genotype are shown in Fig. 13A.

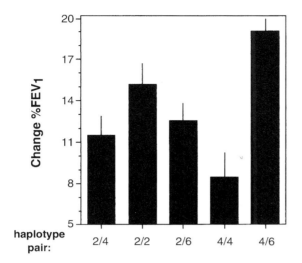

Fig. 12. The acute bronchodilator response to the β-agonist albuterol is associated with β$_2$-AR haplotype. FEV$_1$, forced expiratory volume in 1 s. (From ref. *3*.)

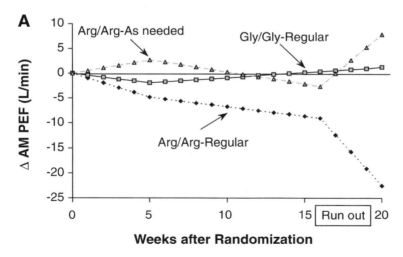

Fig. 13. The response to chronic administration of the β-agonist albuterol is associated with the β$_2$AR allele at position 16: **(A)** fall in peak expiratory flow (PEF) rate as a function of β$_2$-Arg16 genotype and treatment schedule (as needed vs regularly scheduled); **(B)** *(Continued on next page.)*

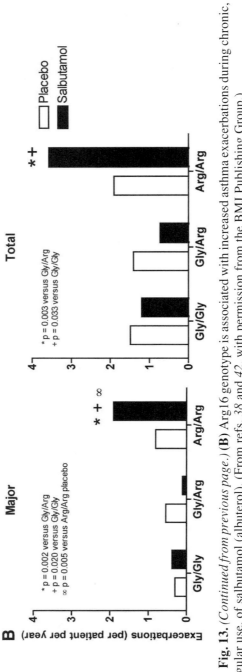

Fig. 13. (*Continued from previous page.*) (**B**) Arg16 genotype is associated with increased asthma exacerbations during chronic, regular use, of salbutamol (albuterol). (From refs. *38* and *42*, with permission from the BMJ Publishing Group.)

Patients who were homozygous for β_2-Arg16 *and* who used albuterol on the regular schedule exhibited a fall in peak flow over the course of the study. In contrast, those who were homozygous for β_2-Gly16 and were on the regular use schedule showed no such loss of lung function. And, as shown, β_2-Arg16 patients who used albuterol on an as-needed basis also showed no decline.

In another study, similar outcome measures were utilized, but the patients included moderate asthmatics; thus, exacerbations were frequent enough to discern if β_2-AR genotype influenced asthma control during β-agonist therapy *(38)*. As shown in Fig. 13B, exacerbations were substantially greater under the conditions of chronic (regularly scheduled) albuterol in the homozygous β_2-Arg16 patients compared to the homozygous β_2-Gly16 individuals. The peak flow data were similar to that of Israel et al. *(42)* but did not quite reach statistical significance. Based on these results, a prospective trial, in which patients are enrolled by homozygous genotype, is now under way.

4.4. Conclusions

A variety of polymorphisms have been delineated for most of the adrenergic receptors. Emphasis has been on the coding regions, but recently the promoter, 5' untranslated and 3' untranslated regions have been investigated as well. Signaling phenotypes have been determined in transfected cells, and to a lesser extent in endogenously expressing cells from humans with various genotypes. The findings thus far with such in-vitro assays must be taken into context, however, because they may be cell-type dependent. Clinical association, sib-pair, and family studies have concentrated on these common variants as risk factors, disease modifiers, or pharmacogenetic loci. The results of such studies are beginning to shed light on the physiologic and/or clinical implications of these polymorphisms.

References

1. Small KM, Forbes SL, Rahman FF, Bridges KM, Liggett SB. A four amino acid deletion polymorphism in the third intracellular loop of the human α_{2C}-adrenergic receptor confers impaired coupling to multiple effectors. J Biol Chem 2000;275: 23,059–23,064.
2. Small KM, Brown KM, Forbes SL, Liggett SB. Polymorphic deletion of three intracellular acidic residues of the α_{2B}-adrenergic receptor decreases G protein-coupled receptor kinase-mediated phosphorylation and desensitization. J Biol Chem 2001;276:4917–4922.
3. Drysdale CM, McGraw DW, Stack CB, et al. Complex promoter and coding region β_2-adrenergic receptor haplotypes alter receptor expression and predict *in vivo* responsiveness. Proc Natl Acad Sci USA 2000;97:10,483–10,488.
4. Mason DA, Moore JD, Green SA, Liggett SB. A gain-of-function polymorphism in a G-protein coupling domain of the human β_1-adrenergic receptor. J Biol Chem 1999;274:12,670–12,674.

5. Moore JD, Mason DA, Green SA, Hsu J, Liggett SB. Racial differences in the frequencies of cardiac β_1-adrenergic receptor polymorphisms: analysis of c145A>G and c1165G>C. Hum Mutat 1999;14:271.

6. Rathz DA, Brown KM, Kramer LA, Liggett SB. Amino acid 49 polymorphisms of the human β_1-adrenergic receptor affect agonist-promoted trafficking. J Cardiovasc Pharmacol 2002;39:155–160.

7. Levin MC, Marullo S, Muntaner O, Andersson B, Magnusson Y. The myocardium-protective Gly-49 variant of the β_1-adrenergic receptor exhibits constitutive activity and increased desensitization and down-regulation. J Biol Chem 2002; 277:30,429–30,435.

8. Perez JM, Rathz DA, Petrashevskaya NN, et al. β_1-Adrenergic receptor polymorphisms confer differential function and predisposition to heart failure. Nat Med 2003;9:1300–1305.

9. Green SA, Cole G, Jacinto M, Innis M, Liggett SB. A polymorphism of the human β_2-adrenergic receptor within the fourth transmembrane domain alters ligand binding and functional properties of the receptor. J Biol Chem 1993;268: 23,116–23,121.

10. Turki J, Lorenz JN, Green SA, Donnelly ET, Jacinto M, Liggett SB. Myocardial signalling defects and impaired cardiac function of a human β_2-adrenergic receptor polymorphism expressed in transgenic mice. Proc Natl Acad Sci USA 1996; 93:10,483–10,488.

11. Green SA, Rathz DA, Schuster AJ, Liggett SB. The Ile164 β_2-adrenoceptor polymorphism alters salmeterol exosite binding and conventional agonist coupling to G_s. Eur J Pharmacol 2001;421:141–147.

12. Green SA, Spasoff AP, Coleman RA, Johnson M, Liggett SB. Sustained activation of a G protein coupled receptor via "anchored" agonist binding: molecular localization of the salmeterol exosite within the β_2-adrenergic receptor. J Biol Chem 1996;271:24,029–24,035.

13. Reihsaus E, Innis M, MacIntyre N, Liggett SB. Mutations in the gene encoding for the β_2-adrenergic receptor in normal and asthmatic subjects. Am J Resp Cell Mol Biol 1993;8:334–339.

14. Green S, Turki J, Innis M, Liggett SB. Amino-terminal polymorphisms of the human β_2-adrenergic receptor impart distinct agonist-promoted regulatory properties. Biochemistry 1994;33:9414–9419.

15. Green SA, Turki J, Bejarano P, Hall IP, Liggett SB. Influence of β_2-adrenergic receptor genotypes on signal transduction in human airway smooth muscle cells. Am J Resp Cell Mol Biol 1995;13:25–33.

16. Moore PE, Laporte JD, Abraham JH, et al. Polymorphism of the β_2-adrenergic receptor gene and desensitization in human airway smooth muscle. Am J Respir Crit Care Med 2000;162:2117–2124.

17. Chong LK, Chowdry J, Ghahramani P, Peachell PT. Influence of genetic polymorphisms in the β_2-adrenoceptor on desensitization in human lung mast cells. Pharmacogenetics 1999;10:153–162.

18. McGraw DW, Forbes SL, Kramer LA, Liggett SB. Polymorphisms of the 5' leader cistron of the human b_2-adrenergic receptor regulate receptor expression. J Clin Invest 1998;102:1927–1932.

19. Clement K, Vaisse C, Manning BSJ, et al. Genetic variation in the β-3-adrenergic receptor and an increased capacity to gain weight in patients with morbid obesity. N Engl J Med 1995;333:352–354.
20. Candelore MR, Deng L, Tota LM, Kelly LJ, Cascieri MA, Strader CD. Pharmacological characterization of a recently described human $β_3$-adrenergic receptor mutant. Endocrinology 1996;137:2638–2641.
21. Pietri-Rouxel F, St John Manning B, Gros J, Strosberg AD. The biochemical effect of the naturally occurring Trp64(ρ)Arg mutation on human $β_3$-adrenoceptor activity. Eur J Biochem 1997;247:1174–1179.
22. Small KM, Forbes SL, Brown KM, Liggett SB. An Asn to Lys polymorphism in the third intracellular loop of the human $α_{2A}$-adrenergic receptor imparts enhanced agonist-promoted G_i coupling. J Biol Chem 2000;275:38,518–38,523.
23. Jewell-Motz EA, Liggett SB. An acidic motif within the third intracellular loop of the $α_2$C2 adrenergic receptor is required for agonist-promoted phosphorylation and desensitization. Biochemistry 1995;34:11,946–11,953.
24. Shibata K, Hirasawa A, Moriyama N, Kawabe K, Ogawa S, Tsujimoto G. $α_{1a}$-Adrenoceptor polymorphism: pharmacological characterization and association with benign prostatic hypertrophy. Br J Pharmacol 1996;118:1403–1408.
25. Buscher R, Herrmann V, Ring KM, et al. Variability in phenylephrine response and essential hypertension: a search for human $α_{1B}$-adrenergic receptor polymorphisms. J Pharmacol Exp Ther 1999;291:793–798.
26. Liggett SB. Pharmacogenetic applications of the Human Genome Project. Nat Med 2001;7:281–283.
27. Rana BK, Shiina T, Insel PA. Genetic variations and polymorphisms of G protein-coupled receptors: functional and therapeutic implications. Annu Rev Pharmacol Toxicol 2001;41:593–624.
28. Small KM, McGraw DW, Liggett SB. Pharmacology and physiology of human adrenergic receptor polymorphisms. Annu Rev Pharmacol Toxicol 2003;43:381–411.
29. Kotanko P, Binder A, Tasker J, et al. Essential hypertension in African Caribbeans associates with a variant of the $β_2$-adrenoceptor. Hypertension 1997;30:773–776.
30. Timmermann B, Mo R, Luft FC, et al. $β_2$ Adrenoceptor genetic variation is associated with genetic predisposition to essential hypertension: the Bergen Blood Pressure Study. Kidney Int 1998;53:1455–1460.
31. Bray MS, Krushkal J, Li L, et al. Positional genomic analysis identifies the $β_2$-adrenergic receptor gene as a susceptibility locus for human hypertension. Circulation 2000;101:2877–2882.
32. Bengtsson K, Melander O, Orho-Melander M, et al. Polymorphism in the $β_1$-adrenergic receptor gene and hypertension. Circulation 2001;104:187–190.
33. Wagoner LE, Craft LL, Zengel P, et al. Polymorphisms of the $β_1$-adrenergic receptor predict exercise capacity in heart failure. Am Heart J 2002;144:840–846.
34. Wagoner LE, Craft LL, Singh B, et al. Polymorphisms of the $β_2$-adrenergic receptor determine exercise capacity in patients with heart failure. Circ Res 2000;86:834–840.
35. Brodde OE, Buscher R, Tellkamp R, Radke J, Dhein S, Insel PA. Blunted cardiac responses to receptor activation in subjects with Thr164Ile β(2)-adrenoceptors. Circulation 2001;103:1048–1050.

36. Liggett SB, Wagoner LE, Craft LL, et al. The Ile164 β_2-adrenergic receptor polymorphism adversely affects the outcome of congestive heart failure. J Clin Invest 1998;102:1534–1539.
37. Small KM, Wagoner LE, Levin AM, Kardia SLR, Liggett SB. Synergistic polymorphisms of β_1- and α_{2C}-adrenergic receptors and the risk of congestive heart failure. N Engl J Med 2002;347:1135–1142.
38. Taylor DR, Drazen JM, Herbison GP, Yandava CN, Hancox RJ, Town GI. Asthma exacerbations during long term β agonist use: influence of β_2 adrenoceptor polymorphism. Thorax 2000;55:762–767.
39. Kraan J, Koeter GH, vd Mark TW, Sluiter HJ, De Vries K. Changes in bronchial hyperreactivity induced by 4 wk of treatment with antiasthmatic drugs in patients with allergic asthma: a comparison between budesonide and terbutaline. J Allergy Clin Immunol 1985;76:636.
40. Sears MR, Taylor DR, Print CG, et al. Regular inhaled beta-agonist treatment in bronchial asthma. Lancet 1990;336:1391–1396.
41. Spitzer WO, Suissa S, Ernst P, et al. The use of β-agonists and the risk of death and near death from asthma. N Engl J Med 1992;326:501–506.
42. Israel E, Drazen JM, Liggett SB, et al. The effect of polymorphisms of the β_2-adrenergic receptor on the response to regular use of albuterol in asthma. Am J Respir Crit Care Med 2000;162:75–80.

14

Microarray Analysis of Novel Adrenergic Receptor Functions

Boyd Rorabaugh, June Yun, and Dianne M. Perez

Summary

The advent of DNA microarray technology has provided a means to identify changes in the expression of thousands of genes simultaneously. This research tool has enabled investigators to study the effects of adrenergic receptor (AR) stimulation on gene expression on a large scale and has led to the identification of many genes that are regulated by adrenergic receptors (ARs). Microarrays have been used to compare the effects of α_{1A}-AR, α_{1B}-AR, and α_{1D}-AR stimulation on gene expression. This work demonstrated that all three α_1-AR subtypes commonly regulate many types of genes. However, genes that are regulated by only one or two α_1-AR subtypes have also been identified. These data provide evidence that the physiological roles of the three α_1-AR subtypes are not redundant despite their activation by the same ligand, use of common signal transduction pathways, and overlapping tissue distributions. Microarray studies have also identified genes that underlie AR-mediated regulation of the cell cycle, apoptosis, neuronal differentiation, cell hypertrophy, and other biological processes that are regulated by ARs. In addition, microarrays have identified changes in gene expression that accompany AR-mediated disease states, including cardiac hypertrophy, neurodegeneration, and hypermetabolism. The purpose of this chapter is to review how microarrays have contributed to our understanding of AR function at the genomic level.

Key Words: Adrenergic; function; gene expression; gene profiling; microarray; mRNA; receptor; transcription.

From: *The Receptors: The Adrenergic Receptors: In the 21st Century*
Edited by: D. Perez © Humana Press Inc., Totowa, NJ

1. Introduction

The existence of nuclear signaling pathways for G protein-coupled receptors (GPCRs) has been well established. GPCRs are known to influence gene expression by activating the serum response element (SRE), cyclic adenosine 5'-monophosphate response element, mitogen-activated protein kinase pathways, and signal transducers and activators of transcription (STAT), and other nuclear signaling pathways *(1–5)*. Some GPCRs also influence the expression of genes by decreasing messenger ribonucleic acid (mRNA) transcript stability *(6)*. Thus, GPCRs use multiple mechanisms to regulate gene expression.

Northern blots, RNA protection assays, and other traditional methods of gene expression analysis have limited investigators to analyzing only one gene or a few genes simultaneously. Consequently, the logistics of evaluating the effects of GPCR stimulation on a large number of genes has historically been an insurmountable barrier. However, the advent of deoxyribonucleic acid (DNA) microarray technology has made it feasible to study changes in gene expression on a large scale. Unlike traditional methods of gene expression analysis, DNA microarrays enable investigators to analyze changes in the expression of thousands of genes simultaneously in a single experiment. The purpose of this chapter is to review how DNA microarrays have contributed to our understanding of the function of adrenergic receptors (ARs) at the genomic level.

2. What Is a DNA Microarray?

A DNA microarray (also known as a gene chip) is essentially a miniaturized dot blot that has been designed for high-throughput analysis of gene expression. A microarray consists of a postage stamp size piece of glass that has many DNA probes uniformly arranged on its surface. Each probe is composed of a polymerase chain reaction product, complementary DNA, or synthetic oligonucleotide that has a unique nucleotide sequence and is located at a specific "address" on the surface of the gene chip. The DNA probe at each address corresponds to a specific gene and can hybridize to RNA that contains the complementary sequence. When fluorescently labeled RNA (prepared from a biological sample) hybridizes with the DNA probes on the gene chip, each address on the chip fluoresces with an intensity that is proportional to the amount of RNA present in the biological sample. Consequently, if two identical gene chips are hybridized with RNA from different biological samples (healthy vs diseased tissue, drug-treated vs untreated cells, two different tissue types, etc.), then changes in the expression of each gene can be measured by comparing the fluorescence of their respective addresses on each gene chip. The results of DNA microarray analysis are generally consistent with those obtained by Northern blotting *(7–10)*, with the microarray often showing increased sensitivity.

The first DNA microarray was synthesized using oligonucleotides complimentary to 45 *Arabidopsis thaliana* genes *(11)*. Microarrays are now available for gene expression analysis in a variety of species, including human, rat, mouse, *Drosophila melanogaster*, *Saccharomyces cerevisiae*, *Caenorhabditis elegans*, *Pseudomonas aeruginosa*, and *Escherichia coli*. These microarrays contain up to 47,000 genes on a single chip. In addition to representing an increasingly large number of genes, DNA microarrays are also becoming more complex. Some microarrays use multiple probes that are complementary to different regions of the mRNA sequence for each gene that is represented on the chip. This enables RNA transcripts that are alternatively spliced into multiple mRNA products to be detected. In addition, some oligonucleotide microarrays also contain a control oligonucleotide for each probe that contains a single nucleotide mismatch. These mismatched oligonucleotides are used to verify the hybridization specificity of each probe.

3. α_1-Adrenergic Receptors

The effects of α_1-AR stimulation on gene expression have been more thoroughly studied than those of α_2-ARs or β-ARs. Microarray studies provide evidence that the three α_1-AR subtypes differentially regulate gene expression. This may provide a mechanism for the sympathetic nervous system to control cell growth, cell differentiation, apoptosis, and other cellular functions by stimulating receptors that are coupled to changes in the expression of different genes. DNA microarray studies have also identified genetic changes that occur during α_1-AR-induced pathological conditions. These studies have provided new insight into the physiological and potential pathological roles of α_1-ARs.

3.1. Transcriptional Regulation by α_1-AR Subtypes

All three α_1-AR subtypes are coupled via the G_q family of G proteins to the activation of phospholipase C. This enzyme catalyzes the hydrolysis of phosphatidylinositol 4,5-bisphosphate into the second messengers inositol 1,4,5-trisphosphate and diacylglycerol. These second messenger molecules trigger changes in cell function by stimulating an increase in cytosolic calcium and activating protein kinase C. In nonmicroarray studies, α_1-ARs also activate mitogen-activated protein kinase, P38 kinase, and Jun kinase, although all α_1-AR subtypes do not activate these pathways with equal efficiency *(12,13)*. Studies using reporter gene constructs have found that α_1-AR subtypes also differentially regulate the expression of genes encoding several transcription factors *(12,13)*. α_{1A}-ARs stimulate transcription of genes encoding activator protein-1, nuclear factor of activated T cells, nuclear factor-κB, and genes controlled by the SRE. α_{1B}-ARs stimulate transcription of activator protein-1 and nuclear factor of activated T cells but have no effect on expression of nuclear factor-κB or genes regulated by the SRE. In contrast, α_{1D}-AR stimulation has no effect on the expression of any of these genes. These studies suggest that the three α_1-AR subtypes might activate different signal transduction pathways that lead to the expression of different genes. However, in these studies the α_{1D}-AR generally had a much smaller effect on gene expression than the α_{1A}-AR or α_{1B}-AR. On a cautionary note, it is possible that these differences are not caused by differential coupling but because α_{1D}-ARs are usually expressed at a lower density or are hardly expressed at all compared to the other two α_1-AR subtypes.

3.2. Genetic Profiling of α_1-AR Subtypes

DNA microarrays have also been used to compare transcriptional responses induced by α_1-AR subtypes. Our laboratory used a DNA microarray containing 7000 rat genes to compare the effects of stimulating α_{1A}-, α_{1B}-, or α_{1D}-ARs in stably transfected Rat-1 fibroblasts. We found that 38 of 7000 genes were commonly regulated (either upregulated or downregulated) by all three α_1-AR subtypes (8). Of these genes, 29 were upregulated at least twofold and 9 were downregulated at least twofold in cells expressing different α_1-AR subtypes compared to cells that do not express ARs. These commonly regulated genes encoded a wide variety of proteins, including cytokines and growth factors, transcription factors, enzymes, and cell matrix proteins. Epinephrine increased the expression of some genes (i.e., *interleukin 6* and *c-fos*) more than 60-fold in cells expressing α_1-ARs compared to nontransfected cells (Table 1). However, most changes were more modest.

Some of the genes that are commonly regulated by all three α_1-AR subtypes have also been previously identified with traditional methods of detection. Common transcription factors such as c-fos and c-jun (14) as well as the early growth response genes (*egr-1*) (15) have been found to increase after α_1-AR activation.

In addition to genes that were commonly regulated by all three α_1-AR subtypes, we also identified genes that were regulated by specific α_1-AR subtypes (Table 1). Stimulation of the α_{1B}-AR caused a 25-fold increase in expression of the *neuritin* gene, involved in neuronal growth. However, α_{1A}- and α_{1D}-ARs had no effect on the expression of this gene. Another interesting neuronal gene that was specifically regulated by the α_{1B}-AR was *synuclein*, a gene associated with parkinsonian syndromes. The α_{1B}-AR decreased its expression by 34-fold. We have also reported that synuclein expression is abnormal in transgenic mice that overexpress the α_{1B}-AR. Interestingly, these mice develop a neurodegenerative disorder called multiple system atrophy that is similar to a human parkinsonian syndrome (16). The α_{1B}-AR also specifically decreased the expression of two genes involved in apoptosis (*caspase 6* and *transforming growth factor-* β3 [*TGF-* β3]) in Rat-1 fibroblasts. We have confirmed in this cell line that the α_{1B}-AR "protects" against apoptosis, and the α_{1A}- and α_{1D}-ARs promote apoptosis

Table 1

Selected Gene Expression Changes in Epinephrine-Stimulated Rat-1 Fibroblasts Expressing α_{1A}-, α_{1B}-, or α_{1D}-Adrenergic Receptors

Gene (accession no.)	Description	α_{1A}-AR	α_{1B}-AR	α_{1D}-AR
Commonly regulated genes				
• Interleukin 6 (M26744)	Growth factor	57 ± 4	62 ± 12	21 ± 3
• c-fos (X06769)	Transcription factor	63 ± 23	43 ± 12	61 ± 13
• c-jun (X17163)	Transcription factor	19 ± 0.1	24 ± 0.1	23 ± 1
• Collagenase (M60616)	Enzyme	5.9 ± 0.2	8.4 ± 0.6	3.6 ± 0.4
• Hexokinase (D26393)	Enzyme	4.9 ± 1.7	4.4 ± 1.0	7.1 ± 1.5
• Fibronectin (M28259)	Extracellular matrix	4.4 ± 1.5	3.7 ± 1.1	3.8 ± 1.3
• Collagen III (M21354)	Extracellular matrix	2.4 ± 0.2	2.1 ± 0.1	4.6 ± 0.2
• egr-1 (M18416)	Transcription factor	2.1 ± 0.1	3.1 ± 0.2	2.7 ± 0.1
• egr-2 (U78102)	Transcription factor	2.0 ± 0.1	2.2 ± 0.1	2.8 ± 0.3
• Cell-adhesion molecule 4 (U23056)	Adhesion	-5.9 ± 2.0	-6.6 ± 2.4	6.0 ± 1.4
• Lysyl oxidase (S77494)	Enzyme	-2.5 ± 0.1	-4.2 ± 0.3	-2.0 ± 0.0
• Dimethylarginase (D86041)	Enzyme	-2.3 ± 0.1	-4.4 ± 0.3	-4.1 ± 0.1
α_{1A}-Specific genes				
• Lactate dehydrogenase (U07181)	Enzyme	6.0 ± 0.9	NC	NC
• Myogenic regulatory factor (M84176)	Transcription factor	3.0 ± 0.5	NC	NC
• Heme oxygenase-2 (J05405)	Enzyme	-5.5 ± 0.9	NC	NC

Continued on next page

Table 1 (*Continued*)
Selected Gene Expression Changes in Epinephrine-Stimulated Rat-1 Fibroblasts Expressing α_{1A}-, α_{1B}-, or α_{1D}-Adrenergic Receptors

Gene (accession no.)	Description	α_{1A}-AR	α_{1B}-AR	α_{1D}-AR
α_{1B}-Specific genes				
• Lumican (X84039)	Connective protein	NC	14.4 ± 0.7	NC
• Caspase 6 (AF025670)	Apoptosis	NC	-5.5 ± 0.1	NC
• TGF-β3 (U03491)	Apoptosis	NC	-2.3 ± 0.1	NC
• Neuritin (U88958)	Neuronal growth	NC	25.3 ± 4.3	NC
• Nucleolin (M55017)	Ribosome biogenesis	NC	8.5 ± 0.8	NC
• Sensory neuron synuclein (X86789)	Neurodegeneration	NC	-33.9 ± 0.6	NC
• Glutamine amidohydrolase (J05499)	Enzyme	NC	-9.9 ± 0.7	NC
• Caveolin (Z46614)	Receptor internalize	NC	-2.9 ± 0.3	NC
α_{1D}-Specific genes				
• Adipsin (M92059)	Acylating protein	NC	NC	20.4 ± 2.2
• Glucose transporter 5 (D28562)	Transport	NC	NC	4.7 ± 0.1
• 90-kDa heat shock protein (S45392)	Chaperone	NC	NC	-3.0 ± 0.1
Differentially regulated genes				
• gp-130 (M92340)	Signal transduction	4.4 ± 0.05	NC	5.2 ± 0.2
• STAT-3 (X91810)	Signal transduction	4.0 ± 0.8	NC	10.1 ± 0.5
• p21-Ras (U09793)	Signal transduction	5.3 ± 0.4	NC	8.4 ± 0.6

Data indicate the fold increase or decrease $\pm$ SEM of gene expression compared to epinephrine-stimulated cells that lack α_1-ARs. NC, no change. (All data derived from ref. 8.)

(unpublished data). The α_{1D}-AR specifically changed the expression of *adipsin* (Table 1), an acylating protein involved in fat metabolism. In general, the α_{1B}-AR influenced the expression of the greatest number of specific genes (17 genes), followed by the α_{1D}-AR (12 genes) and α_{1A}-AR (6 genes).

We also discovered genes that were regulated by two of the α_1-AR subtypes but not by the third subtype. This was always patterned with the α_{1A}- and α_{1D}-ARs showing similar regulation; the α_{1B}-AR showed no coupling. For example, stimulation of α_{1A}- and α_{1D}-ARs significantly increased the expression of gp-130 and STAT-3 at the mRNA and protein levels. However, stimulation of α_{1B}-ARs had no effect on these genes. We also explored these pathways at the protein and biochemical levels, showing that the α_1-AR subtypes were differentially coupled to STAT-3 serine-phosphorylation *(8)*. The mechanism by which the α_1-AR subtypes differentially regulate these genes is not understood. These differences suggest that the physiological roles of the α_1-AR subtypes are not redundant despite the fact that they are activated by the same endogenous ligand, share some common signal transduction pathways, and have overlapping tissue distributions.

Another interesting observation found in this study was that changes in gene expression did not correlate with epinephrine-stimulated inositol phosphate (IP) formation. The α_{1A}-AR is more efficiently coupled than the α_{1B}- or α_{1D}-AR to IP turnover *(8,17)*. However, the commonly regulated genes demonstrated similar fold changes for all three α_1-AR subtypes (Table 1) despite differences in the efficacy of the IP response. A simple explanation for this discrepancy is that IP formation may be at a saturating level for all three subtypes, and any extra production does not result in further changes in gene expression. Alternately, it is also possible that α_1-AR-induced changes in gene expression may be mediated by signal transduction pathways that do not involve the production of IPs.

3.3. Differential Regulation of the Cell Cycle by α_1-ARs

α_1-ARs stimulate proliferation of a variety of cell types, including vascular smooth muscle cells *(18,19)*, prostate stromal cells *(20)*, hepatocytes *(21)*, and neuroepithelial cells *(22)*. α_1-AR stimulation also inhibits the proliferation of some cell types *(23)*. However, the lack of sufficiently selective α_1-AR subtype antagonists and the fact that many cell types express multiple α_1-AR subtypes have made it difficult to determine how each of these receptors influence cell proliferation. Therefore, cell lines that have been transfected with a single α_1-AR subtype have been used to study the effects of α_1-ARs on cell proliferation and cell cycling.

By using microarray technology, our laboratory reported that the α_1-AR subtypes influence the proliferation of Rat-1 fibroblasts by controlling the progression of cells from the G_1 to the S phase of the cell cycle. Stimulation of α_{1A}-

or α_{1D}-ARs decreased the expression of several genes required for cell cycle progression. The α_{1A}- or α_{1D}-AR stimulation decreased the expression of *cyclin E* and *cyclin B* and downregulated the cyclin-dependent kinases associated with cyclins (Table 2). Stimulation of α_{1A}- or α_{1D}-ARs also downregulated the transcription of genes encoding *DNA polymerase α-subunits I–IV*, which are required for DNA synthesis. α_{1B}-AR stimulation did not affect the expression of any of these genes. Rather, stimulation of α_{1B}-ARs increased the expression of *cyclin D1*, which promotes progression of cells from the G_1 to the S phase. Using flow cytometry, we confirmed these changes at the functional level. Stimulation of α_{1A}- or α_{1D}-ARs caused G_1–S phase arrest; α_{1B}-AR stimulation caused unchecked cell cycle progression. We also confirmed the decreased kinase activity of the cyclin-dependent kinases associated with the cyclins and the increased expression of p27 (a kinase inhibitor) when the α_{1A}- or α_{1D}-ARs were stimulated. The α_{1B}-AR showed no regulation of these proteins. Similar effects were also observed in PC 12 cells transfected with different α_1-AR subtypes and in DDT-MF2 cells that endogenously express α_{1B}-ARs *(24)*. These data suggest that α_1-AR subtypes differentially influence cell proliferation by regulating the expression of genes that control the cell cycle.

Another study using α_1-AR-transfected Chinese hamster ovary cells also demonstrated that the three α_1-AR subtypes have different effects on cell proliferation *(25)*. This study was consistent with the results of our laboratory in that G_1–S arrest was an important point of α_1-AR-mediated cell cycle regulation. However, the results of this study differed from our data in that cell cycle arrest was initiated by α_{1A}- or α_{1B}-AR stimulation; the α_{1D}-AR had no effect on the cell cycle. This suggests that individual α_1-AR subtypes may influence the cell cycle differently depending on the cellular environment in which they are expressed.

3.4. Gene Expression Profile of Hearts and Brains That Express Constitutively Active α_{1B}-ARs

The elucidation of functional roles of the α_1-AR subtypes has been hampered by the lack of sufficiently selective ligands. In addition, the inability to produce high-avidity antibodies against the receptor subtypes has also hindered research in this area. Investigators have attempted to circumvent these obstacles by using genetically altered transgenic and knockout mouse models of the different α_1-AR subtypes *(26–30)*. To investigate further the physiological role of α_{1B}-ARs, transgenic mouse lines were generated that systemically express the wild-type α_{1B}-AR or constitutively active α_{1B}-ARs under the control of the mouse α_{1B}-AR promoter *(16)*. The transgenic mouse lines expressing the constitutively active mutant receptor carried either a single-mutant form (C128F) or a triple-mutant form (C128F/A204V/A293E), both of which spontaneously couple to G_q *(31,32)*.

Table 2
α_1-Adrenergic Receptor Subtypes Differentially Regulate the Expression of Genes That Control Progression of the Cell Cycle

Gene (accession no.)	Effect of expression on cell cycle	α_{1A}-AR	α_{1B}-AR	α_{1D}-AR
Cyclin E (D14015)	Required for G_1–S progression	-3.3 ± 0.7	NC	-4.4 ± 0.2
Cyclin-dependent kinase 2-α (D28753)	Required for G_1–S progression	-2.4 ± 0.7	NC	-4.1 ± 1.3
DNA polymerase α-subunit I (AJ011605)	Required for DNA synthesis (S phase)	-2.5 ± 0.1	NC	-3.3 ± 0
DNA polymerase α-subunit II (AJ011606)	Required for DNA synthesis (S phase)	-4.9 ± 1.0	NC	-3.9 ± 1.0
DNA polymerase α-subunit III (AJ011607)	Required for DNA synthesis (S phase)	-2.6 ± 0.5	NC	-4.2 ± 0.2
DNA polymerase α-subunit IV (AJ011608)	Required for DNA synthesis (S phase)	-2.6 ± 0.1	NC	-4.2 ± 0.1
Cyclin B (X64589)	Required for G_2–M progression	-4.0 ± 1.1	NC	-6.7 ± 1.0
Cyclin D1 (D14014)	Required for G_1–S progression	NC	$4.8 + 0.7$	NC

Data indicate the fold increase or decrease $\pm$ SEM of gene expression compared to epinephrine-stimulated cells that lack α_1-ARs. NC, no change. (All data from ref. 24.)

The transgenic mice displayed a cardiovascular phenotype that included mild cardiac hypertrophy with some aspects of heart dysfunction, such as an increased isovolumetric relaxation time and dilated chambers *(33)*. Although displaying a hypertrophic heart, these transgenic mice did not advance into heart failure. Transgenic mice also showed a neurological phenotype that was characterized by neurodegeneration that began in discrete brain regions and spread to encompass many areas of the brain with age *(16)*. These mice had impaired hindlimb movement starting at about 3 mo of age and progressively worsened as the mice grew older. Also, older mice (>8 mo of age) had uninduced grand mal seizures similar to those of human epilepsy *(34)*. Transgenic mice also showed symptoms of autonomic dysfunction, which included reduced plasma catecholamine, corticotropin releasing factor, adrenocorticotropic hormone levels, hypotension, weight loss, and reproduction problems *(16,33)*. Together with cytoplasmic inclusions bodies of α-synuclein in oligodendrocytes, these symptoms were similar to a human disorder, multiple system atrophy, which is characterized by Parkinson-like neurodegeneration and autonomic failure *(35)*. These data suggest a possible role for α_{1B}-ARs in the control of movement disorders.

To identify the molecular mechanisms underlying these symptoms, Yun et al. carried out two microarray studies that compared the gene expression profiles of hearts and brains from mice that overexpress α_{1B}-ARs to those of their normal counterparts *(10,36)*. Because some of the transgenic traits could be age associated, gene expression profiles were also compared at different age points with their age-matched controls. Both studies utilized transgenic mice that systemically expressed the constitutively active triple-mutant α_{1B}-AR and their wild-type nontransgenic counterparts. In the heart study, mRNA was isolated from normal and transgenic mice at 2 mo of age before symptoms were detected and at 12 mo, when transgenic mice had developed cardiac hypertrophy. The mRNA targets were labeled and hybridized to the murine genome U74A oligonucleotide array from Affymetrix, which allowed the screening of 12,656 transcripts of known genes and expressed sequence tags.

As expected, a number of gene transcripts involved in regulating cardiac function were differentially expressed, primarily in the 2-mo-old transgenic hearts (Table 3). These included many genes associated with cardiac hypertrophy. During hypertrophy, cytoskeletal and extracellular matrix alterations lead to the remodeling of the myocardium. Consistent with cytoskeletal alterations associated with classical hypertrophy, changes in the expression of cytoskeletal genes, including *actin* and *tau*, were detected, and several genes encoding collagens were differentially expressed in transgenic hearts (Table 3). It is known that, during cardiac dysfunction, remodeling events in both the cellular cytoskeleton and the extracellular matrix lead to the physical changes associated with

Table 3
Changes in Gene Expression in the Hearts
of 2- and 12-mo-old Mice Expressing
Constitutively Active α_{1B}-Adrenergic Receptors

Encoded protein (accession no.)	Fold changes	
	2 mo	12 mo
Tachykinin I (D17584)	+2.1	NC
Tau (M18775)	+1.8	NC
PKC β1 (X59274)	+1.8	NC
Calbindin-28K (D26352)	−1.0	+2.9
Procollagen IV (X04647)	−1.5	NC
MEF2 (U94423)	−1.6	+0.7
Procollagen III (X52046)	−1.7	NC
Procollagen I (U03419)	−1.8	NC
Actin α1 (M12347)	−2.0	NC
GP130 (X62646)	−2.3	NC
Collagen V (AB009993)	−2.3	NC
CamKII δ (AF059029)	−2.5	NC
Collagen IV (Z35167)	−2.9	NC
Caveolin (U07645)	−3.7	NC
Procollagen-type XVIII (L22545)	NC	+3.3
Ceruloplasmin (U49430)	NC	+2.5
γ-Glutamyl transpeptidase (C76628)	NC	+2.0
Insulin II (X04724)	NC	+1.8
LIM (AF002283)	NC	−1.5

Values represent fold changes compared with age-matched nontransgenic mice. SEM were removed for simplicity. NC, no change. (Data from ref. *10*.)

the hypertrophic heart. These changes are associated with increased expression levels of collagens and structural proteins such as actin. Of interest, the *collagens* and *actin* were downregulated rather than upregulated, primarily in the 2-mo-old transgenic hearts. Similarly, *GP130*, *CamKII*, and *MEF2*, genes associated with signaling of interleukin 6 cytokines (inducers of hypertrophy) also showed reduced transcript levels. These changes indicate a potential subset of genes that are regulated by α_{1B}-ARs and are involved in mediating cardiac hypertrophy; they may also be caused by compensatory responses that attempt to attenuate α_{1B}-AR signaling and prevent further enlargement of the heart.

Another set of genes that were differentially expressed in transgenic hearts was those associated with tyrosine kinase pathways, particularly *cSrc* (Table 4).

Table 4
Changes in the Expression of Genes Encoding
Growth Factors, Tyrosine Kinases, and Associated Genes
in the Hearts of 2- and 12-mo-old Mice That Express
Constitutively Active α_{1B}-Adrenergic Receptors

Encoded protein (accession no.)	Fold changes	
	2 mo	12 mo
Tyrosine Kinases and Associated Proteins		
• Lck (M12056)	+2.7	NC
• PDGF (M29464)	+2.2	NC
• Protein tyrosine phosphatase (X97268)	+1.8	NC
• GM-CSF (X03020)	−1.8	+6.5
• PI3-kinase (U52193)	NC	+3.0
• VEGF (AF022856)	NC	+2.6
• Intestinal tyrosine kinase (Z48757)	NC	+2.2
• Braf (M64429)	NC	+2.2
• cSrc (M17031)	NC	+1.5
• FGF-7	NC	−9.5

Values represent the fold changes compared with age-matched nontransgenic mice. SEM were removed for simplicity. NC, no change. (Data are taken from ref. *10*.)

The transcript for cSrc itself was only increased 1.5-fold in 12-mo-old transgenic hearts. This also corresponded to a 60% increase in cSrc protein levels over that of normal mouse hearts by Western blot analysis *(10)*. Previous studies have shown that other GPCRs can transactivate growth factor receptors, such as receptors for epidermal growth factor and platelet-derived growth factor, which typically signal via Src *(37,38)*. Interestingly, transcripts for platelet-derived growth factor and granulocyte macrophage colony-stimulating factor (GM-CSF) were also differentially expressed in transgenic hearts. The interaction with the Src signaling pathway is also consistent with previous studies indicating that α_1-ARs may exert their growth and mitogenic properties via activation of tyrosine kinases such as cSrc *(12)*. In addition, activated cSrc has been associated with the hypertrophying feline myocardium *(39)* and to induce an increase in cell size in isolated neonatal rat myocytes *(40)*. Thus, Src tyrosine kinases may be involved in the α_{1B}-AR signaling pathway that leads to hypertrophy of these transgenic hearts. This result is not surprising given the fact that β-ARs have been shown to couple to Src after desensitization of the receptor, a result likely to occur in heart failure or excessive catecholamine drive *(41)*.

Table 5
Differential Gene Expression of Inflammatory
and Immune Response Proteins
in 2- and 12-mo-old Mouse Hearts Expressing
Constitutively Active α_{1B}-Adrenergic Receptors

Encoded protein (accession no.)	Fold changes	
	2 mo	12 mo
Inflammatory/Immune Response		
• Complement C3 (K02782)	+1.9	NC
• C1q-related factor (AF095155)	+1.9	NC
• CD3θ T cell receptor (L03353)	+1.8	NC
• Variable heavy chain (X88902)	+0.9	+5.9
• Anti-DNA IgG light chain (U55576)	+0.7	+2.3
• Uteroglobin (L04503)	−2.2	+3.2
• γ-1 Ig (V00793)	−2.5	NC
• Anti-DNA κ-chain (U30629)	NC	+5.9
• Ig active κ-chain V-reg (M13284)	NC	+5.4
• Ig heavy chain (AF036736)	NC	+5.0
• TAX (Z21674)	NC	+4.2
• LY49C (U34891)	NC	+3.4
• B-cell antigen receptor (L28060)	NC	+3.2
• Anti-DNA IgG light chain (U55641)	NC	+3.1
• Toll-like receptor 6 (AB020808)	NC	+3.1
• Ig-κ light chain (U60442)	NC	+2.9
• Ig-V(H)II H18 (X02468)	NC	+2.8
• Ig heavy chain, var (AF025445)	NC	+2.5
• Carboxypeptidase A3 (J05118)	NC	−2.1
• T-cell-specific protein (L38444)	NC	−2.5
• Heavy chain var region (AF035203)	NC	−4.3

Values represent the fold changes compared with age-matched nontransgenic mice. SEM were removed for simplicity. NC, no change. (Data from ref. *10*.)

By far the largest number of gene expression changes detected in transgenic hearts were those involved in the inflammatory or immune response, such as increased production of immunoglobulins and autoantibodies (Table 5). Increased immunoglobulin light and heavy chains were also detected by Western blots, verifying that the increased gene transcription resulted in increases at the protein level *(10)*. These changes were primarily detected in the 12-mo-old hearts, suggesting that the hypertrophic changes associated with this transgenic model leads to inflammation. Alternately, α_{1B}-AR expression may lead to direct proliferation of lymphocytes because mRNAs for α_1-ARs have been localized to these cells (42). Gene expression changes included increases in complement, autoantibodies, and immunoglobulins. It is known from recent investigations that inflammatory responses are associated with heart failure and other cardiac diseases (43), and autoantibodies have also been linked to dilated cardiomyopathy (44,45). In fact, a previous study indicated higher levels of both anti-DNA autoantibodies and complement proteins associated with hypertensive patients presenting with left ventricular hypertrophy as compared with hypertensives without left ventricular hypertrophy or normal patients (46). This may indicate a link between these immune response pathways and cardiac hypertrophy. It is still unclear how the damaged heart evokes the inflammatory response. The α_{1B}-AR transgenic mice also showed increased levels of apoptotic cell death in the myocardium and changes in the expression of a number of genes that are involved in apoptotic cell death (10). Thus, an apoptotic component (i.e., release of self-DNA) may also contribute to the autoantibody response observed in the myocardium of α_{1B}-AR-overexpressing mice.

Genes that may contribute to the neurological phenotype observed in mice expressing constitutively active α_{1B}-ARs were identified by comparing gene expression levels between transgenic and normal brains at three different ages: 2–4 mo (before most disease manifestation), 8–10 mo (when some symptoms begin and some symptoms worsen), and 12–18 mo (when transgenic mice are in a diseased state). Genes that are involved in glutamate or calcium regulation (Table 6), growth and the immune response (Table 7), and transcription or translation regulation (Table 8) were generally changed in older transgenic brains. In contrast, changes in the expression of genes involved in apoptosis (Table 6), synaptic transport (Table 9), and cellular structure (Table 9) were observed in both young and old mice.

Several glutamate receptor genes were also found to be differentially expressed in the transgenic brains. These included the genes that encode three different ionotropic glutamate receptor subunits, N-methyl-D-aspartate (NMDA) receptor R1, and α-amino-3-hydroxy-5-methyl-4-isoxazole proprionic acid 1, all of which were upregulated in older transgenic brains. Accompanying this increase in excitatory glutamatergic signal was a decrease in subunit expression of the inhibitory γ-aminobutyric acid A ($GABA_A$) receptor. Protein levels of the NMDA and GABA receptors were verified by radioligand binding assays and Western blotting. In addition, immunohistochemistry studies indicated increased levels of NMDA receptor subunits in transgenic brains in both the cortex and hippocampus, two regions highly associated with epileptogenesis (47). These findings strongly suggest that glutamate dysregulation is involved in the manifestation of the seizure phenotype and possibly in the etiology of neurodegeneration that is observed in the α_{1B}-AR-overexpressing transgenic mice.

Table 6
Changes in the Expression of Genes Involved in Neurodegeneration Pathways in Mouse Brain Expressing Constitutively Active α_{1B}-Adrenergic Receptors

Encoded protein (accession no.)	Fold changes	
	2–4 mo	12–18 mo
Glutamate regulation		
• Calcium-sensing receptor (AF022252)	+2.8 ± 0.5	NC
• Calmodulin (M27844)	+1.7 ± 0.08	NC
• Cam kinaseII (plasticity; X14836)	–11.0 ± 0.5	+3.9 ± 0.5
• Plasma membrane Ca^{2+}-ATPase (AF053471)	NC	+6.1 ± 0.9
• L-type Ca^{2+} channel (U73487)	NC	+2.6 ± 0.1
• NMDA receptor R1 (D10028)	NC	+2.8 ± 0.1
• Glutamate decarboxylase (D42051)	NC	+2.7 ± 0.1
• Guanylate kinase (U53514)	NC	+2.2 ± 0.05
• $GABA_A$ receptor $\alpha 1$ (X61430)	NC	–1.9 ± 0.03
• $GABA_A$ receptor $\gamma 1$ (X55272)	NC	–3.0 ± 0.1
Apoptotic		
• Bik-like killer (AF048838)	+6.1 ± 2	NC
• Met proto-oncogene (Y00671)	+5.6 ± 2.3	NC
• Transforming growth factor, β (AJ009862)	+5.0 ± 1.0	NC
• Cd40 Ligand (X65453)	+4.2 ± 0.6	NC
• Superoxide dismutase 1 (M35725)	+3.2 ± 0.03	NC
Neurodegeneration		
• α-Tubulin (M13441	+1.7 ± 0.06	NC
• Tau (M18776)	+1.6 ± 0.05	NC
• Apoliprotein E (D00466)	+1.6 ± 0.03	NC
• LR11, ApoE receptor (AB015790)	NC	+5.8 ± 0.3
• Niemann-Pick type C1 (AF003348)	NC	+1.8 ± 0.03

Data represent fold changes ± SEM compared to age-matched nontransgenic mice. NC, no change. (Data from ref. *36*.)

These data also implicate the α_{1B}-AR in the modulation of NMDA and GABA receptors.

Another interesting set of genes that were differentially expressed in transgenic brains was those involved in apoptotic cell death and neurodegeneration. These genes included *Blk* (a proapoptotic Bcl2 family member) and *TGF*-β (a proapoptotic cytokine). Increased levels of activated caspase-3, a mediator of apoptosis, were also detected by immunohistochemistry in the 2- to 3-mo-old transgenic brains, particularly in the white matter. This suggests that caspase-mediated cell

Table 7
Changes in the Expression of Genes Involved in Growth and the Immune Response in Mouse Brains Expressing Constitutively Active α_{1B}-Adrenergic Receptors

	Fold changes	
Encoded protein (accession no.)	2–4 mo	12–18 mo
Growth		
• Inhibin B (U89840)	+5.2 ± 0.9	NC
• Pro-opiomelanocortin α (J00612)	+3.8 ± 0.2	+5.4 ± 0.5
• Brain neurotensin receptor 2 (U51908)	+2.1 ± 0.06	NC
• Calmodulin (M27844)	+1.7 ± 0.09	NC
• Jun kinase (AB005664)	–2.0 ± 0.4	NC
• Carboxypeptidase D (D85391)	NC	+3.6 ± 0.4
• Casein kinase II (U51866)	NC	+4.9 ± 0.2
• Prolactin (X04418)	NC	+53.7 ± 10
• Growth hormone (X02891)	NC	+16.6 ± 0.2
• IRS2 (AF090738)	NC	+7.7 ± 0.2
• Bone morphogenetic prot recept II (AF003942)	NC	+4.1 ± 0.2
• FGF, inducible (U42384)	NC	+3.7 ± 0.4
• Endothelin receptor, B (U32329)	NC	+3.5 ± 0.4
• Brain-derived neurotrophic factor (X55573)	NC	+1.8 ± 0.03
• Thyroid hormone receptor (U09504)	NC	–1.8 ± 0.04
Immune/defense		
• Ig-κ variable (AB007986)	+5.0 ± 0.8	NC
• Interleukin 4 (X035320	+4.6 ± 0.7	NC
• Stress-induced phosphoprotein (U27830)	–1.9 ± 0.09	NC
• Ly49E, Natural killer cell receptor (U10091)	–3.6 ± 0.7	NC
• Tec tyrosine kinase (X55663)	–5.6 ± 0.2	NC
• Natural killer enhancing factor B (U20611)	NC	+2.3 ± 0.04
• Hsp40 (AB028272)	NC	+1.8 ± 0.08
• Interferon-β (V00756)	NC	–1.8 ± 0.2

Data represent the fold changes ± SEM in gene expression compared to brains from age-matched nontransgenic mice. NC, no change. (Data from ref. *36*.)

death occurred in transgenic brains. These findings are consistent with the previous microarray study in the heart because genes involved in regulating TGF-β were also differentially expressed in transgenic hearts *(10)*. This suggests that α_{1B}-AR overexpression may lead to increased apoptotic cell death through a TGF-β-mediated mechanism.

A potentially novel finding is that α_{1B}-ARs regulate the expression of genes that are involved in synaptic or vesicular transport. A number of genes that are

Table 8
Changes in the Expression of Genes Involved in Intracellular Signaling, Transcription, and Translation in Mouse Brains Expressing Constitutively Active α_{1B}-Adrenergic Receptors

Encoded protein (accession no.)	Fold changes	
	2–4 mo	12–18 mo
Transcription/Translation Regulatory		
• Tead4 (U51743)	+7.3 ± 1.3	NC
• Nuclear respiratory factor 2 (M74515)	+6.0 ± 0.7	NC
• Mcm4 (D26089)	+5.2 ± 1.6	NC
• Pbx3b (AF020200)	+1.8 ± 0.06	NC
• Pr264 (X98511)	+1.8 ± 0.05	NC
• Smad3 (AB008192)	–4.1 ± 1.4	NC
• Rck RNA helicase (AF038995)	NC	+5.6 ± 0.1
• Nfatc3 (D85612)	NC	+2.4 ± 0.2
• Protein kinase inhibitor p58 (U284230	NC	+3.5 ± 0.2
• Pbx1b (L27453)	NC	+3.0 ± 0.2
• Ppar γ-binding protein (AF000294)	NC	+2.9 ± 0.1
• Fos (V00727)	NC	+2.1 ± 0.06
• NeuroD (U28068)	NC	+2.1 ± 0.03
• Nuclear factor I/B (Y07685)	NC	–1.7 ± 0.03
• NeuroD2 (D83507)	NC	–3.0 ± 0.04
• Stat1 (U06924)	NC	–2.4 ± 0.2

Data represent fold changes ± SEM in gene expression compared to brains from age-matched nontransgenic mice. NC, no change. (Data from ref. *36*.)

involved in neurotransmitter release (*synaptotagmin*, *SNARE*, and *complexin*) were differentially expressed in the 2- to 3-mo and older transgenic brains. Expression levels of transcripts for a number of axonal transport *kinesin* genes were also changed in transgenic brains. Previous studies have implicated α_1-ARs in glutamate release in the dentate gyrus *(48)* and noradrenaline release from rat renal sympathetic nerve *(49)*. However, more studies need to be carried out to examine further this potential function of α_1-ARs.

4. α_2-Adrenergic Receptors

In contrast to α_1-ARs, the effects of α_2-AR stimulation on gene expression have not been well studied with DNA microarrays. Laifenfeld et al. *(50)* used DNA microarrays to identify gene expression changes that accompany norepinephrine-induced neuronal differentiation in SH-SY5Y cells that endogenously express α_2-ARs. However, much more work is needed to understand fully the effects of α_2-AR stimulation on gene expression.

Table 9
Changes in the Expression of Cell Structure Genes in Mouse Brains Expressing Constitutively Active α_{1B}-Adrenergic Receptors

Encoded protein (accession no.)	Fold changes	
	2–4 mo	12–18 mo
Synaptic/vesicular transport		
• Neurotensin receptor (U51908)	+2.1 ± 0.06	NC
• Synaptophysin (X95818)	−1.8 ± 0.06	NC
• Kinesin heavy chain 1a (D29951)	−2.1 ± 0.1	+2.5 ± 0
• Syntaxin 1B (D29743)	−3.5 ± 1.0	NC
• Girk1 (D45022)	−5.1 ± 1.4	NC
• IGF receptor 2 (U04710)	−9.3 ± 1.7	NC
• SNARE (X61455)	NC	+3.6 ± 0.09
• Kinesin heavy chain 5b (U86090)	NC	−2.0 ± 0.1
• Synapsin IIb (AF096867)	NC	+2.9 ± 0.1
• MB-IRK2 (X80417)	NC	+2.8 ± 0.03
• Trans-Golgi network protein 2 (D50032)	NC	−5.4 ± 0.3
• Kinesin member c2 (U92949)	NC	−2.6 ± 0.1
• RAB7 (X89650)	NC	−1.7 ± 0.03
• Golga 5 (AB016784)	NC	−1.8 ± 0.1
• Synaptotagmin XI (AB026808)	NC	−1.9 ± 0.04
Adhesion/structural		
• Involucrin (L28819)	+4.7 ± 0.06	NC
• Cofilin (L29468)	−1.8 ± 0.3	NC
• Matrin3 (AB009275)	−2.4 ± 0.2	−2.4 ± 0.1
• Eph receptor (X79082)	−3.1 ± 0.5	NC
• Robo1 (Y17793)	−4.8 ± 0.8	NC
• Wasp (U42471)	−5.0 ± 0.4	NC
• P-type ATPase I (U75321)	NC	+7.7 ± 0.3
• Prosaposin (AF037437)	NC	+4.5 ± 0.3
• Microtubule-associated protein 2 (M21041)	NC	+3.6 ± 0.2
• Glial cell adhesion molecule (X16646)	NC	+2.2 ± 0.2
• Ankyrin 3	NC	+2.1 ± 0.01
• Fibronectin receptor-β (integrin; X15202)	NC	−2.2 ± 0.07

Data represent fold changes ± SEM in gene expression compared to brains from age-matched nontransgenic mice. NC, no change. (Data from ref. *36*.)

4.1. Norepinephrine-Induced Neuronal Differentiation

Neuronal differentiation is the process by which neuronal precursor cells develop the morphological, biochemical, and physiological properties of neurons. This is characterized by cell elongation, development of neurites, decreased cell proliferation, development of intracellular neurotransmitter granules, and the production of specific proteins that serve as markers of neuronal differentiation. Norepinephrine stimulates the differentiation of several different cell types of neuronal origin, including PC 12 cells, embryonic frog neurons, and human SH-SY5Y neuroblastoma cells *(51,52)*. The significance of norepinephrine-induced differentiation has not been well studied in vivo. However, deficiencies in norepinephrine-induced neuronal differentiation and synapse formation have been implicated in the development of clinical depression *(50)*.

Human SH-SY5Y cells have been used as a model to study norepinephrine-induced neuronal differentiation. These cells endogenously express α_2-ARs *(50)*. The α_1- and β-ARs have not been identified in these cells, but that does not necessarily preclude their presence. Stimulation of SH-Y5Y cells for 24–48 h with norepinephrine inhibits cell proliferation and induces morphological changes, including cell body elongation, increased dendrites, and formation of granules that contain norepinephrine *(50)*. In addition, norepinephrine also upregulates GAP-43 (a marker of neuronal differentiation) and downregulates Oct 4 expression (a protein that is highly expressed in undifferentiated cells) in SH-SY5Y cells, confirming that norepinephrine causes these cells to differentiate.

DNA microarrays have been used to identify changes in gene expression that accompany norepinephrine-induced differentiation of SH-SY5Y cells. Laifenfeld et al. *(50)* found that norepinephrine modified the expression of 44 neuroassociated genes, including those that encode neurotransmitter receptors, proteins involved in intracellular signal transduction, ion channels, extracellular matrix proteins, and calcium regulatory proteins (Table 10). Norepinephrine also increased the expression of genes that encode laminin, neural cell adhesion molecule, and GAP-43, which are associated with neuronal differentiation, neurite outgrowth, the formation of synapses, and neural plasticity *(51–57)*. Laifenfeld et al. proposed that abnormally low norepinephrine levels in the brain could cause dysregulation of these neurite growth-promoting genes. This could inhibit proper synapse formation and lead to the development of depression. In addition, the antidepressant effects of imipramine, desipramine, amitriptyline, and other antidepressant drugs that elevate synaptic norepinephrine levels may be partially mediated by the norepinephrine-stimulated upregulation of these genes. This is consistent with a nonmicroarray study in which the expression of genes encoding neogenin, synaptophysin, amphiphysin, and other proteins that promote synapse formation was significantly upregulated in the hippocampus of rats chronically treated with antidepressant drugs that increase synaptic norepinephrine concentrations *(57)*. Further investigation of the relationship between AR-stimulated changes in gene expression, synapse formation, and depression may lead to the development of more effective treatments for this disease.

Table 10

Selected Changes in Gene Expression of SH-SY5Y Neuroblastoma Cells Stimulated With Norepinephrine

Gene (accession no.)	Function	Effect of norepinephrine on gene expression
Laminin β-3 subunit (L25541)	Extracellular matrix/neurite outgrowth/differentiation	Increased expression
Laminin γ1 subunit (J03202)	Extracellular matrix/neurite outgrowth/differentiation	Increased expression
Neural cell adhesion molecule L1 (M74387)	Neurite outgrowth/differentiation	Increased expression
Growth-associated protein 43 (GAP-43) (M25667)	Neurite outgrowth/differentiation	Increased expression
Annexin II (D00017)	Calcium regulation	Increased expression
Annexin III (M20560)	Calcium regulation	Increased expression
Annexin IV (X05908)	Calcium regulation	Increased expression
Calcium-binding protein (X78669)	Calcium regulation	Decreased expression
KV11 potassium channel (L02750)	Ion channel	Increased expression
KV34 potassium channel (M64676)	Ion channel	Increased expression
ras-related protein RAB-11B (X53143)	GTP-binding protein	Increased expression
ras-related protein RAB-2 (M28213)	GTP-binding protein	Increased expression
μ-type opioid receptor (L25119)	G protein-coupled receptor	Decreased expression
Prostaglandin E2 receptor EP3 (S69200)	G protein-coupled receptor	Decreased expression

(Data from ref. 53.)

384

5. β-Adrenergic Receptors

DNA microarrays have also been used to study the effects of β-AR stimulation on gene expression. Unlike α_1- and α_2-ARs, DNA microarray studies of β-ARs have only been performed using in vivo experiments. In addition, this is the only group of ARs that has been studied by DNA microarrays in human patients.

5.1. Regulation of Gene Expression by β-ARs in the Parotid Gland

The autonomic nervous system regulates the growth and secretory function of salivary glands. Cholinergic stimulation of salivary glands stimulates ion transport and the copious secretion of saliva. In contrast, sympathetic stimulation increases protein secretion but has little effect on the volume of secreted saliva (*see* review in ref. *58*). Sympathetic stimulation also causes hypertrophy and hyperplasia of salivary glands through β-ARs *(59)*. To identify changes in gene expression that accompany these responses to β-AR stimulation, Ten Hagen et al. *(9)* used a DNA microarray containing 6500 rat genes to identify isoproterenol-stimulated changes in the expression of rat parotid glands in vivo. Rats were given a single injection of isoproterenol, and gene transcription in the parotid gland was analyzed using DNA microarrays 30 min and 2, 6, or 24 h following the injection. Isoproterenol altered (increased or decreased) the expression of 48 genes, which encoded proteins involved in gene transcription, protein synthesis, DNA synthesis, signal transduction, and cell cycling. In general, this is consistent with the increased protein secretion and glandular enlargement caused by sympathetic stimulation of the parotid gland. However, the impact of these data were limited by the fact that this report failed to confirm that these changes in gene expression are related to isoproterenol-induced parotid gland enlargement or secretory function. Consequently, the genetic changes that underlie sympathetic regulation of the parotid gland are still not well defined.

Despite this limitation, this study did provide interesting information concerning the time-course of β-AR-induced changes in gene transcription *(9)*. β-AR stimulation caused rapid (30 min) changes in the expression of some genes; changes in the expression of other genes were not detected until 24 h after isoproterenol stimulation (Fig. 1). β-AR-induced changes in the transcription of genes encoding transcription factors (STAT-3 and activating transcription factor 4) and proteins involved in glycolysis (glyceraldehydes-3-phosphate dehydrogenase [GAPDH] and hexokinase) peaked within 30–120 min after the isoproterenol injection and rapidly returned to prestimulated levels. Changes in the transcription of genes encoding proteins required for protein synthesis (multifunctional aminoacyl-transfer RNA synthetase, lysyl-transfer RNA synthetase, protein synthesis elongation factor 2, protein synthesis initiation factor 5, and protein synthesis initiation factor 4A) peaked 2–6 h after the isoproterenol injection. Expression of genes that regulate DNA synthesis and the cell cycle (cell

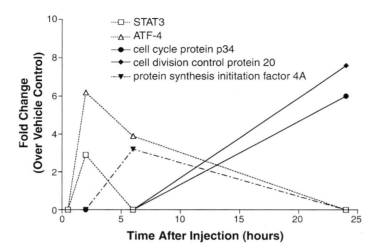

Fig. 1. Temporal variation of gene expression in the parotid gland of isoproterenol-injected rats. Rats were given a single injection of isoproterenol (0.025 g/kg) or vehicle. Parotid glands were isolated 0.5, 2, 6, or 24 h after the injection, and DNA microarrays were used to quantify gene expression in isoproterenol-injected rats to gene expression in rats injected with vehicle only. (Data are from ref. *9.*).

cycle protein p34 and cell division control protein) was not significantly changed until 24 h after the isoproterenol injection. Thus, genes that were upregulated or downregulated by isoproterenol stimulation demonstrated temporal differences in their expression.

Another important finding of this study was that transcription of the *GAPDH* gene decreased threefold within 30 min of isoproterenol stimulation. Similar results have also been reported in brown adipocytes stimulated with isoproterenol *(60)*. This housekeeping gene is commonly used as a control for Northern and Western blots to ensure that equal amounts of RNA or protein samples are loaded into each lane of a gel. However, the discovery that *GAPDH* transcription is significantly decreased by isoproterenol suggests that this gene is not a suitable control for experiments involving β-AR stimulation.

5.2. Gene Expression Changes in Skeletal Muscle of Burn Patients Treated With Propranolol

Severe burn trauma causes an elevation of serum catecholamines and triggers a hypermetabolic response that is mediated by β-ARs *(61–63)*. This hypermetabolic response causes protein catabolism, muscle wasting, and the loss of lean body mass and can persist up to 9 mo after the injury in some patients. Propranolol is one of several drugs that have been used to treat the hypermetabolic response in burned patients. Propranolol significantly reduces energy expenditure, oxygen consumption, and heart rate and decreases muscle catabolism in burned patients *(62)*.

DNA micorarrays were used to identify changes in gene expression that occurred in the skeletal muscle of propranolol-treated burn patients *(63)*. Children 3–18 yr of age with flame or scald burns covering at least 40% of the body were treated for 5 d with propranolol. Skeletal muscle biopsies were obtained before and after propranolol treatment, and DNA microarrays were used to identify propranolol-induced changes in gene expression. Small (1.5- to 2.9-fold) but statistically significant changes in the expression of 14 genes were observed in propranolol-treated patients but not in patients treated with placebo. The affected genes have been associated with stress response pathways, angiogenesis, contractile function, signal transduction, and other cellular processes. However, none of the changes in gene expression identified in this study were conclusively linked to the inhibition of protein catabolism and the preservation of lean tissue mass that has been observed in propranolol-treated burn patients. Thus, it is still unclear whether β-AR-stimulated changes in gene expression are involved in the hypermetabolic response.

6. Conclusion

The unique power of DNA microarrays originates from the ability of microarrays to measure changes in the expression of thousands of genes simultaneously. This allows a large amount of data to be collected in a relatively short time. However, microarray data only provide a starting point for answering biological questions, and many studies have failed to follow up microarray experiments with additional experiments that demonstrate that the changes in gene expression are related to AR-induced changes in cell function. Unfortunately, many of these studies have produced a list of genes that are influenced by AR stimulation but provide no evidence that these changes are physiologically important. It is critical that future DNA microarray studies also use other experimental techniques to confirm that AR-induced changes in gene expression are associated with the physiological changes that are observed on AR stimulation.

Despite this criticism, DNA microarrays have provided insight into the function of ARs that could not be obtained using traditional methods of gene expression analysis. Microarrays have enhanced our understanding of the genetic changes induced by ARs that may be important for the regulation of cell proliferation, cell differentiation, the hypermetabolic response, cardiac hypertrophy, and Parkinson-like neurodegeneration. We anticipate that future DNA microarray studies will continue to advance our understanding of the physiological and pathological functions of ARs.

References

1. Lee EJ, Lee SH, Jung JW, et al. Differential regulation of cAMP-mediated gene transcription and ligand selectivity by MC3R and MC4R melanocortin receptors. Eur J Biochem 2001;268:582–591.
2. Carvalho CR, Carvalheira JB, Lima MH, et al. Novel signal transduction pathways for luteinizing hormone and interaction with insulin: activation of Janus kinase/ signal transducer and activator of transcription and phosphoinositol 3 kinase/Akt pathways. Endocrinology 2003;144:638–647.
3. Naor Z, Benard O, Seger R. Activation of MAPK cascades by G-protein-coupled receptors: the case of gonadotropin-releasing hormone receptor. Trends Endocrinol Metab 2000;11:91–99.
4. Akiyama M, Minami Y, Kuriyama K, Shibata S. MAP kinase-dependent induction of clock gene expression by α_1-adrenergic receptor activation. FEBS Lett 2003; 542:109–114.
5. Zhong H, Lee D, Robeva A, Minneman KP. Signaling pathways activated by α_1-adrenergic receptor subtypes in PC12 cells. Life Sci 2001;68:2269–2276.
6. Tittelbach V, Volff JN, Giray J, Ratge D, Wisser H. Agonist-induced down-regulation of the β_2-adrenoceptor and its mRNA in human mononuclear leukocytes. Biochem Pharmacol 1998;56:967–975.
7. Taniguchi M, Miura K, Iwao H, Yamanaka S. Quantitative assessment of DNA microarrays-comparison with Northern blot analyses. Genomics 2001;71:34–39.
8. Gonzalez-Cabrera PJ, Gaivin RJ, Yun J, et al. Genetic profiling of α_1-adrenergic receptor subtypes by oligonucleotide microarrays: coupling to interleukin-6 secretion but differences in STAT3 phosphorylation and gp-130. Mol Pharmacol 2003; 63:1104–1116.
9. Ten Hagen KG, Balys MM, Tabak LA, Melvin JE. Analysis of isoproterenol-induced changes in parotid gland gene expression. Physiol Genomics 2002;8:107–114.
10. Yun J, Zuscik MJ, Gonzalez-Cabrera P, et al. Gene expression profiling of α_{1B}-adrenergic receptor-induced cardiac hypertrophy by oligonucleotide arrays. Cardiovasc Res 2003;57:443–455.
11. Schena M, Shalon D, Davis RW, Brown PO. Quantitative monitoring of gene expression patterns with a complimentary DNA microarray. Science 1995;270: 467–470.
12. Zhong H, Minneman KP. Activation of tyrosine kinases by α_{1A}-adrenergic and growth factor receptors in transfected PC12 cells. Biochem J 1999;344:889–894.
13. Minneman KP, Lee D, Zhong H, Berts A, Abbott KL, Murphy TJ. Transcriptional responses to growth factor and G protein-coupled receptors in PC12 cells: comparison of α_1-adrenergic receptor subtypes. J Neurochem 2000;74:2392–2400.
14. Garcia-Sainz JA, Alcantara-Hernandez R, Vazquez-Prado J. α_1-Adrenoceptor subtype activation increases proto-oncogene mRNA levels. Role of protein kinase C. Eur J Pharmacol 1998;342:311–317.
15. Iwaki K, Sukhatme VP, Shubeita HE, Chien KR. α- and β-adrenergic stimulation induces distinct patterns of immediate early gene expression in neonatal rat myocardial cells. fos/jun expression is associated with sarcomere assembly; Egr-1 induction is primarily an α_1-mediated response. J Biol Chem 1990;265:13,809–13,817.

16. Zuscik MJ, Sands S, Ross SA, et al. Overexpression of the α_{1B}-adrenergic receptor causes apoptotic neurodegeneration: multiple system atrophy. Nat Med 2000;6: 1388–1394.

17. Theroux TL, Esbenshade TA, Peavy RD, Minneman KP. Coupling efficiencies of human alpha 1-adrenergic receptor subtypes: titration of receptor density and responsiveness with inducible and repressible expression vectors. Mol Pharmacol 1996;50:1376–1387.

18. Erami C, Zhang H, Ho JG, French DM, Faber JE. α_1-Adrenoceptor stimulation directly induces growth of vascular wall in vivo. Am J Physiol 2002;283:H1577–H1587.

19. Hu ZW, Shi XY, Lin RZ, Chen J, Hoffman BB. α_1-Adrenergic receptor stimulation of mitogenesis in human vascular smooth muscle cells: role of tyrosine protein kinases and calcium in activation of mitogen-activated protein kinase. J Pharmacol Exp Ther 1999;290:28–37.

20. Marinese D, Patel R, Walden PD. Mechanistic investigation of the adrenergic induction of ventral prostate hyperplasia in mice. Prostate 2003;54:230–237.

21. Refsnes M, Thoresen GH, Sandnes D, Dajani OF, Dajani L, Christoffers T. Stimulatory and inhibitory effects of catecholamines on DNA synthesis in primary rat hepatocyte cultures: role of α_1- and β-adrenergic mechanisms. J Cell Physiol 1992; 151:164–171.

22. Pabbathi VK, Brennan H, Muzworthy A, et al. Catecholaminergic regulation of proliferation and survival in rat forebrain paraventricular germinal cells. Brain Res 1997;760:22–33.

23. Auer KL, Spector MS, Tombes RM, et al. α-Adrenergic inhibition of proliferation in HEPG2 cells stably transfected with the α_{1B}-adrenergic receptor through a p42MAPkinase/p21Cip1/WAF1-dependent pathway. FEBS Lett 1998;436:131–138.

24. Gonzalez-Cabrera PJ, Ting S, Yun J, McCune DF, Rorabaugh BR, Perez DM. Differential Regulation of the cell cycle by α_1-adrenergic receptor subtypes. Endocrinology 2004; 145: 5157-5167.

25. Shibata K, Katsuma S, Koshimizu T, et al. α_1-Adrenergic receptor subtypes differentially control the cell cycle of transfected CHO cells through a cAMP-dependent mechanism involving p27[Kip1]. J Biol Chem 2003;278:672–678.

26. Milano CA, Dolber PC, Rockman HA, et al. Myocardial expression of a constitutively active α_{1B}-adrenergic receptor in transgenic mice induces cardiac hypertrophy. Proc Natl Acad Sci USA 1994;91:10,109–10,113.

27. Lin F, Owens WA, Chen S, et al. Targeted α_{1A}-adrenergic receptor overexpression induces enhanced cardiac contractility but not hypertrophy. Circ Res 2001; 89:343–350.

28. Cavalli A, Lattion AL, Hummler E, et al. Decreased blood pressure response in mice deficient of the α_{1B}-adrenergic receptor. Proc Natl Acad Sci USA 1997;94: 11,589–11,594.

29. Rokosh DG, Simpson PC. Knockout of the $\alpha_{1a/c}$-adrenergic receptor subtype: The $\alpha_{1a/c}$ is expressed in resistance arteries and is required to maintain arterial blood pressure. Proc Natl Acad Sci USA 2002;99:9474–9479.

30. Tanoue A, Nasa Y, Koshimizu T, et al. The α_{1D}-adrenergic receptor directly regulates arterial blood pressure via vasoconstriction. J Clin Invest 2002;109:765–775.

31. Perez DM, Hwa J, Gaivin R, Mathur M, Brown F, Graham RM. Constitutive activation of a single effector pathway: evidence for multiple activation states of a G protein-coupled receptor. Mol Pharmacol 1996;49:112–122.

32. Hwa J, Gaivin RJ, Porter JE, Perez DM. Synergism of constitutive activity in α_1-adrenergic receptor activation. Biochemistry 1997;36:633–639.

33. Zuscik MJ, Chalothorn D, Hellard D, et al. Hypotension, autonomic failure, and cardiac hypertrophy in transgenic mice overexpressing the α_{1B}-adrenergic receptor. J Biol Chem 2001;276:13,738–13,743.

34. Kunieda T, Zuscik MJ, Boongird A, Perez DM, Lüders HO, Najm IM. Systemic overexpression of the α_{1B}-adrenergic receptor in mice: an animal model of epilepsy. Epilepsia 2002;43:1324–1329.

35. Papay R, Zuscik MT, Ross SA, et al. Mice expressing the α_{1b}-adrenergic receptor induces a synucleinopathy with excessive tyrosine nitration but decreased phosphorylation. J Neurochem 2002;83:1–12.

36. Yun J, Gaivin RJ, McCune DF, et al. Gene expression profile of neurodegeneration induced by α_{1B}-adrenergic receptor overactivity: NMDA/GABA$_A$ dysregulation and apoptosis. Brain 2003;126:2667–2681.

37. Eguchi S, Inagami T. Signal transduction of angiotensin II type I receptor through receptor tyrosine kinase. Regul Pept 2000;91:13–20.

38. Maudsley S, Pierce KL, Zamah AM, et al. The β_2 adrenergic receptor mediates extracellular signal-regulated kinase activation via assembly for a multireceptor complex with epidermal growth factor. J Biol Chem 2000;275:9572–9580.

39. Kuppuswamy D, Kerr C, Narishige T, Kasi VS, Menick DR, Cooper G 4th. Association of tyrosine-phosphorylated c-Src with the cytoskeleton of hypertrophying myocardium. J Biol Chem 1997;272:4500–4508.

40. Fuller SJ, Gillespie-Brown J, Sugden PH. Oncogenic src, raf and ras stimulate a hypertrophic pattern of gene expression and increase cell size in neonatal rat ventricular myocytes. J Biol Chem 1998;273:18,146–18,152.

41. Daaka Y, Luttrell LM, Lefkowitz RJ. Switching of the coupling of the β_2-adrenergic receptor to different G proteins by protein kinase A. Nature 1997;390: 88–91.

42. Tayebati SK, Bronzetti E, Morra Di Cella S, et al. *In situ* hybridization and immunocytochemistry of α_1-adrenoceptors in human peripheral blood lymphocytes. J Auton Pharmacol 2000;20:305–312.

43. Devaux B, Scholz D, Hirche A, Klovekorn WP, Schaper J. Upregulation of cell adhesion molecules and the presence of low grade inflammation in human chronic heart failure. Eur Heart J 1997;18:470–479.

44. Warraich RS, Dunn MJ, Yacoub MH. Subclass specificity of autoantibodies against myosin in patients with idiopathic dilated cardiomyopathy: proinflammatory antibodies in DCM patients. Biochem Biophys Res Commun 1999;259:255–261.

45. Caforio ALP, Mahon NJ, Tona F, McKenna WJ. Circulating cardiac autoantibodies in dilated cardiomyopathy and myocarditis: pathogenetic and clinical significance. Eur J Heart Fail 2002;4:411–417.

46. Lefkos N, Boura P, Boudonas G, et al. Immunopathogenic mechanisms in hypertension. Am J Hypertens 1995;8:1141–1145.

47. Wahnschaffe U, Ebert U, Löscher W. The effects of lesions of the posterior piriform cortex on amygdala kindling in the rat. Brain Res 1993;615:295–303.
48. Scanziani M, Gähwiler BH, Thompson SM. Presynaptic inhibition of excitatory synaptic transmission mediated by α adrenergic receptors in area CA3 of the rat hippocampus in vitro. J Neurosci 1993;13:5393–5401.
49. Murphy TV, Majewski H. Modulation of noradrenaline release in slices of rat kidney cortex through α_1- and α_2-adrenoceptors. Eur J Pharmacol 1989;169:285–295.
50. Laifenfeld D, Klein E, Ben-Shachar D. Norepinephrine alters the expression of genes involved in neuronal sprouting and differentiation: relevance for major depression and antidepressant mechanisms. J Neurochem 2002;83:1054–1064.
51. Taraviras S, Olli-Lahdesmaki T, Lymperopoulos A, et al. Subtype-specific neuronal differentiation of PC12 cells transfected with α_2-adrenergic receptors. Eur J Cell Biol 2002;81:363–374.
52. Rowe SJ, messenger NJ, Warner AE. The role of noradrenaline in the differentiation of amphibian embryonic neurons. Development 1993;119:1343–1357.
53. Kazmi SM, Mishra RK. Identification of α_2-adrenergic receptor sites in human retinoblastoma (Y-79) and neuroblastoma (SH-SY5Y) cells. Biochem Biophys Res Commun 1989;158:921–928.
54. Crossin KL, Krushel LA. Cellular signaling by neural cell adhesion molecules of the immunoglobulin family. Dev Dyn 2000;21:8260–8279.
55. Timpl R, Brown JC. The laminins. Matrix Biol 1994;14:13,729–13,732.
56. Meiri KF, Saffell JL, Walsh FS, Doherty P. Neurite outgrowth stimulated by neural cell adhesion molecules requires growth-associated protein-43 (GAP-43) function and is associated with GAP-43 phosphorylation in growth cones. J Neurosci 1998;18:10,429–10,437.
57. Drigues N, Polytyrev T, Bejar C, Weinstock M, Youdim MBH. cDNA gene expression profile of rat hippocampus after chronic treatment with antidepressant drugs. J Neural Transm 2003;110:1413–1436.
58. Elkstrom J. Autonomic control of salivary secretion. Proc Finn Dent Soc 1989;85:323–331.
59. Brenner GM, Wulf RG. Adrenergic β receptors mediating submandibular salivary gland hypertrophy in the rat. J Pharmacol Exp Ther 1981;218:608–612.
60. Barroso I, Benito B, Barci-Jimenez C, Hernandez A, Obregon MJ, Santisteban P. Norepinephrine, tri-iodothyronine, and insulin upregulate glyceraldehydes-3-phosphate dehydrogenase mRNA during brown adipocyte differentiation. Eur J Endocrinol 1999;141:169–179.
61. Chance WT, Nelson JL, Foley-Nelson T, Kim MW, Fischer JE. The relationship of burn-induced hypermetabolism to central and peripheral catecholamines. J Trauma 1989;29:306–312.
62. Wilmore DW, Long JM, Mason AD, Skreen RW, Pruitt BA. Catecholamines: mediator of the hypermetabolic response to thermal injury. Ann Surg 1974;180:653–669
63. Herndon DN, Dasu HRK, Wolfe RR, Barrow RE. Gene expression profiles and protein balance in skeletal muscle of burned children after β-adrenergic blockade. Am J Physiol Endocrinol Metab 2003;285:E783–E789.

PART VI

SUMMARY AND FUTURE ENDEAVORS

15

Summary and Future Endeavors

Dianne M. Perez

The first half of the 20th century saw the development of the concept of a receptor and the isolation of the first hormone. The last half of the 20th century revealed that there are many subtypes of the adrenergic receptors with different pharmacological properties, and that they are coupled to different G proteins and signal transduction mechanisms. We then basically determined how the ligands bind to the receptor, how G proteins become activated, and how G proteins can selectively couple to receptors through interactions with the intracellular loops of the receptor. We also determined which tissues contain the different subtypes and some of the physiological processes that are regulated by the receptors. The century ended with the cloning of the receptors and the application of basic molecular biological techniques to discern the roles of the individual subtypes. Although much information was garnered in cell lines, there remained a noticeable lack of information in integrated systems and whole animal physiology.

Within each subfamily, the roles of the different subtypes were hard to discern because of the lack of high-avidity antibodies and highly selective antagonists. To avoid these problems, genetically modified mouse models were developed to address the roles of these subtypes in physiological processes. At first, heart-specific overexpression models were developed because of the availability of heart-targeted promoters. Transgenic overexpression models provided the context of what could possibility happen when receptors were overactivated and also provided a pathological model system for exploration into gene therapy targets in heart failure. Next came the knockout models, which provided some more definitive answers in physiological contents. These models are still serving as great model systems and will no doubt continue to be used to address still-unknown questions. In conjunction with the knockouts, double and triple knockouts of the subtypes have also been successfully used. Interestingly, none of these combined knockouts are lethal. Finally, systemic overexpression models using isogenic promoters are now used to determine subtype localization through the

From: *The Receptors: The Adrenergic Receptors: In the 21st Century*
Edited by: D. Perez © Humana Press Inc., Totowa, NJ

use of receptors tagged with green fluorescent protein and to determine possible systemic pathology caused by chronic activation. The use of these tagged receptors in model cell systems and transfected into native tissues is opening new vistas in cellular localization, dimerization, and subtype-specific function.

Although much of the basic signal transduction was worked out in the 20th century, the 21st century is seeing a much more complex involvement of the adrenergic receptors in signal transduction. First, at the level of the ligand, agonist trafficking is being studied to explore the ability of an agonist to drive coupling to specific G proteins and pathways. This may offer some therapeutic benefit in the near future as we try to understand the different conformations of the receptor responsible for this specificity. Besides agonist trafficking, multiple conformations of the receptors are also now being appreciated in other signaling mechanics, such as desensitization, internalization, and phosphorylation. At the level of the receptor, new paradigms in signal transduction and cross talk are constantly being discovered, mostly through novel couplings involving the use of the C-tail and scaffolding domains. Levels of signal transduction specificity are also being seen in the differential regulation of adrenergic receptor function and compartmentalization. New pathways are also being discovered through the use of microarray technology and perhaps in the future proteomics, which may be tailored to clinical applications.

As our knowledge base of these receptors increases, so too will clinical applications. Already, polymorphisms have been discovered that are associated with diseases and compromised function. Together with our understanding of how to manipulate the signaling of these receptors, we may be able to circumvent the signaling alterations associated with these polymorphisms. In clinical medicine, adrenergic regulation is at the center of asthma, heart, and prostate disease. As our knowledge increases in the more unknown regions of the central nervous system, treatment may be possible for debilitating neurological diseases.

Index